Peter C. Olden

MANAGEMENT
of HEALTHCARE
ORGANIZATIONS

Peter C. Olden

MANAGEMENT
of HEALTHCARE
ORGANIZATIONS

An Introduction

SECOND EDITION

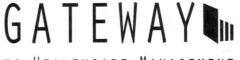

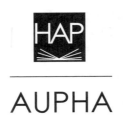

AUPHA

Health Administration Press, Chicago, Illinois
Association of University Programs in Health Administration, Arlington, Virginia

19   18   17   16   15   5   4   3   2   1

Library of Congress Cataloging-in-Publication Data
Olden, Peter C.
  Management of healthcare organizations : an introduction / Peter C. Olden. — Second edition.
    pages cm.
  Includes index.
  ISBN 978-1-56793-690-2 (alk. paper)
  1. Health services administration. 2. Health facilities--Administration. 3. Hospitals—Administration. I. Title.
  RA971.O415 2015
  362.11068—dc23

                              2014030251

The paper used in this publication meets the minimum requirements of American National Standard for Information Sciences—Permanence of Paper for Printed Library Materials, ANSI Z39.48-1984.♾™

Acquisitions editor: Tulie O'Connor; Project manager: Andrew Baumann; Manuscript editor: Sharon Sofinski; Cover design: Marisa Jackson; Layout: Cepheus Edmondson

Found an error or a typo? We want to know! Please e-mail it to hapbooks@ache.org, and write "Book Error" in the subject line.

For photocopying and copyright information, please contact Copyright Clearance Center at www.copyright.com or (978) 750-8400.

Health Administration Press
A division of the Foundation of the American
   College of Healthcare Executives
One North Franklin Street, Suite 1700
Chicago, IL 60606-3529
(312) 424-2800

Association of University Programs
   in Health Administration
2000 North 14th Street
Suite 780
Arlington, VA 22201
(703) 894-0940

To the students who will manage healthcare organizations to help people live healthier lives.

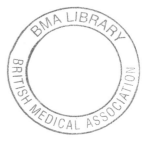

BRIEF CONTENTS

DETAILED CONTENTS

PREFACE

The healthcare field and the number of healthcare organizations (HCOs) continue to grow. So does the need for excellent management of these HCOs. Fortunately, many students and healthcare professionals aspire to management positions in HCOs. Education and training in management for HCOs will help them succeed.

Having been a healthcare management student, healthcare manager, and healthcare management professor, I appreciate good books that help students learn management and how to apply it to HCOs. I studied management at the undergraduate, graduate, and doctoral levels. And I worked in senior management at three hospitals during 14 years as a hospital executive. Since then, for more than 20 years, I have taught undergraduate and graduate courses in healthcare management and related subjects. All that has motivated and enabled me to write this book.

The purpose of this book is to help people learn the body of knowledge we call *management* and then apply it to HCOs. The primary intended audience is undergraduate students who are interested in managing healthcare organizations but have no prior knowledge of this subject. This book will also be useful to students in allied health professions who want to understand management of HCOs. Current supervisors who seek to learn more about management will benefit too. This book can also help healthcare professionals prepare for advancement to management positions.

This introductory-level book has been kept to a reasonable length. There are 15 chapters on 15 important topics for managing HCOs. I have organized and connected the chapters into a cohesive body of knowledge. By the end of this book, students will understand management and how to apply it to HCOs. Because this book is about management, it does not include some other disciplines found in healthcare management curricula such as finance, law, and marketing.

The book is arranged in a logical sequence of chapters that continually builds on and connects with previous chapters. This second edition includes updates to the first edition, more depth, and additional topics. Chapter 1 provides expanded context and background material on health, determinants of health, healthcare services, healthcare organizations, and management jobs in HCOs as well as an updated discussion of trends, issues, and future developments. Chapter 2 covers what management is and how it has evolved as a body of knowledge, theory, and practice. This chapter identifies five basic management functions: planning, organizing, staffing, leading, and controlling. We then study each of these functions in depth throughout the book. New in this edition is a section on institutional theory. In Chapter 3, managers plan the purpose, goals, and work of their HCOs. This second edition expands the project planning discussion with new content for project management and business plans; adds a section on where to get needed data for planning; explains planning at lower levels in more detail; adds Porter's model of competitive advantage; and includes a section on strategic thinking.

After managers complete the planning phase, they must organize to achieve those plans, so we learn about organizing in Chapters 4–6. In Chapter 4, managers organize work into jobs and departments. This edition contains an expanded explanation of systems and open systems and updates the section on how physicians fit into HCOs. Chapter 5 details how managers organize departments into entire organization structures. The chapter has a new section about the governing body and an updated explanation of how the medical staff fits into a hospital. Chapter 6 explains how managers organize groups and teams. Further detail and new trends and developments pertaining to this work have been added in this edition.

Next, managers have to staff positions, departments, and organizations. Chapter 7 explains how managers obtain staff, and Chapter 8 focuses on how managers retain staff. This edition includes onboarding and uses more of a management perspective (and less of a human resources perspective) for these chapters.

After managers staff the HCO, they must lead, direct, influence, and motivate the staff. This is explained in a trilogy of leadership chapters. Chapter 9 presents leadership theories and models, including new material on servant leadership and collaborative leadership. Chapter 10 teaches leading by motivating and influencing, and Chapter 11 explains leading with culture and ethics. New in this edition are more detailed explanations of motivational theories (especially reinforcement theory), updated examples (such as for patient-centered medical homes), more coverage of ethics problems in HCOs, and more detail on how to instill organizational ethics. Following on these three leadership chapters, Chapter 12 teaches how managers control work and performance, and this edition adds information about the purpose of each type of control graph.

After teaching the five basic management functions (planning, organizing, staffing, leading, and controlling) in Chapters 2–12, the book then presents three additional chapters to help apply management to HCOs. Chapter 13 explains how to make decisions and solve problems, which are interrelated. New sections on evidence-based decision making and political decision making have been added. Chapter 14 teaches how to manage change in organizations and includes a new discussion of organizational factors that impede change. Because the management functions and skills in Chapters 1–14 should be done with professionalism, Chapter 15 explains professionalism for managers in HCOs. This edition refocuses the first edition's Chapter 15 to include four sections on professionalism, emotional intelligence, cultural competence, and communication.

References, examples, content, and writing throughout the book are updated. A new case study (about an integrated health system's telehealth services to improve population health) runs throughout the book and introduces each chapter. Three of the case studies at the end of the book are new, and new case study questions for assignments are included with each chapter.

With this content, the book contributes to numerous curriculum requirements for Association of University Programs in Health Administration (AUPHA) undergraduate certification. These include theories of management, organizational behavior, organizational design, functional areas of management, human resources management, strategic planning, managerial skills, leadership, interpersonal skills, managerial ethics, cultural competency, professional development, critical thinking, and communication.

The content includes timeless fundamental principles along with new concepts and current information. There is both theory and practice to learn terms, concepts, theories, principles, methods, and tools—and how to use them. A recurring theme in the book is that management is contingent and the "right" approach depends on changing factors. Students will learn that management problems are not multiple-choice questions with a single best answer. The book teaches the principles, theories, methods, and tools so students can size up situations and develop their solutions. They can practice this skill using the exercises and activities within and at the end of each chapter.

The content and writing style strive to engage students, keep them actively interested, provide a few laughs, and help them understand and remember what they read. It is a style I have been successfully using to teach undergraduate management of healthcare organizations. The publication style uses recurring features and formatting to enhance learning and help make the material appealing. Each chapter opens with a relevant quotation, learning objectives, and part of a continuing real-world case study that we follow through the book. Within each chapter, headings and subheadings organize content and guide the reader. Key points are indicated by **this font.** Key terms are defined in the margins of the pages and included in the book's glossary. Exhibits, bullet lists, examples, activities, and exercises in each chapter keep students engaged and learning. There are sidebars and boxes called Check It Out; Try It, Apply It; and Here's What Happened. At the end of each chapter are One More Time (a summary), For Your Toolbox, discussion questions, and case study questions.

Several features help students see how chapters (and management methods) are interrelated. Chapter by chapter, we follow managers in an integrated healthcare system as they manage their telehealth services to improve quality of care and population health. Their work is featured in the Here's What Happened example that opens each chapter. These examples are drawn from a case study (from The Commonwealth Fund) included as an appendix. When students read these examples that begin the chapters, they may also look at the entire case to appreciate how each chapter's opening case is interrelated with those of other chapters and with management topics. Chapters are further interconnected by end-of-chapter case study questions. These questions pertain to the same six cases included in an appendix, exploring them from different angles. Students see that fully solving a single management problem will require using management principles and tools from many chapters. The writing style in this book further helps students connect chapters and management principles by explicitly stating how things fit together. Finally, an appendix suggests ten real-world applied projects that students can do to further integrate the chapters.

Instructor resources for this book include PowerPoint slides for each chapter, suggested answers to discussion questions, and a test bank. For access to these instructor resources, please e-mail hapbooks@ache.org.

When Enrico Fermi (who later won a Nobel Prize in physics) was a student, he once told a professor, "Before I came here I was confused about this subject. Having listened to your lecture I am still confused. But on a higher level." I hope that after reading this book you will be less confused and on a higher level about the subject of management for healthcare organizations.

Please share with me your feedback about this book. Thank you.

Peter C. Olden, PhD, MHA
Professor of Health Administration
University of Scranton
Scranton, Pennsylvania
peter.olden@scranton.edu

ACKNOWLEDGMENTS

This book and my work on it have benefited from many people. I gratefully acknowledge and deeply appreciate the support of the people noted below, along with others.

At the University of Scranton, I have taught wonderful students who inspired me to keep educating future students. Joanne Reichle and Michele Heenan helped with secretarial tasks. Graduate assistants Caryn Ewbank and James Dalkiewicz helped prepare instructor resources. Professional colleagues at my university and elsewhere offered encouragement and advice.

Staff at Health Administration Press, especially Tulie O'Connor, Janet Davis, Andrew Baumann, Sharon Sofinski, Michael Cunningham, Beth Shomin, Cepheus Edmondson, and Caitlin Aruffo, have helped in more ways than I can list. Health Administration Press kindly gave permission to use selected material from some of its books. This material included cases prepared by Deborah Bender, David Melman, J. Mac Crawford, and Ann Scheck McAlearney and exhibits prepared by Patrice Spath that are all especially useful. The Commonwealth Fund gave permission to use a case prepared by Andrew Broderick. Other publishers and Health Strategies & Solutions, Inc. approved use of their exhibits in this book. Faculty and students who used the first edition of this book gave positive feedback and suggested useful ideas for this second edition.

When I was a student, many professors helped me study and learn about managing healthcare organizations. During my management career, I worked with three hospital chief executive officers—Dana Bamford, Charlie Boone, and Kirby Smith—who each helped me develop practical management experience. What I learned from them has helped me write this book.

My wife, Debbie, and sons, Ryan and Alex, have been supportive and understanding of my professional work and the time and effort needed to write this book. They have also enriched my life in many ways for which I am especially grateful.

And finally, and yet before everyone noted above, my parents, Walter and Helen, instilled in me a passion for reading and learning.

Thank you, everyone. I appreciate your support and could not have written this book without you.

Peter C. Olden, PhD, MHA
University of Scranton

CHAPTER 1

HEALTH, HEALTHCARE, AND HEALTHCARE ORGANIZATIONS

We think it is important not only to be a great performer in the medical model (that is, treating sickness, illness, and injury) but also to be an excellent . . . organization in the health model (that is, keeping people healthy, fit, and vibrant).

Philip A. Newbold, healthcare executive

LEARNING OBJECTIVES

Studying this chapter will help you to

➤ explain what health and population health are;

➤ describe the major forces that determine the health of a population;

➤ identify healthcare services in the continuum of care;

➤ identify types of healthcare organizations;

➤ explain the external environment and how it affects healthcare organizations;

➤ state trends that are shaping the future of healthcare; and

➤ describe the wide variety of healthcare management jobs and careers.

HERE'S WHAT HAPPENED

Partners HealthCare is an integrated healthcare delivery system that combines healthcare organizations (HCOs) such as community health centers, physician practices, hospitals, long-term care facilities, and others. Together, these HCOs offer the continuum of care from prenatal to end-of-life, including preventive, diagnostic, treatment, and long-term services. Thousands of employees perform many different kinds of jobs—including important management jobs. Based in Boston, Partners is committed to its community, and it values innovation, technology, openness, and preparation. Its managers have watched developments in the external environment such as demographic trends, the rise of social media, and the effect of the healthcare reform law on healthcare services and payment. They are transforming Partners HealthCare to better fit the changing external environment in which their HCOs operate. For example, the managers are forming patient-centered medical homes and are striving to keep the local population healthy with prevention (rather than just cure). One important development has been the implementation of its Connected Cardiac Care Program that uses telehealth (healthcare based on information and communication technologies) to connect with remote rural patients to prevent and care for their heart disease.

People are needed to manage HCOs, as the opening example shows. We will follow what happens at Partners HealthCare and use it as a continuing case study throughout the book. (The entire case study is presented in an appendix.) This book will help you learn how to manage HCOs to help people live healthier lives. By doing this, you can do work that has meaning and value (in addition to earning a good paycheck). This chapter explains health, healthcare, health services, and the main forces that determine health. It identifies health services in the continuum of care and then identifies the types of HCOs forming the healthcare sector. The chapter explains the external environment and trends that affect HCOs, the healthcare industry, and the healthcare sector. The chapter ends with information about healthcare management jobs and careers, for which this book will prepare you. After reading this chapter, you will understand better why communities need HCOs—and need people such as you to manage them.

HEALTH AND WHAT DETERMINES IT

Health
A state of complete physical, mental, and social well-being; not merely the absence of disease or infirmity.

What is health? In a well-established definition still used today, the World Health Organization (WHO 1946, 100) says that **health** is "a state of complete physical, mental, and social well-being and not merely the absence of disease or infirmity." **Note that the definition of health is based on being well rather than just not having a disease or problem.**

To further understand health, we can look at Henrik Blum's (1983) classic model (Exhibit 1.1), which shows the dimensions of health and four forces that determine it. Like

Exhibit 1.1
Force Field Model
of Health

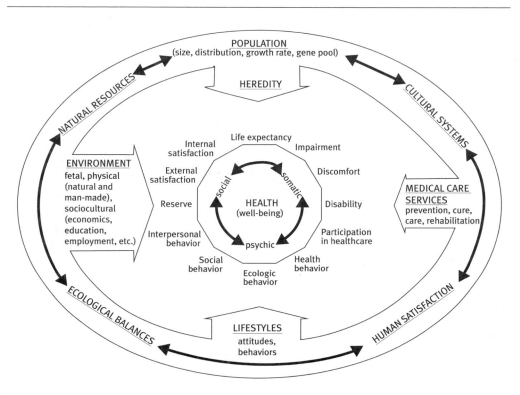

SOURCE: Blum (1983).

WHO's definition, this model also views health as physical (somatic), mental (psychic), and social well-being. Some writers include other types of health, such as spiritual health (Moorhead et al. 2013) or emotional health (Fos and Fine 2005). An individual's health status may be measured by how well that person feels and functions physically, mentally, and socially. Health status can be evaluated through measures of physical disability, emotions, social behaviors, blood pressure, and ability to care for oneself. For a group or population, health status may be measured by birth rates, life expectancy, death rates, commonality of diseases, and group averages for individual measures.

THE FORCE FIELD MODEL OF HEALTH

Four forces—heredity, medical services, environment, and lifestyle—simultaneously determine the health of a population. These forces (determinants) are described in the following paragraphs and shown in Exhibit 1.1.

    Heredity is the starting point of health. Genes and characteristics inherited from parents make a person more likely or less likely to develop certain health problems and to be or not be healthy and well. Perhaps your parents have mentioned some genetic traits

Heredity
Genes, traits, and
characteristics
inherited from parents.

Medical care
Diagnosis and treatment in the care of patients, sometimes limited to care by physicians and sometimes more broadly including care by nurses, therapists, and others who care for patients.

Healthcare
Services that promote health, prevent health problems, diagnose and treat health problems to cure them, and improve quality of life.

Lifestyles
Patterns of attitudes and behaviors that make up one's way of living.

Environment
The world in which one exists and that exists beyond oneself. Environment can include people, organizations, laws, societies, natural events, external forces, and many other elements outside of oneself.

and characteristics that run in your family. Genes were considered fixed until genetic reengineering emerged in the late twentieth century. A manager cannot really change genetics to improve the health of patients and the community.

Medical care (or more broadly, healthcare) refers to the many medical services (and health services) provided by the healthcare system to help people be well. **Medical care** is diagnosis and treatment in the care of patients, sometimes limited to care by physicians and sometimes more broadly including care by nurses, therapists, and others who care for patients (Slee, Slee, and Schmidt 2008, 340). **Healthcare** is services that promote health, prevent health problems, diagnose and treat health problems to cure them, and improve quality of life (Slee, Slee, and Schmidt 2008, 245). Healthcare services exist for all ages and stages of life from womb to tomb. They form a continuum of care that is presented later in this chapter. You have probably used some medical and health services. Medical and health services are important, yet they have the weakest effect of the four forces on health, as shown in Exhibit 1.1 by the reduced thickness of the medical care services arrow.

Lifestyles—attitudes and behaviors such as smoking, seat belt use, diet, exercise, feelings about cancer prevention, and the value one places on health—strongly affect health. Currently, obesity is a prevalent health problem that has been linked to unhealthy lifestyle choices, such as lack of exercise. Although individuals cannot do much to change heredity, medical services, and environment, they can change their lifestyles. For example, some college students are choosing to eat healthier foods and get more exercise. Healthcare managers can improve people's health by helping them improve their lifestyles.

Environment includes the physical and sociocultural setting in which someone lives. Many environmental elements affect health, such as sanitation, violence, sunlight, employment opportunities, neighborhoods, population density, and air pollution. The environment includes elements created by both nature and people. Henrik Blum believed environment has the most powerful effect on health, as indicated by environment having the thickest (strongest) arrow in Exhibit 1.1. That view is still supported today (Kindig 2014). We can understand the importance of environment by considering the life-threatening sanitation problems (and other health problems) caused by floods, hurricanes, and tornadoes. Consider too the differences in health and health problems between safe, wealthy neighborhoods and violent, poor neighborhoods. Notice that in Exhibit 1.1 the environment includes social as well as physical elements. In recent years, some researchers have presented these elements separately as the physical environment and the social environment (Kindig 2014). Doing so emphasizes the social determinants of health (e.g., social support, class, education, income, neighborhood), which have gained importance in the past decade (Shier et al. 2013). According to this approach, five (rather than four) broad forces determine health. The following Here's What Happened reports how an HCO in Newark, New Jersey, improved the local environment to improve health in the neighborhood. Can you think of efforts in your community to improve the environment to improve health?

HERE'S WHAT HAPPENED

A 2012 NOVA Award was given to Newark Beth Israel Medical Center for its success in improving health in the community. The staff had seen that the lifestyles and environment of many people led to unhealthy eating and then obesity, diabetes, and health problems. Like hospitals in other cities, Newark Beth Israel set up school-based education and nutrition programs for healthier diets. The staff also tried something unique by creating a community garden and farmers market in an abandoned parking lot. These became sources of fresh fruits and vegetables, which had been hard to find in the urban neighborhood "food desert." Plans include a greenhouse to enable year-round gardens (Stempniak 2012). The neighborhood had lacked convenient sources of fresh fruits and vegetables, which created a harmful environment for health. When the hospital improved the environment (the neighborhood), it changed a negative determinant of health into a positive one.

Heredity, medical services, lifestyle, and environment interact and affect each other while they also affect health. For example, the environment in which someone lives affects that person's lifestyle and access to medical care services—and all three forces affect the person's health.

Scholars have studied these forces and concluded that specific elements of them (e.g., where one lives, diet, income level) differently affect the health of specific subpopulations (e.g., those based on race, ethnicity, and gender) (Diez Roux 2012; Harris 2013). These **disparities** are common among groups and in communities. Many healthcare managers strive to eliminate disparities so that everyone can live healthy lives. The US population will continue to become more diverse (as shown in the population trends later in this chapter). As a manager, you will have to pay attention to disparities in health status and work to overcome them.

Disparities
Differences in health problems, health status, and use of health services among people who differ in ethnicity, gender, and other characteristics.

Managers should understand that disparities are linked to heredity, environment, lifestyle, and use of medical care services. Knowing this, managers can plan solutions for health problems experienced by groups of people.

How can healthcare managers use Blum's force field model to improve people's health? First, realize that factors other than healthcare services are important. Managers have three general ways to improve people's health: (1) improve their environment, (2) improve their lifestyles, and (3) improve their medical care. **Environment and lifestyle—which can help prevent disease, illness, and injury from occurring in the first**

 CHECK IT OUT

The US Department of Health and Human Services develops health objectives for the country to pursue during each decade. The 2020 national health objectives are available at www.healthypeople.gov/hp2020. The American Hospital Association's NOVA Awards webpage (www.aha.org/aha/news-center/awards/NOVA.html) gives interesting examples of hospitals collaborating with other organizations to improve health by improving people's lifestyles and environments.

place—have a bigger effect on health than does healthcare that is usually provided to treat people after they are ill or injured.

In light of how important lifestyles and environment are for health, many HCOs and their managers have actively improved environment and lifestyles in their communities while also improving healthcare services (Olden and Hoffman 2011). These HCOs have implemented innovative approaches, such as offering wellness programs to seniors, helping children adopt healthy lifestyles, building walking trails and playgrounds, using social media to communicate health information, and other initiatives. These programs have improved nutrition, reduced obesity, and prevented tobacco use, thereby preventing diseases. Think about your community—what have HCOs done there to improve health?

In recent years, healthcare leaders, clinicians, policymakers, and others have become more concerned about **population health**. This approach may be thought of as **measuring a community's health outcomes and the factors that cause them, and then using those measures to coordinate the community's people and organizations to improve health** (Stoto 2013). Population health has gained prominence because of the population health provisions in the Affordable Care Act of 2010. Also, population health is one of the three goals of the Institute for Healthcare Improvement's (IHI 2014) Triple Aim that has been widely presented and accepted by the US healthcare system. Researchers at the University of Wisconsin Population Health Institute report that medical care accounts for only 20 percent of health outcomes; the other 80 percent of people's health is the result of factors such as lifestyle behaviors and the environments in which they live (Kindig 2014). Population health will continue to be important, and managers in many HCOs will try to improve it. The techniques presented in this book will help you manage programs, activities, and services to improve population health in your community. This chapter's opening quote reflects a hospital executive's population health approach to managing his HCO. He and his HCO have earned praise and awards for it. And as we learned in the opening Here's What Happened, Partners HealthCare's managers are also doing more to improve population health.

Population health
Measuring a community's health outcomes and the factors that cause them, and then using those measures to coordinate the community's people and organizations to improve health.

➡ TRY IT, APPLY IT

Suppose you were asked to serve on a college task force to recommend what the college could do to help students improve their health. Using what you have learned in this chapter about the determinants of health, suggest how to improve students' environment, lifestyles, and use of health services to improve their health. Discuss your ideas with other students.

HEALTH SERVICES

There are many different health services. Which ones have you heard of? Some services prevent problems, some diagnose problems, some treat problems, and some support people at the end of life. The hundreds of different health services can be grouped into categories, such as preventive services, diagnostic services, treatment services, rehabilitative services, and so on. These categories can then be arranged in a **continuum of care** to provide womb-to-tomb care as shown in Exhibit 1.2. All of these services must be managed and coordinated to work together for people to be as healthy as possible.

Continuum of care
The full range of healthcare, beginning with prenatal care and continuing to end-of-life care.

HEALTHCARE ORGANIZATIONS

The Here's What Happened at the beginning of the chapter introduced Partners Health-Care—a large, complex HCO (one made up of smaller HCOs) that we will follow throughout the book. What are some HCOs you have heard of, worked at, or given volunteer service to? Some HCOs, such as large general hospitals, provide a wide range of acute care and other services spanning many parts of the continuum of care. Other HCOs, such as hospices, specialize and provide only a narrow range of services in one part of the continuum. Hospitals may also specialize, such as hospitals for only psychiatric care or for only rehabilitation services. Medical group practices and physician offices are another type of HCO. These practices might provide many medical services—such as cardiology, pulmonology, and neurology—or instead focus on a single specialty, such as orthopedics. Many medical groups now offer diagnostic testing, on-site therapy services, outpatient surgery, and other care.

Ambulatory HCOs provide healthcare services to people who come for care and do not stay overnight. One example is an outpatient diagnostic center, which performs lab tests, medical imaging, and other services to diagnose health problems. Other ambulatory options

EXHIBIT 1.2
Continuum of Care

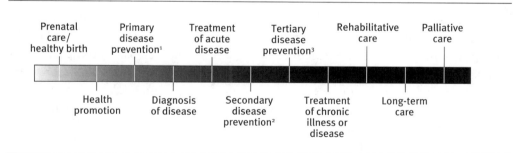

NOTES: 1. Primary disease prevention is preventing agents from causing disease or injury. 2. Secondary disease prevention is early detection and treatment to cure and/or control the cause of disease. 3. Tertiary disease prevention is ameliorating the seriousness of disease by decreasing disability and the dependence resulting from it. SOURCE: Barton (2010).

include ambulatory surgery centers, urgent care facilities for minor problems, mental health clinics, and primary care clinics. Home care organizations provide an array of nursing and therapy services in people's homes. Some organizations, such as nursing homes, provide services for people (not all of whom are elderly) needing care for an extended period of time.

In addition to HCOs that provide hands-on healthcare services to patients and directly affect health, other types of important HCOs indirectly affect people's health. Organizations such as the American Cancer Society and American Lung Association affect people's health by funding research, developing educational programs, and assisting people who need treatment. Medical supply firms and pharmaceutical companies such as Johnson & Johnson produce and distribute the thousands of supplies, drugs, and equipment that other HCOs use to provide healthcare. Companies such as General Electric make high-tech equipment, including magnetic resonance imaging (MRI) scanners and robot surgical systems. Other companies make less sophisticated devices, catheters, intravenous (IV) solutions, wheelchairs, antibiotics, bandages, and many other items. Health insurance companies, such as Blue Cross, are another type of HCO. These businesses assist in the financing of and payment for healthcare services. Trade organizations, such as the Medical Group Management Association, and professional associations, such as the American College of Healthcare Executives, are other types of HCOs. Colleges and universities educate people to work in hundreds of distinct healthcare jobs. Other organizations accredit, license, and regulate HCOs. The list could go on and on. Try to think of other kinds of HCOs. There is no absolute boundary between HCOs and the rest of the economy and society because HCOs overlap and interact with other economic sectors. **Managers should realize that their organization must interact with many other HCOs and organizations that together produce a continuum of care and healthcare services for a population.**

THE ENVIRONMENT OF HEALTHCARE ORGANIZATIONS

An HCO exists in an external environment of people, organizations, industries, trends, forces, events, and developments that are mostly beyond its control. Part of this environment consists of the other HCOs that make up the larger healthcare sector. The HCO's environment beyond healthcare includes citizens, schools, colleges, banks, computer companies, labor unions, stock markets, governments, research laboratories, and more. The environment includes economic, demographic, cultural, legal, and other kinds of developments in society. For example, in the opening Here's What Happened, the environment of Partners HealthCare includes enactment of the healthcare reform law and invention of new devices for mobile technology.

Let's analyze the environment of a nursing home in Baltimore, Maryland. The other nursing homes around the city are part of the environment. They exist in the healthcare sector, which also includes hospitals, home care agencies, health insurers, and all the other

HCOs and health industries in and around Baltimore. This sector exists in the larger society, which includes telecommunications, housing, government, banking, transportation, education, and many other industries and sectors—all part of the environment. In addition, the environment includes potential customers, volunteers, employees, donors, and suppliers. We can also think of this environment in terms of forces and influences—cultural, social, financial, political, and technological—that affect the HCOs.

These other organizations, forces, and people affect HCOs in many ways. For example, the nursing home depends on people to use its services, but those clients may want more weekend activities and social media interaction. They will take their business elsewhere if their preferences aren't met. The nursing home depends on the government to license it and allow it to legally operate. The government could force the nursing home to make improvements to maintain its license and stay open. The nursing home depends on businesses to provide services and supplies, so it will have to contract with an Internet service provider and with a medical supply company.

An HCO exists in, and is influenced by, a larger world. The HCO must be open to its environment and interact effectively with it. To paraphrase an old saying, no HCO is an island unto itself. An HCO depends on people and organizations in its environment just as a person does. The nursing home must be open to its environment to obtain clients, staff, information, funds, equipment, supplies, licensure, and information. When you are a manager, pay attention to your environment!

To better understand the big environment beyond a single HCO, we can divide it into ten distinct sectors (Daft 2013, 149):

1. *Industry sector*: related businesses and competitors that offer products and services similar to what your organization offers

2. *Raw materials sector*: suppliers, manufacturers, and service providers, from some of which your organization obtains needed supplies, equipment, and services

3. *Human resources sector*: employees, labor unions, schools, colleges, employment agencies, and labor markets, from some of which your organization obtains human resources (employees)

4. *Financial resources sector*: banks, lenders, stock markets, and investors, from some of which your organization obtains loans, credit, and other financial resources (this does not include customers who pay your organization for products and services)

5. *Market sector*: actual and potential customers, clients, and users of your organization's products and services

6. *Technology sector*: science and technological methods of producing products and services, some of which your organization uses

7. *Economic conditions sector*: levels and rates of employment, inflation, growth, investment, and other economic circumstances in which your organization exists (this is not financial resources or money for your organization)

8. *Government sector*: laws, regulations, court rulings, political systems, and governments at the local, state, and federal levels, some of which affect your organization

9. *Sociocultural sector*: characteristics of society and culture (e.g., education, values, attitudes) in which your organization exists

10. *International sector*: other countries and globalization of the world in which your organization exists

When you think about an HCO, think too about its environment because that will strongly affect the HCO. Managers must develop good relationships between their HCO and its environment, which is explained further in chapters on planning and organizing. For example, HCO managers use social media tools such as Twitter to interact with their environments (Cooper 2013).

Healthcare Issues, Trends, and Future Developments

Healthcare is always changing—you have probably noticed that. Many powerful trends and developments affect health, healthcare, healthcare organizations, and managers in HCOs. Managers can use the methods, tools, principles, and techniques taught in this book to help their HCOs monitor and adjust to these changes. However, trends sometimes unexpectedly stop, change, reverse themselves, or start anew, making it hard to accurately predict the future. Managers should know "how to create a healthcare organization that can succeed in an unpredictable future" (Olden and Haynos 2013, 1). This book will help you learn how to do that.

Listed here are a few trends occurring in US healthcare and its environment:

◆ What will the US population be like during your career? To whom will your HCOs provide care during your career? Whom in your communities will you help to live healthier lives? Here are projections from the US Census Bureau (2012, 1) for the 50-year period between 2010 and 2060 (students in other countries may check their countries' census bureaus online for similar data):

The population age 65 and older is expected to more than double between 2012 and 2060, from 43.1 million to 92.0 million. The older population would represent just over one in five U.S. residents by the end of the period, up from one in seven today. The increase in the number of the "oldest old" would be even more dramatic—those 85 and older are projected to more than triple from 5.9 million to 18.2 million, reaching 4.3 percent of the total population. . . .

The non-Hispanic white population is projected to peak in 2024, at 199.6 million, up from 197.8 million in 2012. Unlike other race or ethnic groups, however, its population is projected to slowly decrease, falling by nearly 20.6 million from 2024 to 2060. . . .

The Hispanic population would more than double, from 53.3 million in 2012 to 128.8 million in 2060. Consequently, by the end of the period, nearly one in three U.S. residents would be Hispanic, up from about one in six today.

The black population is expected to increase from 41.2 million to 61.8 million over the same period. Its share of the total population would rise slightly, from 13.1 percent in 2012 to 14.7 percent in 2060.

The Asian population is projected to more than double, from 15.9 million in 2012 to 34.4 million in 2060, with its share of nation's total population climbing from 5.1 percent to 8.2 percent in the same period. . . .

All in all, minorities, now 37 percent of the U.S. population, are projected to comprise 57 percent of the population in 2060. (Minorities consist of all but the single-race, non-Hispanic white population.) The total minority population would more than double, from 116.2 million to 241.3 million over the period.

◆ People and organizations are becoming much more connected locally, regionally, nationally, and globally. Communications technology and devices have made wireless electronic communication possible almost anywhere and at any time, and healthcare rapidly is becoming more connected and mobile. Electronic health records are replacing paper medical records (although this transformation is occurring more slowly than expected). Healthcare organizations are using social media, such as Twitter and Facebook, to enable two-way (rather than just one-way) conversations, feedback, interaction, and engagement with stakeholders. All this activity will increase in the future—probably in new and unexpected ways.

◆ Healthcare consumers are becoming more knowledgeable about their own health and more demanding of healthcare organizations. People are more engaged in their health and healthcare including their wellness, health literacy, decision making, and self-management. Employers want employees (as consumers) to be more self-directed with health insurance, wellness, and use of lower cost options. This involvement will escalate in the future (Darling 2014). More patients are actively participating in their care: "Patient-centered care is a method of care that relies upon effective communication, empathy, and a feeling of partnership between doctor and patient" (Ricker 2012, 1).

◆ The healthcare system and HCOs are expected to give more attention in the future to population health and healthy communities. This will involve increased use of epidemiology, risk factors, and public health services. HCOs that have focused on fixing the ill and injured will become more involved in health promotion, disease prevention, and wellness (Jorna and Martin 2014). Doing so will require improving upstream social, economic, behavioral, environmental, and educational factors that affect health. Given the population trends, HCOs will have to do more to reduce disparities in health and healthcare.

◆ The number of uninsured Americans had been increasing for many years, but implementation of the Affordable Care Act—often referred to as the ACA—is reversing that trend. In the future, more Americans will have insurance to pay for more health services. But the multiyear implementation of the ACA has been erratic with successes, failures, and surprises. The ACA will continue to create big challenges for HCO managers.

◆ HCOs will continue to join together in a variety of organizational forms. Hospitals, medical groups, insurers, ambulatory clinics, long-term care companies, community agencies, and other HCOs will form mergers, alliances, networks, integrated delivery systems, accountable care organizations, patient-centered medical homes, and other collaborative structures. These structures are expected to improve coordination throughout the continuum of care, reduce fragmentation of services, share scarce resources, gain economies of scale (size), increase power, and improve quality (Parrington 2014).

◆ More physicians are choosing to be employed by hospitals and health systems rather than to work for their own independent medical practice (Birk 2013). This trend will continue in the future because of declining reimbursements, increasing costs, day-to-day struggles of running a physician practice, and, for new doctors, large student debts (Nester 2014). Hospital managers face many challenges in forming hospital–physician relationships with both employed and independent physicians.

◆ Demand for primary care is increasing—and so is the shortage of primary care physicians, physician assistants, and nurse practitioners. Primary care will continue to become more common in retail settings such as supermarkets, discount department stores, and pharmacies. Consumers will like the convenience, but retail medicine will further fragment healthcare (Nester 2014).

◆ The annual rate of growth of healthcare spending has been declining over the past few years, but total spending is still increasing and the percentage of all spending that goes to healthcare has been increasing—and will continue to increase. Soon, more than 20 percent of all spending in the country will be for healthcare, which will leave less for other needs. Meanwhile, average spending per person for health in the United States continues to exceed that of other countries. People in the United States—on average—spend twice as much per person on healthcare than people in other industrialized countries. Yet, individuals in the United States do not live longer lives, have lower infant mortality, or enjoy better quality of care than people in many other countries (Schoen et al. 2013).

◆ Payers and purchasers have begun to hold HCOs more accountable for performance and value. In the future, payments to providers will be based less on the volume of services and more on the value of services. HCOs' performance will become more transparent (open and visible) with more healthcare assessment and data analytics to guide stakeholders in making health-related choices. This transparency will drive HCOs to further analyze, redesign, and improve processes and reduce waste to create better value, improve quality, and lower cost for customers. In the future, expect more financial incentives to reduce use of expensive inpatient care and expand use of outpatient and wellness services (Tyson 2014; Darling 2014).

◆ Science and technology lead to new methods of health prevention, diagnosis, and treatment. This trend will continue in the future, especially in telemedicine, robotics, genetics, bioengineering, information technology and connectivity, cloud technology, pharmaceuticals, molecular imaging, implantable chips, health monitoring, e-health, neuroscience, customized medicines, gene therapy, tissue engineering, regenerative medicine, data analytics, and smart devices (Kraft 2013).

CHECK IT OUT

Interested in the future of healthcare and healthcare jobs? Trends can be found at the websites of the US Bureau of Labor Statistics healthcare section (www.bls.gov/ooh/healthcare/home.htm) and the American Hospital Association Chartbook (www.aha.org/research/reports/tw/chartbook/ch1.shtml). Check them out—now and throughout your career.

HEALTHCARE MANAGEMENT JOBS AND CAREERS

Earlier we read about the many services and organizations that make up our healthcare system. As a result, many healthcare management jobs exist in settings and specialties such as those shown in Exhibit 1.3. According to the Bureau of Labor Statistics (2014), there were 315,500 jobs in health services management in 2012; by 2022, this number is expected to grow by 23 percent (faster than for all jobs combined). New graduates should expect to begin their careers in entry-level jobs. From there, promotions can lead to middle-management and then upper-management positions. After getting some experience, you will be able to move between different types of HCOs, such as from a hospital to a health insurance company or a medical group practice. There are many opportunities for students to develop exciting, rewarding healthcare management careers. This book was written to help you prepare to enter this profession, yet its lessons, principles, tools, and methods will be useful throughout your career.

Two healthcare management professors have described dozens of careers in healthcare management (Friedman and Kovner 2013). Their work covers jobs and careers in

EXHIBIT 1.3
Types of Healthcare Management Organizations and Jobs

Managers work in these and other types of HCOs:

- Clinics
- Consulting firms
- Health insurance organizations
- Healthcare associations
- Hospitals
- Nursing homes

- Physician practices
- Mental health organizations
- Public health departments
- Rehabilitation centers
- Research institutions

Specialized areas for managers include these and others:

- Finance
- Government relations
- Human resources
- Information systems
- Marketing and public affairs

- Medical staff relations
- Nursing administration
- Patient care services
- Planning and development
- Supplies and equipment management

SOURCE: ACHE (2014).

HCOs for long-term care, ambulatory care, mental health, hospital services, physician and medical care, health insurance, medical equipment, pharmaceuticals, health education, voluntary associations, and other healthcare fields that were briefly described earlier. The range of jobs is enormous and includes the titles listed in Exhibit 1.4. Partners HealthCare (in the opening Here's What Happened) has many of these jobs.

     People who are preparing for a healthcare management job (or who are already in one) likely realize that HCOs offer many types of jobs and career tracks. The demand and supply differ among jobs and careers, so students should follow hiring trends and be alert for new opportunities. For example, the numbers of management jobs in ambulatory care and long-term care are likely to increase more than the number of management jobs in inpatient hospital care will. Healthcare management jobs that focus on quality, process improvement, social media, and population health are likely to increase more than the average for all healthcare management jobs. Further, healthcare evolves so rapidly that new kinds of management jobs will emerge in the coming years (Honaman 2013). There will be an exciting variety of jobs, so a healthcare manager need not be stuck in a dead-end job if she is prepared for a job change. This book can help prepare you for future opportunities.

Titles for healthcare management jobs include these and others:

- Director of materials management
- Chief information officer
- Budget analyst
- Director of physician relations
- Compliance officer
- Director of business development
- Community resource advisor
- Chief quality officer
- Director of environmental services
- Marketing associate
- Project manager
- Director of patient admissions
- Information management specialist
- Education and training director
- Research analyst
- Public health program manager
- Director of finance
- Emergency management coordinator
- Community health center director

- Claims representative
- Administrator
- Director of human resources
- Insurance coordinator
- Risk manager
- Director of government affairs
- Program manager
- Account manager
- Sales representative
- Director of marketing
- Managed care coordinator
- Director of safety
- Volunteer services coordinator
- Billing manager
- Director of utilization management
- Quality assurance coordinator
- Chief executive officer
- Health systems specialist
- Associate administrator

EXHIBIT 1.4
Healthcare Management Job Titles

ONE MORE TIME

Health is more than the absence of disease. It includes complete well-being—physical, mental, and social. People's health is determined by four broad forces: heredity, environment (physical and social), lifestyle, and medical care (which is the least important of the four forces). Healthcare managers improve environments, lifestyles, and medical care to improve a population's health. Healthcare services provide medical care, and these services range from prenatal care to end-of-life palliative care to form a womb-to-tomb continuum of care. Many kinds of healthcare organizations exist. Some of them provide these health services in the continuum of care. Others (e.g., suppliers, insurers) do not directly provide the health services but are essential because they support the service providers. HCOs interact with each other and with many other elements in their (external) environment. All HCOs depend on many other organizations and their environment. The environment strongly affects an HCO, and when the environment changes, it might affect the HCO. Thus, HCOs must monitor and adapt to changes in their environment. Healthcare managers work in a wide variety of jobs and HCOs.

 FOR YOUR TOOLBOX

- Force field model with determinants of health
- Continuum of care
- Environment divided into ten sectors

FOR DISCUSSION

1. Based on what you learned in this chapter, discuss the forces that affect health and well-being in the community where your college is located. Give an example of each force. Which of these forces do you think healthcare managers can control and change the most to improve people's health?

2. What are disparities in healthcare? Why are disparities important for healthcare managers to understand?

3. Why is the external environment so important to healthcare organizations?

4. Discuss several future trends and issues presented in this chapter. Which of these trends and issues do you think will be the most challenging for HCOs?

CASE STUDY QUESTIONS

These questions refer to the Integrative Case Studies at the back of this book.

1. All cases: What kinds of healthcare management jobs are evident in these cases?

2. All cases: What kinds of healthcare services and HCOs are evident in these cases?

3. Taking Care of Business at Graceland Memorial Hospital case: Explain how the external environment has affected the hospital.

4. Decisions, Decisions case: Think about the ten environmental sectors explained in this chapter. Which forces and factors in which sectors of the external environment should the HCO's managers consider when making their decision?

5. Disparities in Care at Southern Regional Health System case: What are some important forces and factors in the HCO's external environment? How is the population health approach evident in this case?

TRY IT, APPLY IT

Name seven to ten healthcare organizations in the community where you grew up, such as specific medical groups and nursing homes. (Do some quick online research if necessary.) List several big changes that are occurring in the community and external environment of those HCOs. Describe how those environmental changes might affect each HCO. Discuss your ideas with a colleague from another community.

CHAPTER 2

MANAGEMENT

The worker is not the problem. The problem is at the top! Management!

W. Edwards Deming, quality expert,
business consultant, and writer

LEARNING OBJECTIVES

Studying this chapter will help you to

➤ define and explain management;

➤ describe how management has evolved as a field of knowledge, theory, and practice;

➤ explain major theories of management;

➤ identify important roles, functions, activities, and competencies of healthcare managers; and

➤ explain how management theory is used in healthcare organizations.

HERE'S WHAT HAPPENED

Partners HealthCare's management team planned, organized, staffed, led, and controlled the HCO and its work. Managers planned new initiatives for accountable care, population health, and financial risk. To accomplish plans, managers organized tasks, authority, division of work, jobs, and coordination. They redesigned care processes for diabetes, heart attack, and colorectal cancer. Specific tasks, responsibility, and authority were assigned to specific jobs such as health coaches, cardiologists, and nurses. A Connected Cardiac Care Team coordinated diverse jobs toward the shared goal of improving cardiac care for remote patients. Managers staffed new jobs by hiring nurses and training them for telehealth responsibilities. When leading employees, managers overcame resistance from some nurses who disliked technology replacing their human touch. Managers led physicians by using financial incentives to motivate them. Performance of the telehealth program was controlled by monitoring enrollment, hospital readmissions, emergency room use, patient satisfaction, and cost savings. When patient enrollment was below target, managers redesigned the enrollment process to increase the number of enrollees. All this planning, organizing, staffing, leading, and controlling by Partners HealthCare's managers—including new, entry-level managers—enabled the managers and HCO to serve their community and improve population health.

Chapter 1 introduced us to HCOs that provide healthcare services. As shown by Partners HealthCare, these HCOs must be managed. In the Here's What Happened, managers demonstrated five essential management functions—they planned, organized, staffed, led, and controlled. Managers of all ages and levels use these and other management skills. This chapter introduces us to the management knowledge, theory, and practice used to manage HCOs. Management has evolved as a profession, and this chapter reviews how management has developed from the early twentieth century to today. We learn how managers today use some classic management approaches while also applying approaches developed in the twenty-first century. This chapter introduces work, skills, functions, roles, and competencies of managers; later chapters will review them in more depth and help you learn how to apply them to HCOs.

This chapter is important because it provides the foundation on which subsequent chapters will build. It explains many management terms, concepts, and principles that are used throughout the book—and in HCO management jobs and careers. As this chapter's opening quote suggests, problems in HCOs sometimes result from managers' actions. Problems can occur when managers do not properly use management principles and methods. Managers, including young professionals on their first day at work, can use this chapter to help them manage their HCOs wisely. With a proper foundation in management principles, you can make a good start in your career and then build on it.

WHAT IS MANAGEMENT?

What comes to mind when you see the word *management*? Do you know someone who works in management? Consider a manager you know. What does she do? What makes him a manager? We may have somewhat different ideas about what management means and what managers do. The word is applied broadly and loosely to work, activities, and people. Some workers might be called managers although they do not perform management activities. We will use a well-accepted definition. **Management** is "the process of getting things done through and with people" (Dunn 2010, 12). **Always remember that management involves people—usually lots of them!**

Management
The process of getting things done through and with people.

THE HISTORY AND EVOLUTION OF MANAGEMENT THEORY

As a field of study, management is younger than some (e.g., biology, mathematics, psychology) but older than others (e.g., computer science, aerospace engineering). While management techniques were surely used before recorded history, writing about management as a body of knowledge is more recent. This section draws from the work of Peter C. Olden and Mark L. Diana (2009) to discuss theoretical approaches that created the foundation of management theory. As you read this section, think about how management has evolved by expanding existing ideas, building on past ideas, and creating entirely new ideas that guide managers today. Although some management theories are from long ago, they are still used today (just as even older theories of Sir Isaac Newton and Sigmund Freud are still used today).

TAYLOR AND SCIENTIFIC MANAGEMENT

Scientific management
A type of management that uses standardization, specialization, and scientific experiments to design jobs for greater efficiency and production.

Management began to develop as a body of knowledge in the early 1900s with the **scientific management** work of Frederick W. Taylor (1903, 1911). Taylor told factory managers they could increase productivity and output not by finding bigger, stronger workers to shovel coal and lift iron but instead by designing the workers' repetitive work for ease and efficiency. He analyzed factory workers' physical motions, postures, steps, and activities and made changes that led to large improvements. For example, standing or sitting a certain way could enable someone to work with less strain on the body, similar to practicing good posture when working with a computer today. Taylor also designed tools that enabled laborers to work with less effort yet accomplish more. (Does this remind you of the saying "Work smarter, not harder"?) Detailed instructions, methods, rules, techniques, training, and time allowances were developed for each job.

Taylor tested his ideas with the scientific method and detailed research in factories. He believed there was "one best way" to perform each repetitive job, and he set out to discover it. Factory managers adopted the one best way rather than let 20 workers do the same job 20 different ways with varying results. Factory production and workers' pay increased. Managers' early efforts to redesign physical work led to redesigning their own management work, because managers now had to identify work tasks, set standards, and plan schedules for workers. Taylor's ideas became known as Taylorism and scientific management, and they were expanded by Frank and Lillian Gilbreth (1917) and Henry L. Gantt (1919).

Scientific management is still applied in many jobs and organizations, including HCOs. Today we use terms such as *ergonomics* and *human engineering* to refer to how jobs, tools, work, postures, and workstations are designed to maximize productivity and minimize injury. When HCO managers design jobs such as emergency nurse, robot technician, or speech therapist, they apply ideas that evolved from scientific management. We will learn more about this approach in later chapters on staffing and production.

FAYOL AND ADMINISTRATIVE THEORY

Henri Fayol (1916) was a pioneer in developing **administrative theory** to improve organizations (rather than improve individual jobs as Taylor did). His ideas were top-down, for top managers to apply to lower levels of the organization. Fayol believed his principles were flexible and applicable to any kind of organization. Although history has shown that his principles work better in some types of organizations than others, they have contributed much to the foundation of theory for managing people and organizations. His work helped develop administrative principles that are still widely used today. We read how managers used some of these principles in the opening Here's What Happened example of Partners HealthCare.

Have you seen an organization chart for a nursing home, health insurance company, or pharmaceutical firm? A typical organization chart (Exhibit 2.1) reflects administrative theory.

Division of work is how work is separated into smaller, more specialized tasks and activities. The work of medicine is divided into orthopedics, neurology, obstetrics, pediatrics, anesthesiology, and other medical specialties.

Administrative theory
An integrated set of ideas to organize work, positions, departments, supervisor–subordinate relationships, hierarchy, and span of control to design an organization.

Division of work
How work is separated into smaller, more specialized activities.

EXHIBIT 2.1
Organization Chart

Specialization refers to the width of the range of tasks done by an employee or department. A data entry clerk is more specialized and has fewer tasks than a nurse.

Coordination refers to how different work units (e.g., departments) are connected to work together toward a common purpose. In a hospital, nursing is coordinated with laboratory, pharmacy, housekeeping, respiratory therapy, and other departments for the common purpose of patient care.

Line work contributes directly to achieving an organization's purpose and main goals. Physical therapy is line work that contributes directly to the patient care goals of a sports medicine clinic.

Staff work uses specialized skills, abilities, and expertise to support line workers. Staff work does not directly contribute to the organization's purpose and main goals. Instead, it indirectly contributes by helping the line workers. Compared to line workers, staff workers have less authority and are expected to advise the line workers who have authority to make the decisions. In a health insurance company, the strategic planning department does staff work to advise the line managers and board of directors (who then create the strategic plan).

The difference between line work and staff work sometimes is fuzzy. Public relations work may be line work in one kind of HCO but staff work in a different HCO, depending on the purpose and goals of each HCO. Top managers should establish which employees are staff workers and which are line workers to clarify who offers advice for decisions and who actually makes the decisions.

Authority is power formally given to a job position (not to the person hired for a position) to make decisions and take actions. The director position of a college student health clinic has authority.

Line of authority refers to the vertical chain of command, authority, and formal communication up and down an organization. In a health insurance company, a billing clerk reports up to the accounts receivable supervisor who reports up to the director of finance who reports up to the vice president of financial affairs who reports up to the president. The president communicates policy down to the director of finance, and so on.

Unity of command means a worker takes commands from and is responsible to only one boss. A webmaster takes commands from and is responsible to only the director of information technology in a large cardiology group practice.

Span of control is how many subordinate workers a manager is directly responsible for—how many workers report up one level (in an organization chart) to that boss. In a medical equipment and supply business, the manager has a span of control over five workers, including one sales supervisor, one delivery team leader, one storeroom supervisor, one accounting team leader, and one administrative assistant.

Centralization (and decentralization) is how high (and low) in an organization the authority to make a decision exists. In a health insurance company, purchasing decisions exceeding $100,000 are centralized at the board of directors level. Purchasing decisions for less than $500 are decentralized at the lower supervisor level.

These ideas help managers determine supervisor–subordinate relationships, group workers into work units such as departments, design levels of hierarchy in an organization chart, arrange who reports to whom, and structure the organization. It would be hard to think of an HCO that does not use some of these administrative principles. We will learn more about these principles in later chapters on organizing, organization structure, staffing, and production.

⊕ TRY IT, APPLY IT

Think about a job you've had, such as a summer job or a current part-time job. Try to apply the administrative theory concepts to your job and the organization. For example, how was work divided? Which departments were coordinated with your department? What, if any, authority did your job have? Share your analysis with classmates.

MAYO AND HUMAN RELATIONS

In the late 1920s and into the 1930s, a team of researchers led by Fritz Roethlisberger and W. J. Dickson (1939) studied workers at the Western Electric Hawthorne Plant outside of Chicago, Illinois. The researchers conducted experiments in which they changed the physical working conditions, such as lighting, of the rooms in which female workers sat and manually assembled telephone components. These experiments, combined with observations, were to help Western Electric managers understand factors affecting workers' productivity, morale, and other aspects of performance. The researchers were puzzled that productivity did not vary as expected. In fact, sometimes the workers were more productive when lighting was decreased rather than increased. Productivity sometimes improved in the experiment room where lighting was increased, yet it also improved in the control room where the lighting was not changed. Do you wonder why? The researchers wondered how that could happen. Eventually, Elton Mayo (1945) and other scientists in the Hawthorne studies determined that social and psychological factors were involved. These experiments affected the women's cooperation, teamwork, feelings of importance, and recognition, which then influenced their morale, work effort, and productivity. The women were not machines or robots; they were humans. They had thoughts, feelings, and personalities, which they brought to work. And Western Electric was not a machine, either; it was a social organization with **norms**, peer pressure, informal leaders, and behaviors.

This work led to the **human relations** approach in management, which was further developed by Chester Barnard (1938), an executive who emphasized cooperation based on communication and social/psychological motivators, not just material/monetary

---

Unity of command
Arrangement in which a worker takes commands from and is responsible to only one boss.

Span of control
How many subordinate workers a manager is directly responsible for; how many workers report directly to that manager. (Sometimes called *span of supervision*.)

Centralization
How high or low in an organization the authority exists to make a decision.

Norms
Behaviors and attitudes expected of people in a group, organization, or society.

Human relations
A type of management based on psychology and sociology that considers employees' feelings and behaviors, especially in groups.

Roethlisberger and Dickson's work at the Western Electric Hawthorne Plant led to the discovery of the Hawthorne effect: We are motivated to change our behavior (e.g., produce more) when we are being watched. However, these researchers from Harvard University discovered much more about human behavior in the workplace. The Hawthorne studies ran from 1924 to 1936. Their deep effect on organizational development and management still strongly influences managers today. You can learn more about the Hawthorne studies, how they were conducted, and lessons for today's managers at www.library.hbs.edu/hc/hawthorne/07.html#seven.

Planning
Deciding what to do and how to do it.

Organizing
Arranging work into jobs, teams, departments, and other work units; arranging supervisor–subordinate relationships; assigning responsibility, authority, and other resources.

Staffing
Obtaining and retaining people to fill jobs and do work.

Directing
Assigning work to workers and motivating them to do the work.

factors. Decades of study have focused greater attention on the human relations aspects of management, such as motivation, organization culture, group behavior, and job design. In recent years, new approaches to human relations have led to innovations, such as using social media to increase employee engagement (Miller and Tucker 2013). We will learn more about human relations in later chapters on staffing, leadership, and communication.

GULICK AND MANAGEMENT FUNCTIONS

Luther Gulick and Lyndall Urwick (1937) studied what executives do and determined that they plan, organize, staff, direct, coordinate, report, and budget (sometimes referred to as POSDCORB). From their work, and from Henri Fayol's before, have come five fundamental management functions: planning, organizing, staffing, directing, and controlling. **Managers plan, organize, staff, direct, and control. In more recent years, the words *influence* and *lead* have been used in place of *direct*.**

In **planning**, managers decide what to do and how to do it. Planning can involve establishing mission, vision, goals, objectives, strategies, and methods. Planning may be short-term, such as a single eight-hour shift in an emergency department, or long-term, such as the five-year strategic plan of a medical school. What kind of short-term and long-term planning have you done in your personal life?

In **organizing**, managers arrange work into jobs, teams, departments, and other work units; arrange supervisor–subordinate relationships; and assign responsibility, authority, and resources. Organizing involves designing an organization chart. For example, five investors build a new assisted-living retirement home and then organize the jobs, departments, and 87 employees as shown on a new organization chart.

In **staffing,** managers obtain and retain people to fill jobs and do the work. Managers also recruit, select, orient, train, compensate, evaluate, protect, and develop employees. For example, a mental health clinic director hires two psychologists and decides how much to pay them.

In **directing** (also called influencing or leading), managers assign work to workers and motivate them to do the work. For example, a lab supervisor assigns different kinds of lab tests to five lab technologists.

In **controlling**, managers monitor performance and make necessary adjustments so that goals and objectives are achieved (or revised if appropriate). Managers also check progress and take corrective steps when needed to ensure completion. Managers may use computerized data collection, analysis, and reports at their digital desktops to control expenses, overtime hours, and medical errors.

It makes sense for managers to do these five functions in the sequence shown, and these functions should be thought of as a cycle rather than a straight line. After all steps are completed, the original plans have been fulfilled (or revised), so new plans must be created. New plans lead to new organizing, staffing, directing, and controlling. The cycle suggests that managers plan goals to pursue, organize tasks to accomplish planned goals, hire staff to perform organized tasks, direct and motivate staff to do the tasks, and then control what happens so that planned goals are achieved. Although managers generally follow a cycle, they might sometimes take two steps forward and one step back to adjust as they proceed. For example, when interviewing applicants for an ethics officer position for a new genetics testing company in Boston, the company president might realize she is unable to clearly explain to applicants the job's authority and reporting relationships. The organization is too fuzzy. The president must return to the organizing function and more clearly organize how the ethics officer will fit into the company. Then the president can interview applicants and hire someone for the job. These five functions are used constantly by HCO managers—as they were used in the opening episode of Partners HealthCare.

Controlling
Monitoring performance and adjusting if necessary so that goals and objectives are achieved.

WEBER AND BUREAUCRATIC THEORY

The word *bureaucracy* may raise negative or cynical feelings because people feel bureaucratic rules sometimes create obstacles and delays. However, when an organization uses bureaucratic principles wisely, they can contribute to effective management. These ideas were developed by economist, sociologist, and political scientist Max Weber (1946, 1947). He used perspectives from economics, sociology, and politics to study organizational management and recommend changes. Here are some of Weber's basic principles:

◆ Staff are subject to organizational authority only in their work for the organization, not in their personal lives.

◆ Employees work in a hierarchy (organization chart) of bureaus, with a higher bureau (office) controlling lower ones.

◆ Control is based on authority rather than on personal relationships.

◆ Each bureau has an established division of labor and duties.

◆ A bureau is managed according to written documents kept in files for continuity.

◆ Workers are hired to fill positions based on open selection rather than election.

◆ Staff are selected based on qualifications and ability rather than personal relationships.

◆ Staff are paid based on position and responsibilities in the hierarchy.

◆ A worker can be promoted in the hierarchy based on seniority and achievement.

◆ Employees do not own rights to the bureau where they work, nor do they own property, equipment, or other resources used for work production.

◆ Staff must follow a system of rules, standards, and discipline that controls their work.

◆ Staff must follow orders given by superiors in official positions.

As you might have realized, the bureaucratic approach makes work and organizations more efficient but less personal. This design was intentional because Weber thought work and organizations were based too much on personal relationships, favoritism, family relationships, and what today is called "office politics." In bureaucracy, rules and authority dominate, and human creativity and personal feelings are stifled. This approach has advantages and disadvantages, as do other management approaches. Bureaucracy makes organizations more predictable, efficient, and stable. However, it also makes them less flexible and less innovative, as Weber realized.

Would you want to work in a bureaucracy? Today, many organizations and HCOs follow bureaucratic principles, some more rigidly than others. Bureaucracy helps you be paid properly, deters your boss from directing you to mow her lawn and wash her car, and lets you be promoted without being the president's nephew. However, bureaucracy might also stifle your creative ideas and control you with many rules. We will learn more about these principles in later chapters on organizing, organization structure, and controlling performance.

CONTINGENCY THEORY

Contingency theory
Theory that there is no single best way to organize; the best way depends on factors that differ from one situation to another.

There is no one best way to organize the structure of an organization, as discovered by management pioneers Joan Woodward (1958, 1965), Tom Burns and G. M. Stalker (1961), and Paul R. Lawrence and J. W. Lorsch (1969). Instead, according to **contingency theory**, the best type of organization is contingent, which means it depends on other factors, such as the organization's environment, purpose, plans, size, and technology used to create products and deliver services. For example, one organization structure works best if the external environment is mostly stable and predictable, whereas a different organization structure is best if the external environment changes quickly and unpredictably. This statement is true not only for an entire organization but also for individual departments and work units in the organization. Different departments face different circumstances, uncertainties, and contingencies and thus should be organized with different centralization, specialization, division of work, vertical hierarchy, coordination, and so forth. **There is no single correct way to organize; instead, "it all depends."**

Think back to the kinds of HCOs identified in Chapter 1. Consider a biotech company, rehabilitation hospital, mental health clinic, and health insurance business. How should these HCOs be organized? Which specialization, division of work, and vertical chain of command would be best? It depends on the unique circumstances and characteristics of each HCO. In a biotech company, should the genetics research department be organized differently than the accounting department or the same way? It depends on the unique circumstances and characteristics of each department.

KATZ AND MANAGEMENT SKILLS

Robert Katz (1974) spent years examining the work of managers. He found that they use three basic kinds of skills—technical, human, and conceptual—to perform three kinds of work. Today in HCOs, a manager's technical work might be preparing a therapist's job description, a dental clinic budget, or an outpatient lab marketing plan. An HCO manager's human interpersonal work might include inspiring mental health counselors or forming cooperative relationships among nurses and pharmacists. A manager's conceptual work might include envisioning future goals for a surgery group practice or considering how relocation to a larger building could affect patients' waiting time.

HERE'S WHAT HAPPENED

The Colorado Beacon Consortium (CBC) enables 51 primary care medical groups in seven rural Colorado counties to improve their services and patient care. The CBC obtained a three-year financial agreement with the federal government to fund its work. Managers used conceptual skills to envision how electronic health records, collaborative learning, and work redesign could enable dozens of rural primary care groups to update and improve how they operated. Managers used human skills to encourage physicians to participate, to resolve disagreements, and to create support for change among community stakeholders. Managers used technical skills to set up analytic tools to measure quality. Early results show better work flow and teamwork within the medical groups and increased preventive and chronic care for patients (McCarthy and Cohen 2013).

INSTITUTIONAL THEORY

John Meyer and Brian Rowan (1977) and Paul DiMaggio and Walter Powell (1983) studied organizations and concluded that they sometimes do things to appear proper to stakeholders rather than to improve organizational efficiency. In fact, managers sometimes do what society says is "the right thing"—even though doing so reduces organizational efficiency. Why would managers do that? Institutional theory (Meyer and Rowan 1977; DiMaggio and Powell 1983) argues that organizations feel compelled to fulfill expected obligations in the external environment although those expectations may cause less efficiency. The external environment creates laws, regulations, customs, beliefs, standards, ethics, norms, and values about what should (and should not) be done. Some of them become firmly established as institutions in society. For example, HCOs must obtain informed consent prior to performing surgery on someone. Businesses should not share confidential information. A not-for-profit charitable organization is expected to act for the good of its community. A medical group's physicians have an obligation to follow the Hippocratic Oath. Dozens of healthcare professions, such as medicine, nursing, and occupational therapy, have their own code of ethics. These codes establish social expectations that become institutionalized as normal behavior. You can look ahead at Chapter 11 on leadership to see a code of ethics for healthcare managers.

Organizations that follow and comply with society's institutions are viewed as more appropriate and legitimate than organizations that do not. If an organization's stakeholders view the organization as legitimate, they will support it in many ways. If an organization loses legitimacy, stakeholders may withdraw support, funding, sales, accreditation, and resources. Then the organization might not survive. Therefore, managers feel pressure to do what is viewed as right even if that action is inefficient (i.e., more costly). Perhaps in some personal situations you too have felt that way.

These social institutions can strongly influence what organizations and managers do or not do. Managers do not want their organizations—or themselves—to lose legitimacy and support. However, compliance with some institutions might decrease rather than increase an organization's efficiency. Why would a health education company buy supplies from a local vendor even though it could buy the supplies more cheaply on Amazon? The health education manager feels external pressure to "buy local" and support the community's supplier even though that is more costly (and thus less efficient). Managers have to judge the pros and cons of complying with institutionalized expectations. Compliance might cost more money, time, or staff and thus be less efficient. **Managers must learn about and understand society's institutions and consider them in their managerial decisions.**

MINTZBERG AND MANAGEMENT ROLES

Henry Mintzberg (1990) helped analyze management by identifying ten roles performed by managers. He grouped the roles into three broad groups: interpersonal roles, informational roles, and decisional roles. The roles are shown in Exhibit 2.2. **Note that leadership is not the same as management, nor is it separate from management: Leadership is a part of management.**

Role	Type	Action	Example of Work
Figurehead	Interpersonal	Symbolically representing one's own organization (or work unit) at ceremonial and social events	Appearing at a groundbreaking ceremony for a new healthcare building
Leader	Interpersonal	Develop, motivate, oversee, and lead subordinate employees to achieve goals	Telling employees that with more teamwork the cancer center could have the best survival rates in the city
Liaison	Interpersonal	Connecting one's own organization (work unit) to other organizations and people outside one's own chain of command	Meeting monthly with the city's youth sports council
Monitor	Informational	Gathering and using information from many sources (internal and external) to know what is happening	Analyzing birth rates in the community
Disseminator	Informational	Sharing information with others in one's own organization (work unit)	Posting the names and job titles of new employees in a company's e-newsletter
Spokesperson	Informational	Sharing information with others outside one's own organization (work unit)	Speaking at a college job fair about plans to increase employment
Entrepreneur	Decisional	Changing, adapting, and improving the organization (work unit)	In a personal fitness business, adding diet/nutrition classes
Disturbance handler	Decisional	Taking care of problems and unexpected events	Arranging extra staffing in the emergency department after a nearby bus accident
Resource allocator	Decisional	Distributing and assigning organizational resources	Budgeting funds to purchase new furniture for the waiting room
Negotiator	Decisional	Working with others to reach agreements and settle disputes	Meeting with a labor union to agree on wages for next year

EXHIBIT 2.2
Mintzberg's Ten Managerial Roles

SOURCE: Adapted from Mintzberg (1990).

Mintzberg emphasized that these roles are interrelated. Suppose Kaitlyn manages a sports medicine clinic in Cincinnati, Ohio. She receives complaints from patients, employees, and the city government about insufficient parking. She will use several interpersonal roles to represent the clinic and connect it with groups of people to resolve the problem. Kaitlyn will use informational roles to monitor the situation, gather information about the problem and possible solutions, and speak to others on behalf of the clinic. As clinic manager, she will handle the problem, negotiate a solution, and probably allocate resources for parking. Kaitlyn will perform several managerial roles shown in Exhibit 2.2. Because managers may perform different roles simultaneously—and may handle several projects at the same time—they need a special skill: juggling. We will learn more about these management roles in the remaining chapters.

 TRY IT, APPLY IT

> External pressures and demands are forcing hospitals to tightly manage expenses. Hospitals must produce their services (e.g., surgeries, CT scans, inpatient days of care, meals) using less money, fewer resources, and fewer staff. Suppose you are a hospital food service department manager who must cut department expenses by 7 percent. Explain in detail how you could use at least five of Mintzberg's managerial roles to do that.

COMPLEX ADAPTIVE SYSTEMS

Throughout much of the twentieth century, management theory generally assumed a mechanistic approach. According to this perspective, the organization is an orderly mechanical system of interacting parts, similar to a machine or car. How the machine (organization) performs can be predicted from history. Managers fix a problem by replacing a broken part or rearranging how parts interact. By the late twentieth century, however, a new perspective emerged that some scientists and managers thought better fit what they were observing and experiencing.

Chaos theory (Gleick 1998) and complexity science (Holland 1992; Waldrop 1992) led to studying **complex adaptive systems**. According to this perspective, as explained by Daft (2010), sometimes a system is too complex and unpredictable to be viewed as a mechanical system. The system is more like a natural biological system. The system's parts have too many interactions to fully predict, understand, and account for; thus, the system may seem chaotic. Yet, while a system's immediate behavior may seem disorderly, over time the behavior may show order. The stock market and a big urban traffic jam are examples. Globalization, cultural diversity, wireless connectivity, and other trends listed in Chapter

Complex adaptive system
A system with so many unpredictable changing parts and interactions that it cannot be fully understood and is thus more like a biological organism (natural system) than a machine (mechanical system).

1 have increased complexity for organizations. The system parts, the relationships among those parts, and the effects of external forces on the parts are not constant or predictable as they are in a machine. Think of humans and groups of humans: Are they always predictable and orderly in their relationships? No, as we have all experienced. Organizations are groups of people, so the complex adaptive systems perspective helps us understand and manage living organizations.

Managers find complex adaptive systems theory useful when the environment changes quickly and unpredictably, because this approach enables organizations to change more quickly and easily. Complex adaptive systems have unique characteristics and require unique approaches to management (McDaniel and Jordan 2009; Weiner and Helfrich 2012):

◆ These systems have many diverse agents (i.e., parts, people) that process information.

◆ Agents share and use information to choose, decide, and adapt.

◆ Relationships among system parts are not constant, proportional, or predictable, so changes among parts can have large effects, small effects, and unpredictable effects.

◆ Relationships among agents may matter more than the agents themselves.

◆ Systems can self-organize and self-manage without external control from higher up in the organization.

◆ Creativity and surprises emerge from the changing relationships among people.

◆ A system and its environment reciprocally affect each other.

Compared to other systems, managing a complex adaptive system requires

◆ more knowledge sharing,

◆ more flexibility (thus fewer rules),

◆ more trust among members,

◆ more experimenting, trial and error, learning, innovation, and "making it up as we go,"

◆ more joint solutions by groups of people,

◆ more comfort with risk and uncertainty, and

◆ more interpreting and making sense of a seemingly chaotic world.

As Hammer (1996) once said, success does not come from predicting the future; it comes from creating an organization that can prosper in an unpredictable future.

DO MANAGERS ALL MANAGE THE SAME WAY?

By now you should know what management is and the roles, activities, and functions that managers carry out. Perhaps you wonder if all managers perform their management work the same way. What do you think? Consider people in general: Do they perform the same role, activity, or function in the same way? You have probably noticed that professors do not all teach the same way. Students do not all study the same way. The same goes for managers: They do not all manage the same way. Managers differ in personalities, attitudes, worldviews, biases, styles, and preferences. **Although managers perform similar roles, they do not perform those roles the same way because of these personal differences.**

Managers manage differently also because of the work and situations they face, which cause a given manager to be more involved in some roles and activities and less involved in others. Lower-level managers, such as team leaders in a nursing home, do more technical work than conceptual work. They follow technical rules and processes to create daily work schedules and order supplies when inventory is low. In contrast, upper-level managers, such as nursing home executive directors, do more conceptual work than technical work. They think strategically about how their nursing home should adapt to future changes in their external environments (e.g., the population becoming more culturally diverse). While both levels of managers plan, they plan for different time horizons, with higher-level managers having to plan farther into the future.

ONE MORE TIME

Management began to develop as a body of knowledge in the early 1900s with the efforts of Taylor and the scientific method to improve work. Fayol pioneered administrative theory to improve organization structure, levels of organization, and supervisor–subordinate relationships. Mayo studied how using psychology and sociology could help managers understand workers' behaviors, norms, feelings, and motivations. Gulick and Urwick identified specific management functions, including planning, organizing, staffing, directing/influencing, and controlling. Weber developed bureaucracy theory to manage organizations with formal structure, bureaus, hierarchy, authority, responsibility, accountability, and consistent rules (rather than personal favoritism). Lawrence and Lorsch argued that the best way to organize is contingent on external factors. Katz asserted that managers use technical, human, and conceptual skills to perform technical, human, and conceptual work. DiMaggio and Powell developed institutional theory to explain that organizations and managers sometimes take actions in order to be viewed as proper and legitimate—even though those actions reduce organizational efficiency. Mintzberg summarized the work of managers into ten interpersonal, informational, and decisional roles. Viewing organizations as natural complex adaptive systems rather than mechanical systems is useful for organizations in rapidly changing, unpredictable environments.

Management is a mix of art and science. A body of scientific research, theories, principles, knowledge, and practice is available to guide managers. Yet scientific methods cannot fully address the many people, situations, and nuances of management. The art of management is also needed, which comes from personal judgment and experience that you will develop during your career.

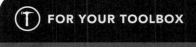

FOR YOUR TOOLBOX

- Scientific management
- Administrative theory
- Human relations
- Management functions
- Bureaucratic theory

- Contingency theory
- Management skills
- Institutional theory
- Management roles
- Complex adaptive systems theory

FOR DISCUSSION

1. How do you think Taylor's work has influenced present-day management of HCOs?

2. Why is Mayo's work important for present-day management of HCOs?

3. The word *bureaucracy* sometimes is used scornfully and cynically. How do you feel about bureaucracy? What are the advantages and disadvantages of bureaucracy in HCOs?

4. Which of Mintzberg's ten managerial roles would come easily to you? Which of these roles would not come naturally to you and would require extra effort and practice?

5. What does contingency theory tell us? How do you feel about this view of management?

CASE STUDY QUESTIONS

These questions refer to the Integrative Case Studies at the back of this book.

1. Ergonomics in Practice case: Explain how this case shows Taylor's scientific management.

2. I Can't Do It All case: Use many of Fayol's administrative theory principles to analyze and describe how Healthdyne is organized.

3. Disparities in Care at Southern Regional Health System case: Explain how Tim Hank could use each of Gulick's five management functions to help his HCO reduce disparities.

4. Nowhere Job case: Referring to Jack's work in the case, explain how Jack uses each of Katz's three management skills.

5. Taking Care of Business at Graceland Memorial Hospital case: Describe how Mr. Prestwood could use at least five of Mintzberg's managerial roles to resolve the situation.

(→) TRY IT, APPLY IT

HCOs are trying to be more green and eco-friendly to help sustain the natural environment. Suppose you are the top manager of a medical group practice. Explain how to use the five management functions discussed in this chapter (planning, organizing, staffing, directing, and controlling) to help make the medical group a green, eco-friendly organization.

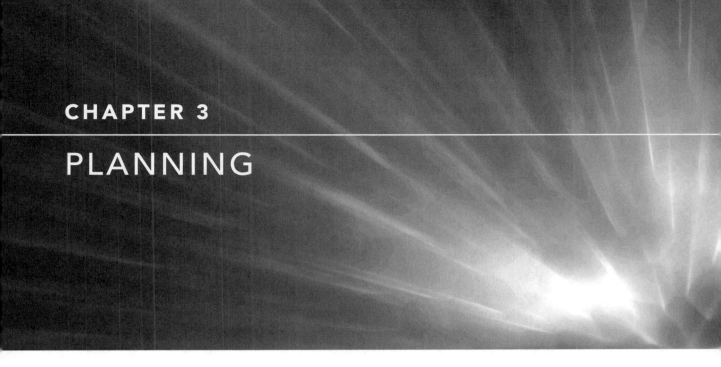

CHAPTER 3

PLANNING

He who fails to plan, plans to fail.

Common business expression

LEARNING OBJECTIVES

Studying this chapter will help you to

➤ explain what planning is;

➤ compare and contrast planning at different levels;

➤ explain a model of strategic planning;

➤ examine two sets of strategies;

➤ describe project planning and project management;

➤ apply a tool for project planning;

➤ explain the contents of a business plan;

➤ identify sources of data and information for planning; and

➤ understand useful ideas about how to plan.

HERE'S WHAT HAPPENED

Managers at Partners HealthCare assessed their external environment and saw both opportunities (e.g., information technology) and threats (e.g., reduced Medicare payments). They also considered Partners's strengths (e.g., extensive electronic health records system) and weaknesses (e.g., discharged hospital patients being readmitted for more care). Based on this and other information, top-level managers planned new strategic goals for Partners. One goal was to reduce the number of readmitted patients. Managers in the Center for Connected Health—a lower-level unit within Partners HealthCare—developed an implementation plan to achieve that goal. It involved using technology to connect with patients at home after hospital discharge. Managers planned which staff members would do which tasks in which sequence to accomplish the goal. They planned to set up information technology, medical technology, and communications technology. They also planned to train discharged patients in self-care and to transmit their health data (blood pressure, weight, and pulse) to the center each day. Via telehealth, staff then could provide just-in-time care and education when needed. This complex project was successfully planned and implemented by managers and staff to achieve Partners's goal.

A s demonstrated in the Here's What Happened, managers plan what their organizations and work units will do in the future and how to do it. Employees at all levels of a healthcare organization (HCO) must plan well to ensure they get their work done. A new manager at a lower level of an HCO can earn respect from higher-level managers by planning wisely for her own department or work unit. This chapter defines planning and explains how it varies at different levels of HCOs. Planning methods are presented to help readers learn how to plan. These methods include strategic planning and project planning for an HCO.

WHAT IS PLANNING?

In simplest terms, planning is deciding what to do and how to it. The planning activity is the first of Luther Gulick's five main management functions discussed in Chapter 2. Planning should precede the other management functions because a manager cannot properly organize, staff, lead, or control an HCO without knowing its goals and what it wants to achieve. We can also relate planning to three of Henry Mintzberg's (1990) ten management roles discussed in Chapter 2: monitor, entrepreneur, and resource allocator.

Planning is, of course, future oriented. When planning, we anticipate and prepare for tomorrow, not the past or present. Students plan which courses to take next year, where to do an internship next semester, and what to do next spring break. Managers plan many aspects of HCOs—can you think of some? Planning enables an HCO's manager to set a direction for the future that employees can pursue. Managers should not be like Alice in Lewis Carroll's *Alice's Adventures in Wonderland* (1946, 71–72):

> "Would you tell me, please, which way I ought to go from here?"
> "That depends a good deal on where you want to get to," said the cat.
> "I don't much care where—" said Alice.
> "Then it doesn't much matter which way you go," said the cat.
> "—so long as I get *somewhere,*" Alice added as an explanation.
> "Oh, you're sure to do that," said the cat.

If a manager does not care where her HCO goes and what it does in the future, the HCO can go anywhere—like Alice. But unlike Alice, good managers do care about where their HCO will go and what it will do in the future. **Managers plan a future direction and goals (where to go) and then plan how to achieve them (how to get there).** We read about Partners HealthCare's planning in the opening Here's What Happened. You have probably done similar planning in your personal life when choosing a college or planning a vacation.

Planning is future oriented—so what must managers do? They must try to predict the future—at least the future that will pertain to their HCO. For example, they need to foresee what their HCO's competitors will do next year and which diseases will be most prevalent in their community three years from now. Review the Healthcare Issues, Trends, and Future Developments section in Chapter 1. Many of these developments will affect your HCO. You will have to face them, anticipate how they will play out in your community, and plan how to adapt your HCO to fit with them. This chapter can help you learn how to do that.

Employees in today's complex HCOs do specific kinds of planning, including financial, strategic, human resources, facilities, and market planning. Addressing all these types of planning is beyond this book's scope. This chapter will describe how to perform **strategic planning** and project planning and how to create business plans that are used to implement strategic plans. These tasks are essential for HCOs in a changing environment.

Managers plan at all levels of the organization. The board of directors plans at the highest level using a broad perspective for the long-term future of the entire HCO. For a hospital in Sacramento, this planning could include a **vision** of where the HCO wants to be in ten years, a five-year strategic plan, a three-year physician recruitment plan, a two-year capital expenditure plan, and a one-year set of **goals** to accomplish. The chief executive officer (CEO) and senior management team assist the board in its planning and also plan for the long term. These activities comprise strategic planning. High-level HCO managers also work with middle-level and lower-level managers and supervisors to plan at these levels of the HCO.

Strategic planning
Deciding how the organization wants to position itself in its future environment and relative to competitors, and then deciding how to achieve that position.

Vision
What the organization wants to be in the long-term future.

Goal
An important, specific, intended target or desired outcome that can be measured to determine how well it was achieved.

Managers at higher levels plan for longer periods, taking a broader view of the HCO. At lower levels, managers plan for shorter periods and for smaller parts of the HCO. Higher-level planning is concerned with *what* to do, while lower-level plans focus on *how* to do it—the methods and steps to achieve the higher-level *what*. Lower-level planning identifies how to achieve higher-level goals by planning who will do what, when, and with which resources.

In larger HCOs that have more specialized staff, managers may be assisted in their planning by a planning department, a planner, a data analyst, a decision support specialist, or other staff. Some new health administration graduates choose planning jobs to begin their careers. Kim did this and has analyzed trends (such as those discussed in Chapter 1), identified relevant developments in her local community, and gathered useful information by talking with stakeholders. Then she assembled and presented that information to her HCO's management team and board of directors.

Smaller HCOs have few staff specialists, so top managers do more planning work themselves or hire planning consultants. Many HCOs avoid purely top-down planning, in which top managers make the plans and determine the goals by themselves. Instead, the planning is partly bottom-up, meaning lower-level work units and staff provide input to top managers for higher-level plans. This method provides important information and perspectives about the HCO's current and future needs, pros and cons of proposals, stakeholders' views, and whether proposed plans are realistic. Also, when lower-level staff participate in the planning process, they are more committed to then **implement** the final strategic plan. They will not feel the plan was imposed on them without their input.

As we learned earlier, planning should precede other management functions. It does not make sense for an orthopedic medical group manager to organize job positions, authority, responsibility, and the organization chart without first knowing the group's goals and strategic direction. The goals and strategic direction affect which tasks, jobs, and positions are needed in the medical group. The orthopedic group manager needs this information to create the organization chart. Then she can organize the necessary work and jobs, staff the positions, direct the staff, and control their performance to achieve the planned goals. The plan becomes the basis for control by showing the manager what is supposed to happen. The manager can then compare what is happening in the group to what is supposed to happen according to the plan. Controlling and improving performance will be explained in more detail in Chapter 12.

Let's learn how managers do high-level strategic planning. Then we will learn how middle- and lower-level managers plan for their departments and work units.

STRATEGIC PLANNING

Strategic planning is a decision-making activity that identifies where an organization is going, sets its direction, and focuses its future efforts. This process results in a vision and strategic goals, which guide everyone in making consistent decisions that move the

Implement
Make happen, carry out, perform, put into effect.

organization toward its planned future (Swayne, Duncan, and Ginter 2009). Strategic planning enables an organization to examine where it is now (Point A), decide where it wants to be in the future (Point B), and make decisions to get there (from Point A to Point B).

In the opening Here's What Happened, we got a glimpse of Partners HealthCare's strategic planning. In a sense, the HCO was at Point A, the managers decided where they wanted the HCO to go—Point B—and they then planned how to move the HCO from Point A to Point B. Strategic planning is an HCO's highest-level planning. It determines how the HCO can succeed in the future, often with an emphasis on beating competitors and satisfying customers. Lower-level planning then guides the HCO in achieving its strategic plans.

When doing strategic planning, managers must use **strategic thinking**, which is the mental process of analyzing and synthesizing information to create a strategy to achieve a goal (McIlwain and Ugwueke 2014). When managers use strategic thinking, they think beyond the data and information. They bring meaning to data. They see many individual trees and then make sense of a forest. They compare and contrast, ponder and wonder, systemize and synthesize, analyze and realize, evaluate and relate. They ask why, how, and what if. They question assumptions. They might annoy people with all their questions. As a result, they sometimes develop unusual insights, revolutionary ideas, and brilliant strategies!

We will use a strategic planning model from Zuckerman (2005) to guide the HCO by answering three questions: Where are we now? Where should we be going? How do we get there? This model is shown in Exhibit 3.1.

Managers begin by analyzing the HCO's current situation (or position) to answer "Where are we now?" They assess the environment beyond the HCO, which we know greatly affects the HCO. They consider, for example,

- technology, such as robot healthcare workers;
- local population changes, such as baby boomers reaching age 65;
- economic trends, such as local unemployment levels;
- laws, such as implementation of the healthcare reform law; and
- many other external factors discussed in Chapter 1.

These factors will affect the HCO and its position. Managers consider the number, size, strength, resources, and plans of competitors and the competitive dynamics of their local community. This environmental analysis reveals **opportunities** to pursue and **threats** to protect against. Managers also assess the HCO's current **mission**, philosophy, and culture along with the HCO's distinctive characteristics, competencies, and shortcomings. They consider the HCO's image, staff, facilities, equipment, quality, workforce, finances, and other elements. By doing so, they can identify the HCO's **strengths** and **weaknesses**.

Strategic thinking
The mental process of analyzing and synthesizing information to create a strategy to achieve a goal.

Mission
The purpose of an organization; why the organization exists.

Strengths
An organization's abilities, assets, and competencies that create strategic advantages.

Weaknesses
An organization's flaws, shortcomings, and liabilities that create strategic disadvantages.

Opportunities
Favorable events, elements, and situations in the environment that an organization could exploit for its strategic gain.

Threats
Unfavorable events, elements, and situations in the environment that could harm an organization.

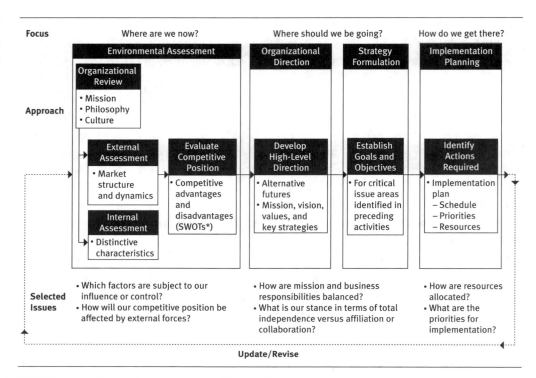

* SWOTs = strengths, weaknesses, opportunities, and threats.
SOURCE: Zuckerman (2005). © 2004 Health Strategies & Solutions, Inc.

(In the earlier Here's What Happened, Partners HealthCare's managers identified some of their strengths, weaknesses, opportunities, and threats, or **SWOTs**.) In the process, strategic planners also identify critical issues to address, such as how to use social media and whether or not to join an accountable care organization.

Managers must consider stakeholders when doing internal and external assessments. Such assessments require identifying key people (inside and outside the HCO)

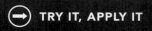

SWOTs
Strengths, weaknesses,
opportunities, and
threats.

TRY IT, APPLY IT

Name a specific campus organization that you are familiar with. Try to list three strengths, three weaknesses, three opportunities, and three threats for that organization. Discuss your organization and ideas with another student.

and organizations (outside the HCO), understanding what they expect of the HCO, and judging how much they could affect the HCO (favorably or unfavorably). Examples of **stakeholders** include employees, the media, financial lenders, business coalitions, patients, other HCOs, governments, special interest groups, accreditors, and labor unions.

Exhibit 3.2 shows common stakeholders and what they often expect of HCOs. Understanding stakeholders helps a manager make internal and external assessments needed to plan future goals.

By the end of this first stage of strategic planning, the HCO managers know the organization's advantages and disadvantages relative to its competitors, its SWOTs, and where it is (Point A). Next, the HCO management must decide where the organization should be going (Point B). This task involves planning the HCO's future direction and forming a strategy to get there. The HCO management decides which opportunities to pursue and how to protect against threats by building on strengths and overcoming weaknesses.

Stakeholders
People and organizations that have a stake (interest) in what an HCO does and that could affect the HCO.

EXHIBIT 3.2
Stakeholders and Their Stakes in HCOs

Stakeholder	Examples of Stakes (Interests) in HCOs and Expectations
Employees	Job satisfaction, good compensation, safe work conditions
Patients, clients	Quality care, compassion, convenience, affordable prices
Media and press	Prompt candid replies to questions, access to top managers
Creditors	Repayment as scheduled
Physicians	Superb patient care, new equipment, convenient scheduling
Businesses	Affordable healthcare, lower insurance premiums and prices
Other HCOs	Cooperation for transfers of patients
Governments	Compliance with laws and regulations
Special interest groups	Support for their interests (e.g., hiring minorities, caring for people with diabetes)
Accreditation commissions	Compliance with accreditation standards
Vendors and suppliers	Prompt payment
Neighbors	Respect for neighbors and their property

✓ CHECK IT OUT

Many organizations post their mission, vision, **values**, and goals on their websites. They want stakeholders to know what they are doing. The American College of Healthcare Executives (ACHE) is the leading professional association for healthcare leaders and has more than 40,000 members. The ACHE website lists this HCO's mission, vision, values, and goals as follows:

- *Mission:* To advance our members and healthcare management excellence

- *Vision:* To be the premier professional society for healthcare executives dedicated to improving healthcare delivery

- *Values:* Integrity, lifelong learning, leadership, diversity

- *Goal Areas:* Membership, knowledge, career advancement, leadership, service excellence

Learn more about this HCO and its mission, vision, values, and goals at http://www.ache.org/abt_ache/mission_2013.cfm. Then research online the mission, vision, values, and goals of other HCOs.

Values
Deeply held fundamental beliefs and ideals.

Strategy
A pattern of ideas used to attain and sustain competitive advantage over rivals.

In this second stage of strategic planning, managers also consider possible alternative futures for the organization. For example, they might consider these two "futures":

1. Implementation of the Affordable Care Act (ACA) will proceed smoothly and enable 90 percent of our community to have good health insurance.

2. Implementation of the ACA will be delayed and partly blocked so that only 75 percent of our community will have good health insurance.

STRATEGY

There are many ways we can think about strategy. After all, people have written about it for centuries. We will think of **strategy** as a pattern of ideas used to attain and sustain competitive advantage over rivals (Luke, Walston, and Plummer 2003). Strategy helps managers and their organization to survive and thrive in the environment. Strategy is conceptual—it is ideas conceived by strategists and managers. And it is not just a single idea—it is an ongoing cluster of ideas that form a consistent pattern. Managers use this pattern to guide their decisions and actions and thereby create competitive advantage. To be effective, strategy must be sustainable. If competitors can easily duplicate an HCO's strategy, the advantage over rivals will be lost.

One approach to strategy offers a group of five strategies (patterns of ideas) that can guide an HCO to attain and sustain advantage over competitors—if the HCO implements the strategy well (Luke, Walston, and Plummer 2003):

1. *Pace:* timing and intensity of action (e.g., the HCO is always first to adopt a new kind of medical technology)

2. *Potential:* resources and abilities that potentially could enable advantage (e.g., the HCO has the most advanced information systems)

3. *Performance:* operational performance (e.g., the HCO achieves the best survival rates for lung cancer patients)

4. *Position:* image in the minds of others (e.g., consumers think of the HCO as caring and compassionate toward elderly patients)

5. *Power:* mass and clout (e.g., the HCO is an enormous academic medical center with more workers than any other employer in the city)

Another approach to strategy presents two broad patterns of action (Porter 1985). A business may gain competitive advantage to succeed in its market by using either the *low-cost* strategy or the *differentiation* strategy.

Using the low-cost strategy, an HCO would drive down its costs as low as possible (to sell products and services at prices lower than its competitors'). For example, the HCO would not offer high-end features and upscale comforts. The HCO's facility would not be spacious and attractive, but its costs and prices would be low.

An HCO using a differentiation strategy would add features that make its products and services different and more appealing to customers. For example, the facility would be spacious and attractive—complete with high-definition TVs—but prices would be high. An organization should not try to use both strategies, nor should it switch back and forth between the strategies. HCO managers should pick one type of strategy, stay with it, and use it consistently so customers know what the HCO offers and stands for.

Each of Porter's two broad strategies can be applied to a wide or a narrow market. A business might use the low-cost strategy with a wide customer market (e.g., all people aged 18 or older) or with only a narrow customer market (e.g., only college students). Thus, there are four possible strategies:

Low-cost for a wide market	Differentiation for a wide market
Low-cost for a narrow market	Differentiation for a narrow market

Although these strategies are useful for HCOs, they were not originally developed for HCOs. Managers should be careful about using the low-cost strategy. While many people want lower prices for healthcare, some equate low prices with low quality. An HCO with a low-cost strategy that advertises "We have the lowest-cost care in town" might not pass "the mother test" in some people's minds (i.e., you wouldn't want to take your mother there). When their health is involved, many people want the best, especially when insurance pays for it. Rightly or wrongly, they may take low cost as a sign of low quality. The low-cost strategy can work for some healthcare services, but managers need to think carefully about how it will be perceived.

After developing the organization's mission, vision, and strategy, HCO managers form specific goals to help the HCO achieve its mission and vision. For example, a home health care business may set a goal of increasing its market share by 6 percent in Hamilton County by the end of its next fiscal year. As in the first stage of strategic planning, the HCO identifies critical issues it must address, such as how much to collaborate with other HCOs. After finishing this second stage, the HCO has decided where it should be going—what its new position in its market will be. It has decided Point B.

In the third stage of planning, the HCO's managers plan how to get from Point A to Point B. They ask, how do we accomplish the goals needed to achieve our mission and vision and implement the strategy needed to survive and thrive in our environment?

They develop implementation plans that, compared to the plans in the prior stage, are less abstract and have more concrete tasks and actions. Creating detailed plans involves more lower-level planning by managers, departments, and individual work units. For each task, a detailed work plan may be prepared that outlines who will do what, when, and using which resources. Partners HealthCare developed an implementation plan detailing what it must do to achieve its goal of reducing hospital readmissions. A medical group in the city of Scranton, Pennsylvania, might set a goal of opening a clinic in a nearby rural area. The implementation plan should name the people responsible for specific actions, such as who will lease office space by February 1, who will hire staff by February 15, who will purchase exam tables and clinical equipment by February 20, and so forth. An implementation plan can identify resources needed, such as $3,000 for advertising to recruit applicants for new staff positions. A useful planning tool is the Gantt chart, which is discussed at the end of this chapter. The planners also address critical issues at this stage, such as how to best allocate available staff to achieve multiple goals.

Finally, the strategic planning model shows an arrow at the bottom. The arrow indicates that after the plans are implemented, the results then feed back into the cyclical planning process to influence future planning. The outcomes that follow implementation will answer managers' questions, such as: How well did our strategies enable us to gain advantage over rivals? Did our medical group gain advantage by opening a rural clinic? How well did we achieve our goals? Did our hospital reduce its readmissions? Answers will affect future planning and create a new "where we are now" (Point A).

Managers must constantly plan. They must continually gather information about their organization's performance, results, opportunities, threats, and problems. Managers respond to this information by planning what to do next. While managers usually create a strategic plan annually, they do other planning more often. Many plan daily, weekly, and monthly.

PLANNING AT LOWER LEVELS

Lower-level managers plan annual goals, projects, and work in their departments that, when accomplished, will help the HCO achieve its higher-level mission, vision, and goals. Top-level managers in the HCO determine how much to involve lower-level managers—who analyzes data, who gives input, who decides goals, and so forth. In some HCOs, top-level managers work with departments to forecast relevant future trends, events, and workloads. In larger HCOs, specialized staff such as planning analysts help to gather data, interpret it, and assist department managers.

A department's workload forecast becomes the basis for a department's plans. Department managers plan their annual and monthly workloads, such as lab tests performed, healthy lifestyle classes taught, wheelchairs sold, or computer workstations installed. Based on planned workloads, managers forecast the resources needed to produce those workloads—staff, equipment, space, supplies, training, and other resources. They prepare schedules to show when during the year staff will be hired, equipment will be bought, new services will be begun, seasonal workloads will vary, and so forth. Then the cost of each resource is calculated and used to prepare annual and monthly budgets for the coming year. Department managers can get cost data from vendors, finance staff, human resources staff, and procurement staff. The workload forecast, anticipated resource requirements, and budget are plans that guide future action and provide targets to reach. Managers use these targets in the control process that we will study in Chapter 12.

Within each department, managers (supervisors) of smaller work units cooperate with department managers to plan for even shorter periods of time. The supervisor of the cytology section in the lab may create monthly work schedules for staff, weekly estimates of supplies needed, and daily task lists. The histology supervisor, microbiology supervisor, and hematology supervisor do the same. Shift supervisors plan how to divide the work of an eight-hour shift among the staff and may have to adjust plans if the work unit is short-staffed on a particular day.

Individual divisions, departments, and lower-level work units within the HCO prepare their own plans to support the higher-level plans and HCO mission. Managers of these units may follow a similar approach to that described previously for strategic planning, although planning at lower levels is more specific to each work unit and focused on implementation plans. For example, at Valley Medical Supply Company, the sales department is responsible for selling medical equipment and supplies. After Valley Medical Supply makes its strategic plan, its sales department prepares annual sales plans for products and customer groups that must be achieved for the company to reach its strategic plan goals.

The Valley Medical Supply sales manager, Fernando, plans by answering the three key questions: Where are we now? Where should we be going? How do we get there? He does this for his specific work unit, the sales department. Fernando assesses the relevant external environment and his current situation and analyzes the sales department's SWOTs. The answer to the second question will likely come from the higher-level plan that calls for a 7 percent increase in sales to hospitals, a 5 percent increase to nursing homes, a 5 percent increase to medical groups, and a 4 percent increase to all other HCOs. As sales manager, Fernando breaks these targets into smaller targets—for example, dividing them by geographic area. Breaking down the targets helps him plan how to assign his sales team so his department can achieve the sales target increases. He creates an implementation plan to answer the third question: How do we get there? In this case, how do we increase sales to hospitals, to medical groups, and so on according to the higher-level plan?

At this focused level, planning provides answers regarding who will do what, when, and with which resources to achieve the target increase in sales. Fernando plans how to assign his sales staff for each month of the year, when to do sales training, when to buy which new equipment (e.g., cars, iPads, cell phones), and how much to expect in sales for each potential customer each month.

The main point is that lower-level work units may plan implementation of higher-level goals set by top management's strategic plan. After higher-level plans are approved by upper management and the board of directors, they are shared with middle- and lower-level managers. These managers are responsible for departments where the day-to-day, hands-on work is done to produce the products and services. They may prepare the implementation plans that, when executed, will bring to life the higher-level managers' ideas and goals. Lower-level department managers draft departmental implementation plans that detail what their departments must do to help achieve the strategic plan and goals. Lower-level managers review plans with higher-level managers and reach agreement on priorities, staff requirements, supplies and equipment needs, budgets, and timelines. Sometimes, a higher-level or lower-level project manager and project team might develop the implementation plan, as explained later in this chapter.

In addition to determining what his department must do to help achieve the organization's larger plans and goals, a manager must plan for his own department. In Fernando's case, he and his sales department will identify what they will achieve as departmental goals next year. The goals might include renovating existing space to create a better employee break room and devising a better scheduling system for department staff. A Gantt chart could be prepared to plan how to achieve each goal.

Similar to a senior manager, a lower-level manager constantly gathers and analyzes information about his department and its SWOTs. Based on this information, the manager plans what to do.

PROJECT PLANNING AND MANAGEMENT

The third stage of the strategic planning process—implementation planning—typically requires planning for different projects needed to achieve the goals and objectives set in the second stage. For example, suppose a sports medicine clinic has been providing services to local schools and athletic leagues in Grand Rapids. In the strategic planning process, the clinic managers might decide to also offer fitness classes to businesses for employee wellness. This project is approved in the second stage of the strategic plan. In the third stage, the clinic managers plan a project: the start-up of this new service for businesses. They plan how to get there: how to begin offering exercise classes for businesses. To do so, they could use the methods and steps that follow.

Managers often use projects to implement and achieve goals in an organization's strategic plan. This approach is good for the implementation stage of strategic planning because it identifies a goal and then plans in much detail how to accomplish that goal. According to the Project Management Institute (PMI 2013), a project is temporary work done to create something new or improved, such as a product, service, process, document, or result. Unlike ongoing routine activity, a project has a start and a finish. Think of an HCO you know. What projects might have been done there? Perhaps its projects included a new diabetes treatment program, a new warehouse, the conversion to electronic health records, the installation of energy-efficient lighting, or a policy for employees' rights and responsibilities.

A project does not just happen; someone has to plan and manage it to make it happen. Project planning can be simple or complex. At a minimum, the manager should state the purpose of the project, identify specific outputs the project will deliver, list the tasks that must be done, schedule the tasks, assign people to do the tasks, and list resources needed to carry out the plan. For complex projects, an HCO is likely to use a more comprehensive approach called project management. The Mayo Clinic often uses project management to implement projects that improve medical care (Winterhouse Institute 2010). Project management is one way that managers add value to their organizations—and help people live healthier lives.

"**Project management** is the application of knowledge, skills, tools, and techniques to project activities to meet the project requirements" (PMI 2013, 5). Organizations—including HCOs—believe project management helps them achieve many benefits, including better control of resources, customer relations, development times, costs, quality, profit margins, productivity, coordination, worker morale, and reliability (Schwalbe and Furlong 2013, 3). To start a project, a senior-level manager appoints a project manager with responsibility to initiate, plan, execute, monitor and control, and close the project. Each of these actions is briefly defined as follows (PMI 2013, 5):

Project management
The application of knowledge, skills, tools, and techniques to project activities to meet project requirements.

- ◆ *Initiate:* Define a new project or new phase of an existing project by obtaining authorization to start the project or phase

- ◆ *Plan:* Establish the scope of the project, refine the objectives, and define the course of action required to obtain the objectives

- ◆ *Execute:* Complete the work defined in the project management plan to satisfy the project specifications

- ◆ *Monitor and control:* Track, review, and regulate the progress and performance of the project; identify any areas in which changes to the plan are required; and initiate the corresponding changes

- ◆ *Close:* Finalize all activities to formally close the project

Innovative HCOs depend on project managers to bring to life the organization's goals and plans (PMI 2013; Schwalbe and Furlong 2013). Project managers work to ensure assigned projects are completed within established constraints of time, budget, risks, scope, quality, and available resources. This work involves much thought and action.

Project managers analyze the organization's structure, culture, processes, and people, and the influence each might have on a project. They determine key individuals—stakeholders—who have interests in and expectations for the project. Some stakeholders might have conflicting interests (stakes) that must be resolved so that the project is not "pushed and pulled" in different directions.

To accomplish this work, a project manager carefully forms a team of people for the project. The size, membership, and structure of the team will vary depending on the project, the organization, and other factors. (Forming a team—such as a project team—requires careful thought and choices, which are explained in Chapter 6.) The project manager and team use management skills (many of which are presented in this book) as well as project management tools, software, and apps to plan and manage the

- ◆ scope (expected results) of the project;

- ◆ schedule and timing of detailed tasks and activities required to complete the project;

- ◆ resources needed for the project;

- ◆ cost and budget for the project;

- ◆ procurement of supplies, equipment, and services for the project;

- ◆ risks involved in the project; and

- ◆ work of other people and stakeholders to accomplish the project.

Many HCO managers like the excitement, involvement, and achievement that come with project management. Some earn special certifications from the PMI, such as Certified Associate in Project Management (CAPM) or the more advanced Project Management Professional (PMP). Project management requires many of the same tools, methods, and competencies as general management, although it applies them to specific, time-limited projects. Recall from Chapter 2 Gulick's five management functions and Katz's three types of management skills. As a project manager, you would use all of them. Interpersonal skills are important, especially for "leadership, team building, motivation, communication, influencing, decision making, political and cultural awareness, negotiation, trust building, conflict management, and coaching" (PMI 2013, 19). These skills reflect what project managers do—they lead, build teams, motivate, make decisions, and so on. You will learn many of these skills in later chapters of this book on team building, motivation, decision making, leading, and other management functions. As you read this book, think about how you can apply what you learn to project management.

Project managers in HCOs should realize that healthcare is different from many other products and services. Healthcare projects often directly affect people's health and may have life-and-death consequences. Healthcare is often personal and emotional, especially for patients. Finances are usually complex, hard to measure, and difficult to assign within a project. Compared to outcomes in other industries, healthcare outcomes are hard to measure, quantify, and link to a specific project, although outcome measurement has been improving. Thus, managing healthcare projects can involve unique challenges (Schwalbe and Furlong 2013).

Perhaps you realized that managing a project includes managing change. We will return to project management when we study change management in Chapter 14. By then, you will have learned more tools, methods, theories, and concepts that can be used to manage projects and change.

A **Gantt chart** can be used as a project planning tool to show who will do what, and when, to accomplish a project on time and achieve the project purpose. One example of a Gantt chart is shown in Exhibit 3.3; Gantt charts can have many variations. Simple Gantt charts can be made in Microsoft Excel by inserting a bar chart. For more complex charts, managers use commercial software designed specifically for project planning and management.

Gantt chart
Graphic arrangement of tasks (needed to complete a project) in sequence with start and end dates for each task.

EXHIBIT 3.3
Gantt Chart for a Clinic Registration Change Project

	March	April	May	June	July	August	September	October
Develop project charter	■							
Appoint improvement team		■						
Kickoff project— first team meeting		◆						
Analyze current practices			■					
Gather performance data				■				
Identify improvement opportunities— second meeting				◆				
Solicit solution ideas from colleagues					■			
Finalize solutions— third meeting					◆			
Implement solutions on a trial basis						■		
Evaluate the effect of solutions— fourth meeting							◆	
Roll out successful solutions								■
Redesign ineffective solutions— fifth meeting								◆

SOURCE: Spath (2013).

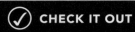

CHECK IT OUT

You can find many examples of Gantt charts online. Some are simple with just basic information, while others are complex with detailed layers of information. Some charts become so large that they are then divided into subcharts that combine to portray an entire project. Search online for the term *Gantt charts* to see many variations of this useful planning tool.

The Gantt chart shows the tasks or activities needed to complete the project. A good practice is to state each task using a verb followed by a noun: for example, *create* (verb) *a registration form* (noun). Each task can be broken down into smaller tasks; managers decide how much subtasking to include. Managers set anticipated start and end dates for each task, considering constraints, deadlines, work schedules, and other factors. When managers decide how tight to make the timeline, allowing some flexibility is usually a good idea. Tasks are generally arranged by start date in descending order. A horizontal bar shows the start and end dates for each task. Different shapes may indicate different tasks and activities; for example, a diamond indicates a meeting. The shapes can be color coded to signal importance, risk, or other characteristics. If more than one person will be responsible for tasks, planners should insert names or job titles to show who will do which tasks. Once the project begins, managers monitor progress and gradually darken each task bar to show progress on each task. Actual (versus planned) start and end dates may be added, and managers can revise the chart if necessary. We will return to Gantt charts in Chapter 12.

BUSINESS PLANS

As part of the long-range (i.e., beyond one year) planning process, an HCO might develop a business plan. This plan could be for the entire organization, especially if the HCO is small. Or, the plan could be for a part of a large HCO, such as a separate ambulatory surgery center owned by a large hospital. While an in-depth explanation of business plans is beyond the scope of this book, this chapter briefly outlines the contents of a business plan and its relationship to strategic planning.

A business plan can help managers implement the HCO's goals and can serve as a guide for starting and operating a business to achieve preset goals and objectives. A business plan uses a lot of information from the strategic plan but requires additional information, such as data from financial plans.

What is in a business plan? The US Small Business Administration (2014) provides a model business plan for three to five years. It includes the following elements:

- *Executive summary:* Provides a quick look at the entire business plan

- *Company description:* Describes the company, business, or organization with information on what it does, how it differs from others, and which markets it serves

◆ *Market analysis:* Describes the industry, customer market, and competitors

◆ *Organization and management:* Explains how the organization will be structured and managed, similar to what is shown by an organization chart

◆ *Service or product line:* Details the products and services offered and their benefits for intended customers

◆ *Marketing and sales:* Explains the marketing, sales, and promotion of the business

◆ *Funding request:* Gives the information needed when seeking outside funding, such as a grant or loan

◆ *Financial projections:* Provides financial analyses and forecasted profit-or-loss statement, cash flow, and balance sheet

◆ *Appendix:* Optional; contains resumes of key staff, contracts, leases, or permits

A useful online resource for business plans is Bplans (2014), which is owned and operated by Palo Alto Software (a company that serves entrepreneurs and managers). Bplans has hundreds of online sample business plans with extensive narratives, charts, and data. The plans include 26 sample plans for healthcare businesses, such as chiropractic clinic, health club, medical equipment business, dental office, family medicine clinic, laboratory, home health services company, medical billing company, nursing home, and occupational health business. The business plan for home health care services includes the following items:

1. Executive summary with the overall mission, objectives, and keys to success for the business

2. Company summary

3. Services offered

4. Market analysis with market segmentation, market targets, and competitor analysis

5. Strategy and implementation with marketing strategies and target dates for key events

6. Management summary with staffing plan

7. Financial plan with projected balance sheet, cash flow, profit-or-loss statement, break-even analysis, and key financial ratios

Data and Information for Planning

How do managers find data and information for planning? What are some sources you can think of? One option is by searching online. On the Internet, you can find

- local demographic and epidemiological data to describe the population and identify trends (data in county or state department of health and census bureau),

- information about HCOs and health trends in your community (data in local newspapers and HCO websites and reports), and

- trends and predictions for HCOs (data from professional associations such as the American College of Healthcare Executives and the Healthcare Financial Management Association).

Another important source is your HCO. It has lots of data stored digitally and in paper files, reports, surveys, and other documents. Your HCO continually captures data about customers, supplies bought and used, workloads, numbers of products and services, staff hours worked, and much more. Many HCOs store digital data in data warehouses that employees may search for specific types of data. Some also combine their data with hundreds of other large data sources and then perform data analytics to better understand their organization, customers, competitors, and external environments. Ask your HCO's chief information officer what types of data are available and how to access them.

People are another source of data and information. Talk with stakeholders to obtain qualitative information that is not captured well digitally. Gather opinions about what might happen next year. Ask others what they think your main competitor will do. Be sure to talk to people who use your products and services and people you coordinate with. They can help you learn about your department's strengths and weaknesses. Your manager will have valuable opinions, as will your department's workers. Talk with people outside your HCO too—vendors and sales representatives, staff in relevant local government agencies, and employees of health organizations that your HCO works with. These sources will get you started. You will surely discover others during your career.

Concluding Thoughts About Planning

The strategic planning model and the planning topics discussed in this chapter are often used in an HCO to plan and implement its full mission, vision, and goals. Managers plan for market share, quality, cultural diversity, finances, and many other aspects of HCOs. We should realize, however, that the planning process and topics can be used to plan for a single aspect of an HCO.

For example, the Lehigh Valley Health Network (LVHN) used strategic planning specifically for cultural competence (Gertner et al. 2010). LVHN includes two hospitals, ten community health centers, and thousands of physicians and employees who provide a full range of healthcare services. The senior vice president of human resources led a multidisciplinary task force for cultural competency that did strategic planning, lower-level planning, and project planning. It gathered data from relevant stakeholders and assessed LVHN's external environment and internal cultural competency situation. This information enabled the task force to evaluate LVHN's cultural competency position and issues. Then the task force planned a cultural competence mission that was consistent with and supported LVHN's overall mission. From there, the task force planned cultural competence goals and objectives to achieve its new cultural competence mission. Lower-level planning and project planning—including planning tasks and methods discussed earlier, such as the use of Gantt charts—were then used to implement the plans, goals, and objectives of cultural competency.

In concluding this chapter, here are useful guidelines to keep in mind when you plan:

◆ Managers should view planning as a process, not as an event.

◆ Managers should value the process of planning and the actual plan.

◆ Managers should realize that planning is orderly yet messy, sequential yet circular.

◆ Managers should allow for flexibility in the planning process and in the plan.

◆ Managers should combine objective analysis with subjective judgment in planning.

◆ Managers should use—but not overuse—historical records and data in planning.

◆ Managers should look inward (at the organization) and outward (at the environment) when planning.

ONE MORE TIME

Planning is deciding what to do and how to it. Planning is future oriented, is continual, and is done at all levels of an HCO. Planning must be done well because it sets the stage for the other management functions—organizing, staffing, leading, and controlling. Managers at higher levels plan for the long term with a broad perspective of the HCO. At lower levels, managers plan for a shorter period and for a smaller part of the HCO. Higher-level planning is concerned more with what to do, while lower-level plans are concerned more with how to do it.

Strategic planning is essential for an HCO to prepare for its future. This type of planning enables an HCO to examine where it is now in its environment, where it wants to be in the future, and how it will get there. Strategic planning should include analysis of SWOTs, stakeholders, and critical issues. This analysis leads to the HCO's mission, vision, values, goals, objectives, and strategy. An HCO then uses project plans to help determine how to implement its goals. Project planning can include the use of a Gantt chart to identify tasks, timelines, and assignments to accomplish a goal or project. Managers use project management methods and business plans to plan and implement complex projects to achieve organizational goals.

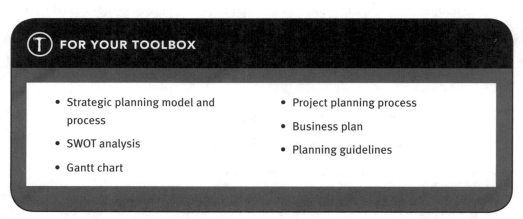

(T) FOR YOUR TOOLBOX

- Strategic planning model and process
- SWOT analysis
- Gantt chart
- Project planning process
- Business plan
- Planning guidelines

FOR DISCUSSION

1. What is planning? What is strategic planning?

2. Referring to Exhibit 3.1, discuss how strategic planning is done. Which part of the model do you think would be most challenging for managers?

3. How could a manager determine the SWOTs for an HCO?

4. Compare and contrast planning at higher levels of an HCO with planning at lower levels.

5. Discuss how project planning is done and why it is important in HCOs.

CASE STUDY QUESTIONS

These questions refer to the Integrative Case Studies at the back of this book.

1. Disparities in Care at Southern Regional Health System case: Apply the first stage of the strategic planning model (shown in Exhibit 3.1) to describe "where we are now" for SRHS. Then apply stage two of the model to describe "where we should be going" for SRHS.

2. Taking Care of Business at Graceland Memorial Hospital case: Identify the stakeholders and their stakes in this case (as in Exhibit 3.2).

3. Decisions, Decisions case: Assume the HCO decides to develop a new day-care center. Create a Gantt chart (as in Exhibit 3.3) for that project.

4. Ergonomics in Practice case: Explain how project management methods could be used to implement the lift system at Riverlea Rehab.

⊙ TRY IT, APPLY IT

Suppose you are the student health and wellness coordinator at a university. In its strategic plan, the university has set a goal of offering students more places on campus to exercise and more incentives to do so. You must prepare an implementation plan to achieve this goal. Brainstorm tasks and activities needed to increase the number of exercise places and incentives. Then prepare a detailed Gantt chart to show the sequence and timeline of your proposed tasks and activities. Assign job titles to show who will be responsible for each task in your Gantt chart. Carefully think through the dozens of tasks that would have to be done and show much detail.

CHAPTER 4

ORGANIZING: JOBS, POSITIONS, AND DEPARTMENTS

For every minute spent organizing, an hour is earned.

Benjamin Franklin, author, printer,
scientist, inventor, diplomat

LEARNING OBJECTIVES

Studying this chapter will help you to

➤ explain organizations;

➤ define systems and explain why systems are open to their environments;

➤ relate organizing to planning;

➤ organize work tasks into jobs, positions, and departments;

➤ coordinate work among jobs, positions, and departments;

➤ compare and contrast mechanistic and organic structures;

➤ examine complications that might arise when organizing work; and

➤ explain how to organize medical positions.

HERE'S WHAT HAPPENED

Throughout Partners HealthCare's long history and extensive growth, managers had been organizing work into tasks, jobs, positions, departments, divisions, and other groupings to achieve the HCO's mission and goals. When Partners's managers developed new strategic plan and goals, they had to reorganize the HCO's work. They assigned specific responsibilities to specific jobs: primary care physician, cardiologist, diabetes educator, telehealth nurse, pharmacist, equipment technician, project specialist, Center for Connected Health director, and many others. Managers decided how much decision-making authority to decentralize to lower levels of the hierarchy (organization chart). Many positions and work groups were specialized with a narrow range of tasks. Thus, managers had to integrate (coordinate) all the jobs, departments, teams, divisions, and groups into one organization or system working toward a shared purpose and goals. Figuring out how to organize work among the staff—and then how to coordinate it—is one way that managers added value to Partners HealthCare. By doing that, managers helped the organization run smoothly, achieve goals, satisfy employees and patients, and improve population health in the Boston region.

In Chapter 2, we learned terms and concepts for organizing work that are important parts of management theory. This chapter will further apply those concepts, showing how they are used in the wide variety of HCOs. (You might want to quickly review those terms.)

After managers at Partners HealthCare developed plans for their organization, they faced a complex question: How should they organize work and workers to accomplish those plans? It was not a multiple-choice question with just one correct answer. It was a complex puzzle for which different managers might choose different answers based on their unique interpretation of the situation. Remember contingency theory from Chapter 2? The best way to organize is contingent (depends) on factors such as organization size, environment, plans, and technology, which managers must try to perceive and interpret. There is no one best way to organize. There are many possible ways to organize—and each has pros and cons. Managers must consider the pros and cons of different organizational forms and decide which would be best for the HCO now. Later, they should reconsider the HCO's organization when its size, environment, plans, and other factors change.

Organizing is the second of the five main functions of management that we study. Several of the management roles described by Henry Mintzberg (discussed in Chapter 2) involve organizing: liaison, entrepreneur, disturbance handler, and resource allocator.

Managers at all levels must organize the work and workers for which they are responsible. Even managers of small departments or sections of a department must understand how to formally organize work so that they can achieve their area's goals. This chapter first defines organizations and systems and then explains how hundreds of work tasks are organized into jobs and positions, which are then organized into departments. The chapter also describes how to coordinate jobs in departments.

Organizing work in HCOs is too complex a subject to address in one chapter. After learning how to organize jobs and departments in this chapter, in Chapter 5 you will learn about structural designs to organize departments into an entire organization and link to the external environment. Chapter 6 discusses groups and teams and how to coordinate positions and departments. These chapters also explain complications that arise when organizing HCOs. Together, these three chapters provide a practical introduction to how managers organize HCOs.

ORGANIZATIONS

Organizations
Social entities that are goal directed, designed as deliberately structured and coordinated activity systems, and linked to the external environment.

Organizations are "social entities that are goal-directed, designed as deliberately structured and coordinated activity systems, and are linked to the external environment" (Daft 2013, 642). What does this mean?

- ◆ An organization is a social entity—it has people.

- ◆ An organization is goal directed—it pursues a purpose.

- ◆ An organization is deliberately structured and coordinated—it is intentionally set up, organized, and arranged.

- ◆ An organization is an activity system—it has actions and parts that interact and thus affect each other.

- ◆ An organization is linked to the environment—it connects and interacts with what is out there beyond itself.

SYSTEMS

System
A set of interrelated parts that function as a whole to achieve a common purpose.

A **system** is a "set of interrelated parts that function as a whole to achieve a common purpose" (Daft 2013, 33). For example, a university is a system with many interrelated parts that work together to achieve the mission or purpose of the university. A motorcycle is a system, and so is a town, a cell phone, and a medical clinic. Can you identify the purpose and some parts of each of these systems?

Within a system, some components may work together as a subsystem to achieve a common, smaller subpurpose. For example, an office of alumni affairs is a subsystem in a university—it has components that work together to achieve a smaller subpurpose pertaining to alumni. A motorcycle has a braking subsystem, and a medical clinic has a staffing subsystem for hiring employees. Because we are concerned with organizations, and organizations are made up of people, for the rest of our discussion we will focus on social (people) systems rather than mechanical systems such as a motorcycle. Organizations are social systems, as was first explained by Katz and Kahn (1966).

The system perspective is important for managers because it emphasizes interrelated parts working toward a common goal. Think about what that means. If one part of an organization falters, grows, evolves, or in some way changes, then its relationships with other interrelated parts will change. The changed interrelationships may then cause other parts to evolve, falter, or change and no longer work toward the common purpose. For example, if a registration clerk in a public health clinic falters in her work one day (perhaps because of a stressful event that morning), then the interaction between the registration staff and the nursing staff may also change, resulting in communication problems, delays, and misunderstandings. The changed relationship between the two system parts (registration and nursing) will alter how the staff works. Even if one system component changes for the better, it can cause a different interaction with other system components that could upset the system. For example, if the clerk works more quickly one day so that she can leave early, that change could affect how the registration and nursing staffs (subsystems) interact. Nurses might feel that the system has sped up and struggle to keep up.

The systems perspective reminds us to always think ahead and proactively consider how a change (good or bad) in one system part might affect other system parts and how they interact. If Joe, the budget analyst, retires and Darrell, the finance manager, hires Chelsea to replace him, the interaction between the budget analyst and the finance manager—two system parts—is likely to be different (at least for a while). The finance manager should anticipate this and try to adjust so that all system parts work together toward the common purpose.

OPEN AND CLOSED SYSTEMS

Managers and management scholars originally thought of organizations as closed systems. This meant the organizations were closed off from external forces and did not interact with their environments. Organizations were viewed as existing separate from and independent of their environments. Is that possible? Not really.

Scholars and managers then developed the open system perspective (Bertalanffy 1968). They argued that organizations are affected by their environments (whether they want to be or not) and must interact with them. Organizations have to be open systems—open to their environments—to acquire resources, staff, supplies, equipment, information, technology, and other inputs from the environment. These inputs are brought into the organization and used to produce services and products. This production occurs within the production subsystem of an organization and transforms inputs into outputs by mixing, arranging, connecting, combining, and processing inputs in many different ways to create many different services and products. Then organizations must be open to the external environment to give, sell, provide, and deliver their products, services, and outputs to customers, clients, and people in the environment outside the organization.

EXHIBIT 4.1

Organizations
Are Open to
Environment

| Inputs from environment brought into HCO | HCO transforms inputs to outputs | HCO sends outputs out to the environment |

An HCO that is open to its environment imports inputs and exports outputs as shown in Exhibit 4.1. For example, a medical lab in Tuscaloosa, Alabama, is open to its environment to acquire lab equipment, test reagents, lab technicians, waiting room chairs, technical advice, lab certification, paper clips, blood tubes, and other inputs. The lab is open to its environment to sell its services and outputs to patients, businesses, and health insurance companies.

Another reason organizations are open systems is that organizations are affected by their environments. They cannot seal themselves off from external forces such as economic conditions, new technological inventions, people's attitudes, and competitors' actions. An organization is open to (i.e., affected by) its environment because external forces act on the organization; recall the discussion of changes and trends in Chapter 1. External forces can strongly affect an HCO, and the HCO must recognize those forces and adapt to them (or else suffer). HCOs have been affected by such external forces as laws, hurricanes, multiculturalism, economic recession, aging baby boomers, and people's desire for around-the-clock availability of healthcare. HCOs cannot close themselves off from the environment. Social media enable stakeholders in the environment (e.g., vendors, patients, job hunters, government agencies, and others) to interact directly and easily with HCOs. This increases the extent to which HCOs are open to their environments and to which managers must use an open-system approach.

Taking this discussion one step further, recall from Chapter 2 that organizations may be complex, adaptive systems. This approach views organizations not only as open to their environment but also as natural, dynamic, evolving organisms (not rigid machines) able to adapt to unpredictable environmental change. How open, complex, and adaptive an organization is depends on how managers design the organization.

In summary, an HCO chooses to be open to its environment to import inputs and to export outputs. An HCO is open to (affected by) the environment because of how environmental forces exert themselves on the HCO.

Formal organization
The official organization as approved by managers and stated in written documents.

Organization structure
The reporting relationships, vertical hierarchy, spans of control, groupings of jobs into departments and an entire organization, and systems for coordination and communication.

ORGANIZING WORK IN HEALTHCARE ORGANIZATIONS

An organization (as defined here) includes deliberately structured activity. Managers intentionally organize (structure) the activities, tasks, and work into systems that become the **formal organization**. This creates the **organization structure** of reporting relationships, vertical hierarchy, spans of control, groupings of jobs into departments and an entire organization, and, systems for coordination and communication (Daft 2013).

This structured activity can involve managers at various levels performing five types of organizing:

1. Work tasks must be grouped into job positions. Managers at all levels do this for their particular work units and areas of responsibility.

2. Jobs must be organized (grouped) into work units such as departments. Middle and top managers do this.

3. Departments must be organized (grouped) into an entire organization. Top managers do this.

4. Work must be coordinated among and across job positions and departments. Managers throughout the organization do this.

5. Because it is an open system, the organization must be linked to other organizations and people in its environment. All managers do this.

Managers do not necessarily organize work in this sequence one step at a time. Nor do they always use all five types of organizing to achieve every goal or plan. Entrepreneurs who start an entirely new diagnostic testing business—with lab, computed tomography (CT), magnetic resonance imaging (MRI), electrocardiogram (EKG), and other tests—will have to do all five types of organizing. Years later, in the same organization, the managers might do only the first and second types of organizing when they want to add one new position in one existing department. Because these five types of organizing interact, managers may use several of them simultaneously until everything fits together.

HCO managers do not always first organize tasks into jobs and then jobs into a department. They might decide to add a department and then decide which jobs and positions are needed for it. Let's consider a hospital that wants to recruit physicians. First, suppose the hospital adds one new physician recruiter in its existing medical staff affairs office. That works out well, so another recruiter is added, and then a secretary, and then another recruiter. Eventually, managers organize those four positions into a new, separate department of physician recruitment. Alternatively, suppose that in the strategic planning process, managers decide the hospital must become more active in physician recruiting. They decide to create a new department of physician recruitment. Later, to implement this goal, managers decide which tasks, jobs, and positions are needed for the new department.

After organizing HCOs in these five ways, managers are not done organizing forever. They will occasionally need to reorganize to better achieve the HCO's mission, vision, goals, strategies, and plans. Recall that HCOs are open systems—open to their environments. Changes in the external environment force changes in how HCOs should be organized. For example, accreditors, health insurers, businesses (which pay for health insurance), and government agencies in the external environment have demanded that HCOs reduce medical errors and improve patient safety. This external pressure has led many HCOs to reorganize their tasks, jobs, departments, and work coordination (Olden and McCaughrin 2007).

Organizing Tasks into Jobs and Positions

Managers must decide which work tasks and responsibilities to assign to which jobs and positions, along with the authority, reporting relationships, and qualifications for each job. These elements interrelate, so it is hard to determine one without the others. A good starting point is to consider which tasks to combine into a certain job, and then figure out the other parts of the job.

In this chapter, **job** and **position** have been used somewhat interchangeably. We should realize these two terms have slightly different meanings. "A job consists of a group of activities and duties that entail natural units of work that are similar and related" (Fottler 2008a, 163). Some jobs, such as president, are performed by just one person. Other jobs, such as nurse, might be performed by two, three, or more people because of the volume of nursing work. In that case, there would be two, three, or more nurse positions, with each position filled by a separate person. "A position consists of different duties and responsibilities that are performed by only one employee" (Fottler 2008a, 163). Thus, five people may fill five nurse positions who all perform the nurse job.

Organizing particular tasks into a job creates division of work and specialization. Think of a job you had and list specific tasks you did. Also think of the tasks workers did when you went to a doctor's office for a checkup, an urgent care facility for a minor injury, or a hospice to visit a relative. Hundreds of tasks are done in HCOs, and managers design jobs to organize all these tasks into specific jobs. As a result, tasks are not randomly done or left to chance. They are assigned to certain jobs that are accountable for completing those tasks. (After managers divide the work into specialized jobs, they will have to coordinate and combine all these specialized jobs to work together toward common goals. Methods for doing this are explained later in this chapter.)

When assigning tasks to jobs, managers decide how wide or narrow to design a job. A job with many tasks is wider and less specialized than a job with fewer tasks. There is no "one best way" rule for how wide or narrow managers should make a job. One manager might follow the "practice makes perfect" guideline and have a narrow range of repeated tasks that someone presumably becomes very good at (the scientific management approach discussed in Chapter 2). This division of work would have separate, narrow jobs for carpentry, plumbing, electrical work, and painting in a nursing home. But narrow, repetitive jobs can become boring, and workers may eventually feel less motivated doing them day after day. A manager may therefore decide to add tasks to broaden a job (the human relations approach described in Chapter 2). Thus, a nursing home manager might assign all maintenance tasks to all maintenance jobs and have less division of work and specialization.

The question of how much to specialize and how many tasks to include in jobs occurs throughout an HCO with maintenance workers, nurses, physical therapists, human resources staff, food service workers, and managers themselves. Vice president titles in large hospitals reflect specialization and division of work: VP of financial affairs, VP of human resources, VP of patient care, and others. A C-suite of hospital executive offices may include specialized executives such as chief executive officer, chief operating officer,

Job
A group of activities and duties that entail natural units of work that are similar and related; may be performed by more than one person.

Position
Consists of duties and responsibilities that are performed by only one person.

chief finance officer, chief nursing officer, chief information officer, chief medical officer, chief quality officer, and others. Small hospitals may have only one VP, without specialization. Where and when tasks are performed also affects division of work, specialization, and how tasks are organized. Tasks for a weekend nurse may be similar but not completely the same as tasks for a nurse working weekdays. The tasks of a physical therapist in a nursing home may differ from the tasks of a therapist in a sports medicine clinic.

HERE'S WHAT HAPPENED

When Oxford Pediatrics began using a standard child developmental screening survey, here is how it divided work to be done and how it assigned tasks to jobs (Hostetter 2008):

- Clerical staff identifies families scheduled for future visits and mails them the survey to complete and bring to the visit.
- Medical assistants score the surveys and record the results on children's medical charts.
- Physicians (and nurse practitioners) review the survey results and discuss them with parents.
- Physicians (when necessary) refer parents/children for speech therapy, physical therapy, occupational therapy, or audiology service, and enter referral information in a referral book.
- Clerical staff mail the medical records of a referred child to the therapist.

Along with assignment of specific tasks to specific jobs, managers decide other elements of each job:

◆ How much authority (power) to delegate to a job—for example, to spend money, to enter notes in medical records, to sign contracts, or to give flu shots to patients (Each job must have sufficient authority to take actions, use resources, make decisions, and perform tasks that have been assigned to the job. Delegation is explained in more detail later in this chapter.)

◆ The reporting relationships in the vertical chain of command or hierarchy (explained further in the next part of this chapter)

   – The position (boss) one level up in the hierarchy to which a lower position reports

   – Position(s) (if any) one level down the hierarchy that report up to a higher position (boss)

◆ Qualifications needed to perform a job, such as education, experience, licensure, behaviors, and other characteristics (explained in more detail in Chapter 7)

ORGANIZING AN HCO's JOBS AND POSITIONS INTO DEPARTMENTS

Another step in organizing work (to accomplish goals) is **departmentalization**, which organizes jobs and positions into departments or other work groups. A manager must decide on what basis to group positions. A department (or bureau, division, section, office) may contain jobs that have something in common (Dunn 2010). The jobs

◆ perform the same kind of work (e.g., housekeeping),

◆ serve the same group of customers (e.g., women),

◆ create the same health service (e.g., surgical care),

◆ work in the same place (e.g., the downtown site), or

◆ work at the same time (e.g., third shift).

Departmentalization
Organization of jobs into departments, bureaus, divisions, sections, offices, and other formal work groups.

Organization chart
Visual portrayal of vertical hierarchy, departments, span of control, reporting relationships, and flow of authority.

As a department manager, you will apply management theory principles you learned in Chapter 2 to design your department's reporting relationships (vertical hierarchy), span of control, line/staff positions, unity of command, and (de)centralization.

We will study the application of management theory principles by using an example of positions in the sales department of a health insurance company. The sales manager, Kayla, must decide the *reporting relationships* of workers in her department. She decides that all four sales representatives will report directly to her, as shown in the **organization chart** in Exhibit 4.2. This creates *vertical hierarchy* for the department.

When deciding reporting relationships and vertical hierarchy, the department manager is also deciding the *span of control* (how many workers will report directly to a manager). If all four sales reps and one secretary report to Kayla, her span of control is five, which is reasonable. Suppose that over time, the department grows and hires nine more

EXHIBIT 4.2
Department Organization Chart with Two Levels in the Vertical Hierarchy

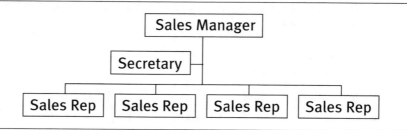

sales reps who also report to Kayla. Her span of 14 could be too many for her to effectively manage. She would not have enough time to manage all the workers, her decisions would be delayed, and the sales reps would feel their boss is unavailable and uninterested in them. As department manager, Kayla should consider adding another level of management—a supervisor level—between the sales reps and the department manager. This adds a level to the vertical hierarchy, as shown in Exhibit 4.3. All sales reps now report to either the East Region Supervisor or the West Region Supervisor. The manager's span of control is now only three (two supervisors and one secretary). Kayla will have to delegate sufficient authority and responsibility to the supervisors so that they can make decisions without having to consult her too often. Delegation of that authority to the supervisors will enable closer supervision of sales reps, which might be needed to achieve the planned sales goals.

Like many aspects of management, the "best" approach is contingent on several factors. Recall from Chapter 2 that researchers found that different departments face different contingencies and thus should be organized with different degrees of centralization, specialization, division of work, chain of command, and so forth. The tasks workers do, workers' education levels, and external pressures all affect span of control.

If all the workers do similar work that is simple, repetitive, and easily explained in procedural rules, a manager might capably supervise ten or more workers. However, if workers do many different tasks that are complex, hard to explain, unpredictable, and nonroutine, then more supervision is needed, and a manager should have a smaller span of control. If the department's environment changes often and unpredictably, a smaller span of control will allow more frequent supervision to help workers adjust. More education, training, and professionalism of workers also enable less supervision per worker and thus a wider span of control. Smaller spans require more personnel, because more supervisors are required. This becomes costly and may not be feasible.

Organizing jobs into a department also involves deciding which jobs are *line* positions and which are *staff* positions. In Exhibits 4.2 and 4.3, we see the sales reps are line positions in the vertical chain of command because they contribute directly to accomplishing the sales goals of the department. The secretary is in a staff position outside the vertical chain of command. That job supports the line positions and indirectly helps to achieve

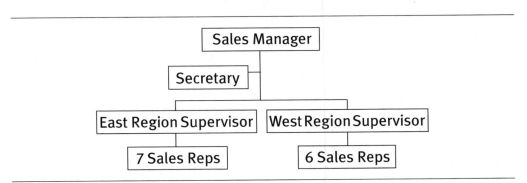

EXHIBIT 4.3
Department Organization Chart with Three Levels in the Vertical Hierarchy

the department's sales goals. Staff positions may provide assistance to relieve the workload of line positions, or staff may provide a specialized ability that line positions do not have.

The *unity of command* is considered when organizing jobs in a department. According to this principle, a worker reports to—and takes directions from—a single boss. This approach makes sense, and most workers would like it. But it is not always realistic, even in a sales office—and especially in HCOs, as we will see later. In Exhibit 4.2, four sales agents all report only to the sales manager and follow unity of command. However, the secretary reports directly to the sales manager yet most likely also takes direction from the four sales reps whom the secretary helps. Direct contact between the sales reps and secretary enables them to work together rather than by communication through the sales manager. This makes better use of the sales manager's time and reduces miscommunications, delays, and other problems. However, it places more demands on the secretary and may require more meetings to resolve conflict if all four salespersons tell the secretary their work should be done first.

The manager must also decide how much to *centralize* and *decentralize* authority. Recall that decentralization **delegates authority** to a lower-level position to make decisions. Decentralizing authority empowers the lower position by granting it authority to make decisions and take action necessary to perform the job. How much to decentralize depends on the people involved, type of work, and other factors. Certainly, the manager must delegate enough authority to enable subordinates to perform tasks assigned to their jobs. Kayla, as sales manager, can keep all authority centralized for some decisions and tasks (e.g., hiring new sales reps) so that only she will handle them. Yet she can simultaneously decentralize authority to sales reps for other decisions and tasks (e.g., scheduling sales calls and preparing contract proposals). The manager must delegate enough authority to lower-level positions—and share enough information with them—so that those employees at lower levels can do the jobs they are responsible for (as assigned by the manager). In delegating authority, however, the manager must realize that sales reps probably will not all do their work the same way, apply rules the same way, or make the same decisions.

Decentralization increases variation and decreases standardization at lower levels of the organization (Charns and Young 2012). Is that OK? Can the manager accept that? Each manager must consider these questions when organizing her work unit.

Beyond decentralization, Kayla might assign more tasks and delegate more authority to one sales rep (Josh) so that he may try new tasks for professional growth and cover for Kayla when she is on vacation. However, other sales reps may feel left out and think Kayla is unfair. Now employee morale and teamwork are declining! Kayla must delegate carefully and consider the pros and cons of delegating. Later chapters on leadership will offer advice for delegating work fairly.

In summary, when delegating authority, the following things must happen: A manager must ensure that the employee knows what the manager expects to be done and grant the employee authority for the necessary tasks, decisions, resource use, and actions. Then the employee must accept the responsibility and authority needed for the job, and agree to perform the job as expected. After authority is delegated to lower positions, the

Delegate authority
Share authority from
one position to a lower-
level position.

manager position still has the authority too. Delegating authority is like sharing knowledge—it increases the number of positions and people that have it, rather than taking it
from one and giving it to another (Dunn 2010). The manager is still responsible for the
work assigned to lower-level employees. If those employees slack off, drop the ball, and do
not fulfill their assignments, the manager is ultimately responsible and must do it herself.

Returning to the Here's What Happened at the beginning of this chapter, notice
how Partners HealthCare used these organizing principles. Managers brought together
specialized jobs (e.g., diabetes educator, telehealth nurse, equipment technician) and created a Center for Connected Health with responsibility for developing patient-centered
telehealth services. A director was given authority for the center, and authority for patient
care decisions was delegated to lower-level patient care staff.

COORDINATING JOBS AND POSITIONS IN AN HCO

Have you ever had to deal with two different nurses in a physician's office and neither
seemed to know what the other one had done? Sometimes organizations lack coordination.

In HCOs, there is too much work for just one person, so it is divided up among
many workers. Some workers are specialized and differentiated by their skills, training,
values, professional culture, and jobs. Yet somehow these workers must all work together
toward a common mission. Managers must link together many separate jobs so that they
all work toward a common purpose. To do so, they can use coordination mechanisms
vertically, horizontally, and sometimes even diagonally across the organization. That is part
of organization structure. Henry Mintzberg (1983b, as cited by Longest and Young 2006)
identified five coordination mechanisms. A sixth mechanism (groups) has been added
(Daft 2013). These mechanisms are listed and defined below. Examples for an outpatient
surgery center are included to illustrate each mechanism.

1. *Standardized work process:* a specific, consistent method of how to perform
   work that is often written in policy manuals, rule books, plans, standard
   operating procedures, and other documents. The surgery center has a written
   nine-step process for how to register a new patient for surgery.

2. *Standardized worker skills:* specific education, training, and skills needed for
   a job that lets other workers know what to expect from someone doing that
   job. All the surgeons know what they can expect of an anesthesiologist based
   on the education, training, and skills needed to be licensed and hired as an
   anesthesiologist.

3. *Standardized work output:* specific, consistent contents of completed work that
   other workers know to expect. A finance director prepares a budget report
   each month, and the executive director and board of directors know what
   kind of financial information to expect in the report.

Supervision
Workers have a supervisor–subordinate relationship in the chain of command, and they inform each other.

Mutual adjustment
Workers who do not have a supervisor–subordinate relationship exchange information and alter their work if needed to fit with each other.

4. ***Supervision:*** workers have a supervisor–subordinate relationship in the chain of command, and they inform each other about important matters. The nursing supervisor in the morning tells a nurse which surgery cases she will do today. During the day, that nurse informs the supervisor of progress on the cases and about an equipment problem in Room 4.

5. ***Mutual adjustment:*** workers do *not* have a supervisor–subordinate relationship in the chain of command (because they work in different departments), and they exchange information about important matters as coworkers. A maintenance worker and nurse confer to decide when to replace light bulbs in the recovery room.

6. *Groups:* workers from multiple work units and departments exchange information in meetings, patient rounds, conferences, committees, and task forces. Employees from six different departments meet and exchange information weekly to plan the summer picnic.

In the opening case, Partners HealthCare used telehealth patient care protocols for remote patients. This method standardizes care processes among health professionals to coordinate their tasks and activities. Some healthcare professionals feel that standardizing medical care is "cookbook medicine" that interferes with their professional judgment. However, as we will learn in Chapter 12, more HCOs are using standardized medical processes to reduce variation in care and reduce mistakes. It really works!

Besides these methods, managers form groups such as committees, councils, task forces, and project teams to coordinate tasks and work among many workers—and often many departments. Managers use these organizational structures to bring together workers who must coordinate work by planning schedules, exchanging information, rearranging their own work if necessary, and monitoring progress. (Have you ever served on a task force or committee at your college, during high school, or in a summer job? Which people did it bring together and for what purpose?) At the beginning of this chapter, we read that Partners HealthCare had to coordinate workers. Chapter 6 explains more about groups and how to make them effective.

Coordination largely depends on information exchange. Mobile text messaging, company intranets, websites, iPads, social media, FaceTime, and other information technologies enable widespread, fast coordination. Technology continually evolves, and HCOs must work hard to keep up. New, younger managers can help their HCOs determine how best to use new technology to coordinate work vertically, horizontally, and diagonally among jobs.

FACTORS THAT INFLUENCE ORGANIZING WORK

The HCO's environment (external factors) and the organization itself (internal factors) affect how managers organize work. Prior strategic planning, discussed in Chapter 3, analyzed both types of factors. Managers should already know the environment, its opportunities and threats, and whether it is stable or changing. They also should know the organization and its strengths, weaknesses, mission, goals, and type of work. Take a few minutes to jot down some examples of how the environment and the organization itself could affect how work is organized. Then read the following examples.

◆ Newly invented technology (for medicine and communication) creates new ways of performing existing tasks—and sometimes, entirely new tasks—that must be organized into jobs. Invention of digital communication out in the environment led to redesign of jobs to use digital health records. Digital "writing" slows down emergency physicians in hospital emergency departments, so many of those departments hire digital scribes. The scribe is in the emergency room with the physician and patient and writes all the digital medical records in real time while the physician treats the patient. After caring for the patient, the physician reviews, edits, and signs the digital record.

◆ Changes in HCO size (number of employees) alter how work is organized. Growth generally leads to more specialization. Conversely, if an HCO downsizes during an economic recession, the fewer remaining workers may be expected to do whatever needs to be done and will thus be less specialized.

Mechanistic Emphasizing specialized, rigidly defined tasks; strict hierarchy, control, rules, and authority; and vertical communication and interaction.

Organic Emphasizing shared common tasks; teamwork; loose hierarchy, control, rules, and authority; and horizontal communication and interaction.

EXTERNAL FACTORS

Recall from Chapter 2 that contingency theory arose from studies that found one type of organization structure works best if the external environment is mostly stable and predictable, whereas a different organization structure works best if the external environment changes quickly and unpredictably. There is no single best way to organize.

A mechanistic organization fits best with a stable, predictable environment, while an organic organization fits best with an unstable, changing environment. Characteristics of **mechanistic** and **organic** organizations are shown in Exhibit 4.4.

These two structures are idealized types; most organizations are in between them yet tend toward one type. Many managers feel their environments have become more unstable and unpredictable, so they have reorganized their HCOs to become more organic. The organic model seems more alive and natural than the mechanistic form. Many organizations are becoming more organic with more horizontal structure, looser rules, more teamwork, and fewer solo jobs. In addition, organizations are collaborating more and adapting more (Daft 2013; Olden 2012).

 CHECK IT OUT

Healthcare workers often use care protocols that list standardized work processes for specific health problems. These protocols are based on scientific evidence and help coordinate work among healthcare workers. Do a Google search for "standard care protocols" or "hospital care protocols" to find examples of standardized work processes in healthcare.

Exhibit **4.4**
Environment and
Structure

Stable, Predictable Environment	Unstable, Unpredictable Environment
Mechanistic structure is best	*Organic structure is best*
Separate specialized tasks	Shared common tasks
Rigidly defined tasks	Tasks adjusted with teamwork
Strict hierarchy, control, rules, authority	Loose hierarchy, control, rules, authority
Vertical communication, interaction	Horizontal communication, interaction

SOURCE: Information from Daft (2013).

You might want to quickly review the ten sectors of the external environment described in Chapter 1. Thinking about these sectors will help you understand the many external factors that affect how work and jobs are organized. For example, professional norms, labor supply, state laws, reimbursement, and other external forces influenced the design of pharmacist jobs. Years ago, the task of filling a prescription in a hospital pharmacy was designed into a pharmacist job. However, stakeholders pressured hospital managers to reduce costs. Also, because of a pharmacist shortage, hospitals struggled to fill pharmacist jobs and had to pay more to do so. Managers then reorganized some tasks done by pharmacists into a new pharmacy technician job that required less education, skill, and pay. Working under the supervision of pharmacists, technicians count pills, label containers, and perform other minor tasks that pharmacists had been doing. Meanwhile, external licensure laws required that certain tasks still be done by a pharmacist.

These changes enabled hospitals to perform required tasks less expensively while adapting to external factors. Similar job redesign has occurred for other jobs and continues today as HCOs redesign workers' jobs to enable (and require) them to use social media with customers. This job redesign entails more than just knowing how to use new digital devices—it also includes thinking like customers (Baird and Parasnis 2011). Staff must understand and respect customers' desire for more participation, information, dialogue, control, and partnership in their healthcare, such as for long-term diabetes (Cooper 2013).

INTERNAL FACTORS

An HCO's size, goals, worker motivation, and coordination are internal factors to consider when organizing tasks into jobs. In a small HCO there may only be enough work to require two maintenance positions, which does not allow much division of work into specializations such as carpentry, plumbing, and painting. Larger HCOs have more work so more workers are hired, which allows for more specialization. In a small HCO, there will not be enough medical imaging work for a full-time CT tech, a full-time MRI tech, and so forth. So the HCO may have broader unspecialized imaging technicians that do CT, MRI, and radiology.

An HCO's goals also influence how work is organized. If the HCO has a goal to improve quality in medical imaging, managers may create narrower medical imaging jobs that specialize in just one modality (e.g., CT, MRI) and staff those jobs with workers who are experts in just one modality. Assuming practice makes perfect, this specialization would improve quality.

Some HCOs have goals that mainly involve providing services, such as chemotherapy and surgery. In other HCOs, goals mainly involve making products, such as bandages or CT scanners. These examples are two ends of a continuum; most organizations are somewhere in between. These different goals require different ways of producing outputs for customers—either performing services or manufacturing products. Services often involve customer interaction.

Managers may organize jobs flexibly to allow workers to interact with customers and adjust to their needs. Doing so calls for more decentralization of authority to frontline service workers so that they can make decisions quickly for customers. It also calls for fewer rigid rules and more professionalism.

When designing jobs, managers must think about worker motivation. If jobs are too repetitive and only follow a simple step-by-step process, workers may become unmotivated. Jobs with tasks performed alone may demotivate people who need social interaction. Jobs with rigidly organized narrow tasks and no opportunity for creativity demotivate people who need growth or self-expression. We will learn more about motivation in later chapters about staffing, leading, and motivating.

Managers must bear in mind coordination of jobs when designing and dividing work. Coordination is the flip side of division of work. If tasks are divided into narrow, specialized jobs, then more time, effort, meetings, and expense are needed to coordinate those jobs toward a common purpose. Increased specialization of healthcare has increased fragmentation of work and jobs. To provide excellent healthcare, managers must coordinate specialized (but fragmented) jobs toward the common purpose of quality healthcare.

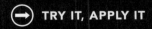 **TRY IT, APPLY IT**

Suppose you are the assistant manager of a medical equipment and supply company that operates a store and warehouse in Columbus, Ohio. You sell, rent, and install medical supplies and equipment for home use throughout the city. Brainstorm and list at least 20 tasks that your workers should perform. Then decide which jobs should perform which tasks. Compare your ideas with those of other students.

There are multiple ways of organizing jobs. Some focus on getting the work done, producing the products and services, and achieving the goals. Other approaches focus on keeping workers satisfied, enabling employees to grow, and fulfilling human needs. Each approach has advantages and disadvantages, and a manager must try to balance all considerations when organizing work. After deciding on an approach and implementing it, the manager should evaluate it and reorganize if necessary.

A FEW COMPLICATIONS

Managers can use the methods and principles explained earlier to organize work in HCOs. When doing so, they should also consider several possible complications—informal organizations, contract workers, unionized workers, and medical positions.

INFORMAL ORGANIZATIONS

Informal organization
Workers' own unwritten rules, procedures, expectations, agreements, and communication networks (e.g., the grapevine).

This chapter has focused on the formal organization—the organization shown in the official bylaws, charts, policies, and other documents of the organization. However, workers do not always follow the formal organization. They may create their own **informal organization** that coexists with the formal organization. This unwritten organization uses workers' own informal rules, procedures, expectations, agreements, and communication networks (e.g., the grapevine). The informal organization is common and often reflects how things are really done (White and Griffith 2010).

Unofficial arrangements arise from social relationships among people who work together, such as the third-shift personnel in a skilled nursing facility, the information technology staff at a health insurance firm, or the therapists in a rehabilitation center. Coworkers with common interests or friendships outside the HCO may also create informal groups at work. Members of these groups talk, gossip, share opinions, support each other, and report what they have heard (true and untrue) elsewhere in the organization.

The informal organization and its leaders can be influential in supporting—or opposing—the formal organization. Formal organization leaders should realize this and work with informal leaders. This subject is addressed in more detail in Chapter 15.

CONTRACT WORKERS

Sometimes an HCO does not hire all its workers and have all its workers on its payroll. For example, when a hospital has many vacant nurse positions and has been unable to hire nurses to fill them, it may contract with a temporary agency for nurses. The temp agency hires its own nurses and then contracts for them to temporarily work at HCOs. The hospital pays a fee to the agency for workers to fill in at the hospital. Temp agencies often provide nurses and other workers, sometimes for a few days and sometimes for much longer. The contract between the agency and the hospital formally addresses work responsibilities, supervision, authority, and so forth. Yet questions and conflicts can arise in these contract arrangements. In a hospital, an agency nurse might feel like saying, "I don't work for you; I work for the Nurses 'R' Us Agency." Department managers should be attentive to temporary worker arrangements and confer with the workers and the agency to reach and follow formal (written) agreements to prevent such problems.

Another type of contract worker is someone, usually with specialized expertise, who negotiates a contract with an HCO rather than being hired as an employee. Biomedical engineers, medical physicists, and speech therapists are examples. These arrangements can be useful in some situations, but they complicate the formal organization of a department and an HCO. When a hospital in Spartanburg, South Carolina, began a new radiation treatment center for cancer, it contracted with a full-time medical physicist. Along with job responsibilities, the written contract described how that position fit into the organization. The contract stated which manager the position reported to, defined the position as staff with no line authority, and explained coordination requirements for the position with management, employees, and the medical staff.

UNIONIZED WORKERS

Some workers may vote to join a labor union, which is explained more in Chapter 8. Nurses, maintenance workers, clerical workers, and physicians sometimes join unions. Although the union is not part of the official organization, it controls unionized workers and their work. Unions obtain authority through employees' elections and negotiated contracts (backed by labor laws) to control aspects of who works when, where, and how. Union rules also control how managers and employees communicate with each other and how union representatives may participate and intervene. Unions complicate how work is organized into jobs and departments and must be considered and managed by managers.

PHYSICIANS AS WORKERS

In hospitals, medical practices, health insurance companies, and other HCOs, some tasks, jobs, and positions must be done by a physician. Some of these jobs involve medical patient care work, such as surgeon, radiologist, anesthesiologist, hospitalist, and pediatrician. Others are administrative, such as vice president of medical affairs, medical director of quality care, and EKG medical director. For these jobs, the HCO may hire and pay a physician, may contract with and pay a physician (see the Contract Workers section above), or may grant the physician privileges to work in the HCO without being paid by the HCO. (In the last case, the physician is paid by patients and their insurance plans.)

Medical positions filled by physicians can make HCOs quite unlike other organizations. These arrangements complicate organization structure because they often do not fit neatly into the traditional chain of command and organization chart.

Let's consider hospitals because they are the most complicated. To begin with, a hospital may not hire a physician through the human resources department the way it hires most staff. A physician applies to the hospital for medical staff privileges in a specialty such as neurology, orthopedics, or cardiology. She specifies the kinds of medical work and procedures for which she is requesting privileges. She submits her credentials (e.g., medical school degree, years of residency training, recommendation letters) and provides evidence of competency to perform her specified medical work. The board of directors decides whether or not to grant the physician privileges based on her credentials.

Hospitals have hospital-based physician (HBP) positions, such as radiologist, pathologist, emergency physician, and hospitalist. Although there are variations, physicians in these positions work mostly in the hospital rather than in their own private medical practice in the community. Physicians in these jobs might be employed by or contract with (and be paid by) the hospital to provide their services. Or, they might provide services in hospitals but bill patients and insurers for their services. HBPs have authority and responsibility for medical work but do not have authority over administrative matters unless administrative tasks are specifically assigned to them by managers. The administrative managers have authority and responsibility for administrative matters but not for medical work.

Where does medicine end and administration begin? Good question. **The boundary between medicine and administration can be fuzzy.** Unity of command is routinely violated as HBPs and administrative managers both direct the same radiology technicians or the same emergency nurses. Rather than decide alone, a radiology department manager usually includes the HBP radiologist when deciding whom to hire as a new radiology technologist. The manager and physician also share responsibility for quality of patient care. But problems arise when physicians feel that anything affecting medical care is a medical matter and within their sole authority. If a radiologist claims authority to fire a technologist who made a serious mistake, the manager would say that is an administrative matter. On the other hand, managers must be careful about how involved they get in medical matters. If a physician asks a nonphysician administrative manager, "And where did *you* go to medical school?" the physician is thinking the manager has become too involved in something that requires medical expertise. Yet, the administrative manager can—and must—require physicians to comply with hospital medical staff bylaws, rules, and standards.

Usually boundaries, turf, and responsibilities are understood and respected so that work proceeds smoothly. When managers take the lead with candid, open dialogue, HBPs can be designed into the hierarchy with agreement on authority, coordination, organizing, and other matters. Because these physicians are in the hospital, they and managers see each other and usually know each other well enough to work out disagreements.

Then there are physicians who work in the hospital but, unlike HBPs, are not hired, contracted by, or paid by the hospital. The hospital grants privileges to these physicians to practice medicine on the hospital's patients and then bill the patients (or insurance plans) for payment. For example, a surgeon is granted surgical privileges to perform surgery on a hospital's patients and then be paid by the patient or insurance plan.

Do managers have authority over the surgeon? Well, not entirely. In the hospital organization chart, the surgeon does not report to the operating room (OR) manager as the scrub nurses do. In some hospitals, surgeons are shown in a medical hierarchy separate from the usual organization chart. This medical hierarchy (explained more in Chapter 5) usually reports to the chief of the medical staff or perhaps to the CEO and ultimately is accountable to the board of directors. Physicians have more autonomy than other workers to decide how they will perform their work. The manager can specify how the OR custodian should clean the room after a surgical case, but the manager cannot specify how the surgeon should perform the surgery. Yet the manager does have authority to ensure the surgeon complies with hospital bylaws, policies, and standards. When the hospital grants a physician privileges to practice in the hospital, the privileges require this compliance.

To varying degrees, medicine and management are becoming more blended with less separation of medical and administrative matters. Many variations of this relationship are reflected in hospital organization charts. Regardless of how integrated or separate medicine and management are, the physician has medical expertise for medical matters. The manager cannot direct and assign tasks to the surgeon the way she would assign tasks to an OR scrub nurse or other workers. Collaborative, collegial management is needed. Remember that physicians are physicians—which means they have autonomy, influence, and expectations based on medical expertise and status.

ONE MORE TIME

Organizations are "social entities that are goal-directed, designed as deliberately structured and coordinated activity systems, and are linked to the external environment" (Daft 2013, 642). As a system, an HCO has interacting parts that affect each other. As an open system, it acquires resource inputs from the environment, transforms them into healthcare products and services, and discharges those outputs to the external environment. It is influenced by the environment and must adapt to it.

Managers deliberately structure HCOs by organizing tasks into jobs, organizing jobs into departments, and organizing departments into an organization. Work must be coordinated among and across jobs and departments. To accomplish this, managers use management theory, concepts, and principles including specialization, division of work, authority, reporting relationships, vertical hierarchy, chain of command, span of control, line and staff positions, unity of command, (de)centralization, and coordination devices. These elements are used to organize work. Later they are used to reorganize work and adjust the organization to improve performance.

There is no one best way to organize—it is contingent on external factors in the environment and internal factors in the HCO itself. Mechanistic structure works best in a stable environment, while organic structure is best for unstable environments. Organizations usually blend both approaches to fit with their environments and other contingency factors. Managers must consider the informal organization, contract workers, unionized workers, and physicians—all of which can complicate organizing and managing HCOs.

(T) FOR YOUR TOOLBOX

- Organization charts
- Principles of specialization and division of work
- Principles of vertical hierarchy, span of control, line and staff positions, unity of command
- Principles of authority
- Coordination mechanisms

FOR DISCUSSION

1. What is a system? How is the open-system perspective useful for managing HCOs?

2. Organizing work into distinct jobs requires managers to make decisions about authority, specialization, reporting relationships, and other matters. Which of these decisions do you think would be easiest to make? Which would be hardest?

3. Compare and contrast how you would organize work in stable and unstable environments.

4. Think about work (paid or unpaid) that you have done in an organization. Explain which coordination methods were used to link your work with other people's work.

5. Discuss internal factors and external factors that influence how work is organized.

CASE STUDY QUESTIONS

These questions refer to the Integrative Case Studies at the back of this book.

1. Taking Care of Business at Graceland Memorial Hospital case: Review the definition of *organizations* and the five elements of that definition. In this case, how are the five elements of organizations evident for Graceland Memorial Hospital?

2. Nowhere Job case: Analyze Jack's job by examining tasks, authority, qualifications, reporting relationships, and other characteristics of the job.

3. Taking Care of Business at Graceland Memorial Hospital case: Draw what you think the hospital organization chart would look like. Include all positions named in the case.

4. Nowhere Job case: Does Jack's company have a mechanistic structure, an organic structure, or a mix of mechanistic and organic structures? Justify your answer.

5. Ergonomics in Practice case: How is the informal organization apparent at Riverlea Rehab Hospital? Why do you suppose staff follow the informal organization rather than the administrative director Tim Montana?

⊙ TRY IT, APPLY IT

Suppose you are hired to start a new website design department in an existing consulting firm. Use what you have learned in this chapter to organize the work for this new department. You are the department manager and will need to address the following questions: Which tasks must be performed? How will tasks be organized into jobs? How will jobs be organized into a department? How specialized will the jobs be? How will work and jobs be coordinated? What will the vertical hierarchy look like? How much authority (and for what purposes) will you decentralize to different jobs? Which external and internal factors will affect how you organize jobs and the department?

CHAPTER 5

ORGANIZING: ORGANIZATIONS

Form follows function.

Louis Sullivan, architect

Studying this chapter will help you to

➤ organize positions and departments into complete organizations;

➤ describe, compare, and contrast five different organizational forms;

➤ examine the purpose of a governing body atop the organization;

➤ coordinate work internally throughout a healthcare organization;

➤ link healthcare organizations with external organizations; and

➤ explain medical staff organization, authority, and coordination in a hospital.

HERE'S WHAT HAPPENED

Partners HealthCare is a large, complex organization governed by a board of directors. The corporate-level senior management includes the president/chief executive officer (CEO), executive vice president of administration and finance, vice president (VP) of graduate medical education, VP of population health management, VP of human resources, VP of communications, chief clinical officer, chief strategy officer, chief information officer, chief quality and safety officer, senior medical director, and others. Below them are middle managers and lower-level managers responsible for an array of departments. Each department has employees; larger departments also have levels of management. Partners owns and operates academic medical centers, hospitals, physician practices, managed care plans, community health centers, rehabilitation facilities, clinics, hospices, research institutes, and other HCOs. Each has an organization structure of managers, departments, and positions. Dozens of committees, teams, and groups—such as transitions teams and a strategy implementation group—coordinate the many parts into a whole. Besides this internal organization structure, Partners also organizes itself externally to connect with its environment. Partners forms interorganizational relationships to link with colleges and universities, insurance companies, suppliers, city government, grant funders, and others in its environment. Managers decide how to organize internally and externally to fulfill their mission and goals.

As we continue to study the real-world example of Partners HealthCare, we learn that it created organization structures to achieve its goals and mission. Many managers organize work tasks into positions and departments. Higher-level managers organize departments into an entire organization. Managers also decide how to organize work and positions to connect with the external environment.

Managers must decide which functions and departments should be grouped near each other for close interaction and which departments can be more dispersed. They must arrange coordination of departments vertically and horizontally in the organization. Managers apply the principles of hierarchy, span of control, delegation of authority, centralization, line and staff positions, and departmentalization to create the whole organization. Newer and lower-level managers must understand this organization to know how their own work unit or department fits into the bigger picture and interacts with other parts of the organization. No department exists independently of other departments!

This chapter first provides background information about organizing entire HCOs and what managers should consider during that process. Five forms of organization structure are presented, along with their advantages and disadvantages. The chapter then explains methods for coordinating departments within an HCO and for coordinating an HCO's activities and functions with external organizations. Finally, this chapter describes complications that might arise in HCOs and affect how the organization is designed. The discussion includes the organized medical staff—a unique organization structure found in hospitals.

Organization Structures

Much (but not all) of an organization's structure is reflected in its organization chart. This chapter explains five different forms of organization structure (with organization charts) that are used in HCOs:

1. Functional

2. Divisional

3. Matrix

4. Parallel

5. Modular

Each of these general models has pros and cons. In reality, many HCOs mix elements of these structural forms to create their own unique, combined form.

Recall from Chapter 4 that organizations may be organic or mechanistic—or a mixture of both types. Variation in organization forms occurs as each HCO adjusts how mechanistic or organic it will be, considering its environment, mission, goals, size, work technology, and culture (Daft 2013).

Which structural form is best? It depends, as you might have guessed. This chapter's opening quote suggests that the form depends on the function or purpose of the organization. As the form of a building depends on the purpose of the building, the form of an organization depends on the purpose of the organization. That is why managers must first plan the mission, goals, and purpose of the organization. The form of a university organization is different from the form of a health insurance organization partly because of their different purposes.

When determining organization structure, managers must also consider differentiation among departments and work units. Each department is specialized to perform work that differs from other departments' work. Because the emergency, housekeeping, and administration departments do different work, each department interacts with different parts of the external environment, pursues different department goals, uses different resources and production methods, and organizes with different department structures. Further, employees in each department have different knowledge, skills, attitudes, behaviors, values, and ways of thinking. **Differentiation**—differences among departments in how the departments are set up and how their workers think and feel (Charns and Young

Differentiation
Differences among departments in how the departments are set up and how their workers think and feel.

2012)—helps to achieve specialized types of work. However, differentiated departments eventually must be integrated (coordinated) to work together toward the organization's overall purpose. Without integration, differentiated workers and departments will work only toward their own department goals and not toward overall organization goals. Integrating departments is explained further in this chapter's section on coordination.

The five organization charts (see the exhibits in this chapter) show five different approaches to organizing departments into a formal organization. Vertical lines in a chart show the vertical hierarchy (chain of command), reporting relationships, authority, and communication up and down the hierarchy. Higher boxes in a chart represent positions with more authority and responsibility. Of course, just drawing boxes and lines on a piece of paper does not make an organization. Organization charts simply represent managers' ideas about how they want the organization to be structured. To create the desired organization in real life, managers must implement their ideas. Managers create the organization by staffing, leading, directing, resolving conflict, managing change, and other work explained throughout this book.

Planning and organizing are closely connected. First, Chapter 3 taught us that managers must assess changes, opportunities, and threats in the environment and adapt the HCO to those changes. Adaptation often requires a change in organization structure, such as from a functional to a divisional form. Second, in the planning process, managers assess the HCO's strengths and weaknesses, which may reveal that the HCO is not working well because of organizational problems. Perhaps middle managers do not have enough authority to act quickly, or perhaps departments are isolated rather than coordinated. If so, then managers will have to redesign the organization. Third, as Chapter 3 explained, managers establish goals and then develop plans to implement them. Implementation often includes redesigning the organization structure so that the HCO can achieve the goals. In Chapter 3, we read that Partners HealthCare set a goal to reduce the number of readmitted patients. To achieve that goal, managers had to apply organizing principles to redesign tasks, positions, departments, and Partners's organization structure.

FUNCTIONAL

The **functional form** organizes departments and positions according to the functions workers perform and the abilities they use. In Exhibit 5.1, we see the finance functions organized with a VP of finance, health services functions organized with a VP of health services, and so on. The functional form is often used by smaller HCOs with few services in stable environments. This form is not effective for larger, diversified HCOs in rapidly changing environments because decision making is too centralized (at the top) and would be too slow. Horizontal coordination methods should be added to improve collaboration between workers under each functional VP. For example, liaisons could be assigned between the finance and health services functions to help manage costs of health services.

Functional form
Organizes departments and positions according to the functions workers perform and the abilities they use.

EXHIBIT 5.1
Functional
Organization Chart

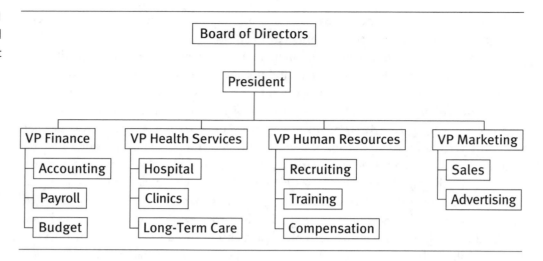

EXHIBIT 5.1
Functional
Organization Chart

The advantages and disadvantages of the functional form are as follows (Daft 2013; Leatt, Kimberly, and Baker 2006):

Advantages

◆ Specialized positions grouped in departments

◆ Efficiency and cost control

◆ Development of in-depth knowledge and abilities

 CHECK IT OUT

The American Hospital Association is involved in many interesting issues on behalf of hospitals. You can check out these issues at www.aha.org/advocacy-issues/index.shtml. Other associations work on behalf of other types of healthcare organizations. These associations include the Medical Group Management Association (www.mgma.com) and America's Health Insurance Plans (www.ahip.org). Look at these websites to learn more about issues facing HCOs. While you study the five organization forms in this chapter, think about how external issues of hospitals, medical groups, and health insurance companies might influence which organization forms their managers use.

Disadvantages

◆ Slow decision making

◆ Slow adaptation to changing environment

◆ Functional "silos" focus on their functional work

◆ Inadequate horizontal departmental coordination

DIVISIONAL

The **divisional form** organizes departments and positions to focus on groups of customers or services, rather than on types of workers. When an

HCO in Savannah, Georgia, grows and broadens its range of services, it may change from a functional to a divisional form. Compare and contrast these two forms in Exhibit 5.2. What changed?

Positions and departments in the company were reorganized into a hospital division, a clinics division, and a long-term care division. Each division is designed to focus on one type of customer, such as customers who need hospital services. Each division is headed by a separate VP with the accompanying stature and authority. What else do you see? Each division now has its own finance staff, health services staff, human resources staff, and marketing staff. The finance experts are no longer grouped together as they were in the

Divisional form
Organizes departments and positions to focus on particular groups of customers or services.

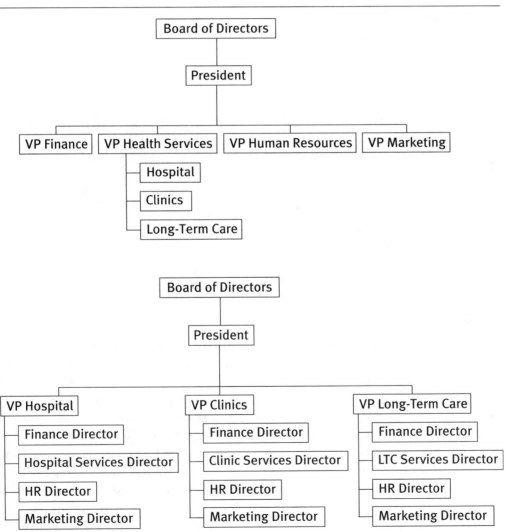

EXHIBIT 5.2
Change from Functional to Divisional Form

functional form. Each division now has its own finance knowledge, abilities, and expertise to quickly respond to its own financial affairs and those of its customers. Changes in the environment do not affect hospital, clinic, and long-term care services the same way. The divisional structure recognizes this issue and gives each division the staff and decentralized authority to monitor its environment and adjust itself. Of course, doing so increases the size and expense of staff. The HCO expects the increased cost of staff will be offset by increased customer satisfaction, sales, market share, and revenue.

The advantages and disadvantages of the divisional form are as follows (Daft 2013; Leatt, Kimberly, and Baker 2006):

Advantages

◆ Adaptation to changing environment

◆ Better customer satisfaction

◆ Decentralized, faster decisions

◆ Coordination of functions within divisions

Disadvantages

◆ Inefficiency resulting from more staff and expense

◆ Products/services "silos" focus on their own services

◆ Less coordination and synergy among all products and services

◆ Less development of in-depth functional expertise

MATRIX

Matrix form
Combines the functional and divisional organization forms to obtain advantages of both forms.

The **matrix form** combines the functional and divisional forms. It strives for efficiency (using the vertical functional form) while focusing on specific groups of customers, products, and services (using the horizontal divisional form). A matrix organization obtains some advantages of both the functional (vertical) and divisional (horizontal) forms. This approach is useful when an HCO must make efficient use of costly resources yet also decentralize decisions to quickly adapt and innovate for different groups of customers.

Look at Exhibit 5.3. What's going on in this organization? Functional management positions exist for functions such as human resources, marketing, and finance. The functional managers report up the functional vertical hierarchy to the president. They each have authority over their own staff of lower-level positions, such as a staff of marketing positions under the VP of marketing. On the left side of the organization chart are several divisional managers, who may be called product (or service) line managers. Each of these managers is responsible for a specific group of products or services. To meet the goals set for those service divisions, the divisional managers use workers hired by functional managers. There is no unity of command for these workers. The VP of marketing assigns Sara (a marketing employee) to work on cardiology services. Sara works for the cardiology manager and the VP of marketing. Some employees may even report to more than one divisional manager. A nurse who works for the functional VP of nursing could be assigned three days per week to the cardiology manager and two days per week to the neurology manager.

Often, HCOs that adopt product (service) line management organize into a matrix form. For each unique service division, service line managers can adapt to unique changes in service technology, customer preferences, reimbursement, and other factors that affect that unique service. These managers horizontally coordinate the marketing, finance, service production, and other functions across the HCO to achieve their divisional goals. The functional and divisional managers all lead workers, which requires effective interpersonal, conflict resolution, and communication skills. Diana took a job as the gastroenterology service line manager at a hospital in Denver, Colorado. She was responsible for the success (or failure) of this service yet lacked full control over the staff and resources, which made her job challenging.

Top managers might also use a variation of the matrix design for project management in an HCO. Senior managers would assign a project manager to each project. The project managers would appear in place of the service line managers in the matrix chart.

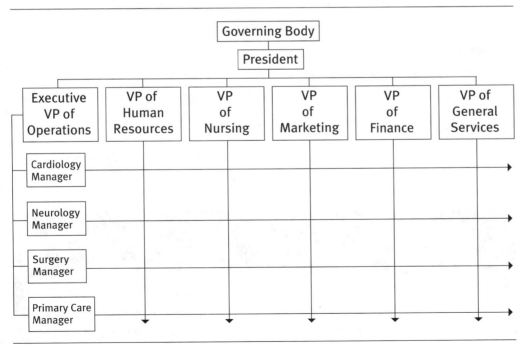

EXHIBIT 5.3

Matrix
Organization Chart

SOURCE: Adapted from Daft (2013).

Each project manager would form a project team to implement each project using functional employees from finance, marketing, and so forth. Employees would work their "regular" job while also serving on project teams led by project managers. Outside stakeholders, such as an architect or supply vendor, might also be on project teams, which would present a different matrix than that for ongoing service line management. HCOs can and do create structural variations to fit their unique organizational needs.

As mentioned earlier, managers sometimes blend two structural forms to create a mixed form that they think is best for their situation. Thus, managers might blend a mostly functional form with the matrix form just for a few medical service lines. When you are a manager, remember that there are many possibilities and you can be creative. You will have to decide which organizational form is best for your HCO and situation.

The advantages and disadvantages of the matrix form are as follows (Daft 2013; Leatt, Kimberly, and Baker 2006):

Advantages

◆ Development of both functional and product expertise

◆ Efficient use of staff while improving customer satisfaction

◆ Adaptation to external changes affecting individual products

◆ Coordination and communication across the organization

Disadvantages

◆ No unity of command; workers have more than one boss

◆ Workers may become confused and stressed and experience conflict

◆ Well-developed skills required for communication and resolving conflicts

◆ Much time and expense required to train staff to work in a matrix

◆ Conflict is frequent, which requires staff training, time, and effort to resolve

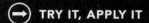 **TRY IT, APPLY IT**

How would you feel about working for two bosses in a matrix organization? Think about it and write down your likes and dislikes about this arrangement. Describe what managers could do to help overcome your dislikes. Discuss your ideas with colleagues.

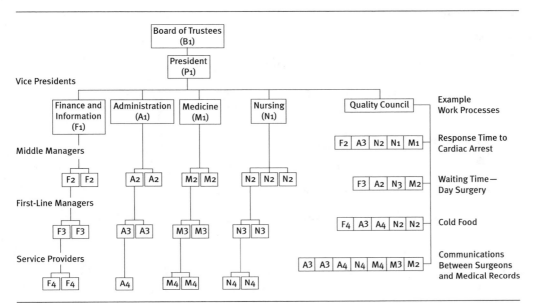

SOURCE: From Shortell/Kaluzny: *Healthcare Management*, 5/e. © 2006 Delmar Learning, a part of Cengage Learning, Inc. Reproduced by permission, www.cengage.com/permissions.

EXHIBIT 5.4
Parallel
Organization Chart

PARALLEL

The **parallel form** starts with a functional structure to produce the routine work, products, and services (Leatt, Kimberly, and Baker 2006). This structure is seen in the traditional vertical hierarchy on the left side of Exhibit 5.4. Then, a parallel structure is added on the right side to organize positions when needed for multidepartmental approaches to solving complex problems. Workers throughout the basic functional organization are assigned additional responsibilities in the parallel organization to help solve these problems. For example, the parallel structure has a group of workers responsible for improving waiting time for day surgery in the HCO. Someone (F3) from the third level of the finance function has been assigned to this parallel structure, and so have workers (A2, N3, M2) from the second level of administration, third level of nursing, and second level of medicine. The parallel structure organizes necessary workers from throughout the HCO to come together for joint problem solving. Notice that a top-level council of members appointed from the basic functional organization manages the parallel structure. Many HCOs use this approach to improve performance (although they might not show the parallel structure in their organization chart). Disputes sometimes arise between the two structures, such as when frontline nurses (service providers) have to leave their patients to attend committee meetings. The nursing supervisor may feel the nurses should stay and care for patients.

The advantages and disadvantages of the parallel form are as follows (Leatt, Kimberly, and Baker 2006):

Parallel form
Starts with a functional structure to produce the routine work and then adds a parallel structure to organize for multidepartmental approaches to solving complex problems.

Advantages

- ◆ Coordinated problem solving
- ◆ Better performance (such as quality)
- ◆ Opportunity for workers' professional growth

Disadvantages

- ◆ Staff spend more time in meetings
- ◆ Meetings result in an increased cost of operations
- ◆ Conflicts arise between two structures over resources, power, and control

MODULAR (VIRTUAL NETWORK)

Modular form

Outsources much work to other organizations and connects them with contracts and electronic information systems.

Managers of organizations using the **modular form** or virtual network form (Daft 2013) outsource functions and departments to other organizations and connect them with contracts and electronic information systems back to the main organization. The top manager is similar to a general contractor who subcontracts (outsources) much work to other organizations. The organization might decide to do only what it specializes in and outsource everything else. For example, a surgical group practice may focus on doing what it excels at—surgery. The physicians could contract out financial management, information systems, legal services, human resource work, marketing, and administration. An example of the modular form is shown in Exhibit 5.5.

The modular structure is a matter of degree: Most HCOs contract out at least some work. For a new surgical group practice, this approach enables a fast start, flexibility, and quick growth through partner organizations such as a law firm, an accounting firm, and an advertising firm. Years later, when it is much bigger, the surgical group will still probably outsource some work (e.g., legal work) rather than hire its own staff (e.g., an attorney). Even large HCOs contract out some work, such as contracting with language interpretation companies to communicate with patients who do not know the local prevailing language. A manager should always remember that the modular approach creates dependencies. Success depends on other organizations. If any one of the outside firms performs badly, the surgical group practice will suffer and may even fail. This principle is true for all HCOs that use the modular form.

The advantages and disadvantages of the modular form are as follows (Daft 2013):

Advantages

- ◆ Fast start-up of a new organization

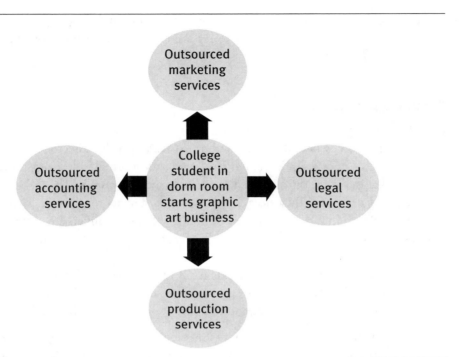

Exhibit 5.5
Modular
Organizational
Form

◆ Quick access to expertise, systems, facilities, and equipment (with minimal investment)

◆ Flexibility to grow, shrink, and adjust

◆ Less time spent on managing a large, complex organization

Disadvantages

◆ Dependence on other organizations for critical services

◆ Risk of failure if outsource partner fails

◆ Time and expense to find partners and negotiate contracts

These five organization structures and charts are just a starting point. Managers often create custom structures by combining elements of more than one organization form. They may start with a functional form and then make exceptions for the independent OB-GYN service line and the outpatient surgery service line—each with a service line manager. Or, top managers might create a divisional structure in which each division has its own finance staff and marketing staff, but then put all human resources in a functional approach for the entire HCO to ensure consistency of employment practices. The possibilities and variations are endless. If you've seen one HCO organization chart, you sure haven't seen them all!

GOVERNING BODY

Most HCOs (except for very small ones) have a governing body at the top of the organization structure. It may be called the board of trustees, board of directors, governing body, board of governors, or a similar name. The board acts on behalf of the organization's owners to do what is best for the owners. The owners may be investors, shareholders, citizens, a city, a church, or others. They elect or appoint a board to act for the owners and to ensure the organization fulfills the owners' responsibilities. Board members are entrusted with the following responsibilities to govern an HCO for the owners (White and Griffith 2010):

1. The board appoints the president/CEO, who leads and manages the HCO to fulfill the HCO's mission, goals, vision, and strategy. The board then monitors the CEO's performance and provides appropriate, candid feedback.

2. The board approves the HCO's mission, goals, vision, and strategy each year. It also approves the HCO's major policies (e.g., on hiring for diversity, accepting gifts from vendors) that provide guidance and direction to the staff to achieve the mission, goals, vision, and strategy.

3. The board approves the annual budget and other key elements of the financial plan each year. This action may include approving all expenditures above a preset level, approving the overall increase in prices, approving the overall increase in workforce salaries, and approving all loans.

4. The board monitors the HCO's performance compared to preset targets (e.g., 5 percent increase in cardiology market share, 0 patients readmitted within 30 days). When target performance levels are not met, the board requires explanation and corrective action by the CEO or medical staff.

5. The board ensures compliance with laws and regulations pertaining to governance and the HCO, such as the Sarbanes-Oxley law. Stakeholders now demand more accountability from boards and expect them to provide accurate information to the public.

6. The board helps connect the HCO to the external community and gathers information from the external environment to help the HCO.

7. If an HCO has a medical staff, the board appoints the physicians, monitors their performance, and holds them accountable for the quality of medical care in the HCO.

Most boards have some members from outside the HCO, such as a realtor or banker, and some from inside the HCO, such as the CEO (and chief of staff if there is a medical staff). The board chooses and appoints its own members. A board might seek people who can bring a certain perspective to the board, such as a physician or a patient. Boards also seek people who can contribute particular expertise, such as in strategic planning or fundraising. To fulfill its responsibilities, the board appoints members to committees such as for finance, strategic planning, and quality.

COORDINATION WITHIN AN HCO

Managers link departments vertically, horizontally, and diagonally as needed throughout the HCO so that they all work together toward the shared mission. To link departments, managers use the coordination mechanisms presented in Chapter 4 for linking jobs: supervision, mutual adjustment, standardized work processes, standardized work output, standardized worker skills, and coordinating groups (e.g., committees, councils, task forces, patient rounds, project teams). The linking methods in Chapter 4 involve mostly workers whose jobs are not specifically for coordinating work among departments. In this chapter you will now learn about jobs and positions that have specific responsibilities for linking departments. These jobs—liaison and integrator—are more formally involved in coordinating than are jobs such as nurse or plumber, in which people only occasionally do a few things to coordinate their work with others.

A **liaison** coordinates one department with another department (Daft 2013). Departments have to link themselves when the work of one department affects the work of a second department. (Sometimes the second department also affects the first department, so there are reciprocal effects.) For example, the work of the pharmacy affects the work of pediatric nursing (and vice versa). Thus, a pharmacist may be assigned the task of attending the monthly meetings of the pediatric nursing department to serve as a liaison between pharmacists and pediatric nurses to coordinate their work. The pharmacist explains her work to pediatric nurses and also learns about the nurses' work, which she later explains to her pharmacy department. Reciprocally, a pediatric nurse may be appointed to serve as a liaison to the pharmacy department. The pharmacist liaison does pharmacy work and coordinating work. The pediatric nurse liaison does nursing work and coordinating work.

An **integrator** works full-time coordinating the work of several departments toward a common purpose (Daft 2013). The integrator does not also do other types of work such as nursing, accounting, or marketing. In Exhibit 5.3, the service line managers for cardiology, neurology, surgery, and primary care are full-time integrators. The cardiology integrator coordinates work from the departments of human resources, nursing, marketing, finance, and general services to achieve cardiology goals. A project manager is another type of integrator.

On a grander scale, managers use the five organization structures described in this chapter to coordinate among departments up, down, across, and throughout the organization. The organization chart reflects who supervises whom, which provides coordination

Liaison
A job that includes responsibility to coordinate one department with another department.

Integrator
A person who works full-time coordinating the work of several departments toward a common purpose.

✓ CHECK IT OUT

The Committee on Quality of Health Care in America at the Institute of Medicine published a landmark study in 2001, *Crossing the Quality Chasm: A New Health System for the 21st Century*. The study calls for redesign of healthcare to be more timely, safe, efficient, effective, equitable, and patient centered. The committee's report includes recommendations for reorganizing and coordinating healthcare tasks to achieve these six aims. Managers are still striving to accomplish all the recommendations. A summary of the report can be found by searching online for "IOM quality chasm PDF". The report is an influential document that all healthcare managers should read.

up and down the organization. The chart may also reflect integrators who provide coordination. Other structures for coordination—such as task forces, committees, and teams—are shown in the parallel organization chart and sometimes in other charts. Even if managers do not show these other structures in organization charts, managers always use them. Managers also use standardized work processes (protocols, procedure, rules), communication systems and networks (personal, digital), and the other coordination mechanisms explained above and in Chapter 4.

Coordination is essential for bringing together the many specialized work units, departments, and sections of an HCO so that they work toward the HCO's common mission and goals. Also, coordination is needed because some individual departments affect other departments. Suppose the human resources department of a health insurance company in St. Louis, Missouri, does not do its job well. That will affect other departments, such as sales and enrollment, that depend on the human resources department to recruit and compensate employees. Thus, the sales department and the enrollment department will coordinate their work with the human resources department to ensure adequate staffing. When departments share resources (e.g., staff, equipment, office space, information), coordination is essential. Think back to the matrix and parallel organization structures, in which staff members are shared among parts of the organization. The departments must coordinate carefully to share workers.

LINKING AN HCO WITH OTHER ORGANIZATIONS AND ITS ENVIRONMENT

As we learned earlier, an HCO must be open to and interact with its environment. An HCO in Fayetteville, North Carolina, must acquire labor, supplies, information, perhaps governmental approvals, and other resources needed to fulfill its mission and goals. And, it must have customers, clients, and others who use its products and services. The HCO must organize jobs and departments to connect with parts of the environment. Can you think of examples? List jobs and departments that link a health insurance company to its environment. Then read these examples:

◆   A human resources recruiter connects the insurance company to the environment to acquire workers from colleges, vocational schools, labor unions, and job recruiters.

- ◆ An attorney connects the insurance company with a government agency to learn how to comply with a new law.

- ◆ A procurement department connects the insurance company with office supply companies, computer vendors, and other businesses to acquire needed supplies and equipment.

- ◆ A finance department connects the insurance company with bankers to raise funds for expansion.

- ◆ A sales department connects the insurance company with small businesses that might want to buy health insurance for their workers.

Within departments, specific positions are assigned responsibility for linking the department (and the HCO) with a certain part of the environment, as in the foregoing examples. Recall from Chapter 1 that the environment may be thought of as having sectors for labor, supplies, funds, customers, and so forth. Managers can assign tasks to specific jobs to link the HCO to specific sectors of the environment. Employees at all levels of the HCO can help link the HCO to the environment. As a manager, you will have to interact with the environment to connect your HCO to it.

Cardinal Health (2014) is a healthcare supply company with thousands of HCO customers. An HCO can buy its medical supplies from Cardinal. In a more open systems approach to link with the environment, an HCO can also outsource inventory management to Cardinal. In that case Cardinal takes responsibility for monitoring usage of dozens of different medical supplies, delivering and restocking supplies "just in time" to minimize costs, and distributing supplies throughout the HCO to departments that use them. These actions form a tighter connection between Cardinal and its customers (HCOs) in the environment.

Managers can also formally connect their HCO with other organizations and create interorganizational structures such as alliances, mergers, joint ventures, hospital systems, supply chains, networks, and independent practice associations. We will not explore these organizational forms in depth. Realize that interorganizational structures are ways of linking an HCO with one or more other organizations in its environment. These structures connect organizations—sometimes two, sometimes 100 or more—with a new organization (e.g., joint venture) or an expanded original organization (e.g., hospital system) that helps the individual organizations achieve their goals. As we read in Chapter 1, many HCOs are joining with others, and this trend will continue. At the beginning of this chapter, we saw that Partners HealthCare is actually made up of numerous HCOs that together form an integrated health system. Blue Cross companies throughout the country are members of the national Blue Cross federation. In addition, independent physician practices sometimes form associations that help them negotiate better deals with health insurers. To make these arrangements successful, independent HCOs give some of their power and resources to the alliance, joint venture, or network. In return, they expect to gain benefits from the alliance, such as cheaper prices on equipment, access to innovations, or better reimbursement payments. An HCO uses legal documents, bylaws, and other mechanisms to structure these new organizations and coordinate work among the member HCOs.

COMPLICATIONS

Managers can use the models and principles explained earlier in this chapter to organize HCOs. When doing so, they should consider two types of complications that are explained next.

PHYSICIANS AND THE MEDICAL STAFF IN AN HCO

The five organization structures in this chapter involve traditional bureaucratic principles, such as vertical hierarchy with authority. As we learned in Chapter 4, this approach does not always work neatly with medical positions for physicians, which complicates how managers organize HCOs. In this chapter, we study two more aspects of physicians in HCOs:

1. The professional bureaucracy

2. The organized medical staff of a hospital

Professional bureaucracy
Organization, coordination, and authority are based on highly specialized education, training, and expertise, with less reliance on authority from a job position.

In HCOs such as medical group practices and hospitals, physicians produce the core services. For some aspects of this work, a **professional bureaucracy** may work better than a traditional bureaucracy. In this professional organization structure, the coordination and authority are based on highly specialized education, training, and expertise (Mintzberg 1983b; Daft 2010). **This professionalism theoretically influences work performance so strongly and consistently that detailed bureaucratic standards and rules are not needed.** Instead, standardized skills and outputs (explained in Chapter 4) create the coordination among these physicians who—by their extensive professional education, training, and socialization—know what to do and what to expect of colleagues. Physicians' performance is controlled by professional norms, values, and culture from outside the HCO. Physicians expect more autonomy and less managerial oversight than they would receive in a traditional bureaucracy, as long as they work within their professional norms and training (Flood, Zinn, and Scott 2006). Bureaucratic authority defers to professional training and expertise.

Should a hospital be organized as a traditional bureaucracy, a professional bureaucracy, or a combination of both? While not all hospitals are alike, the following discussion will offer a general answer to this question. Keep in mind that because of external forces, hospitals are trying new approaches to integrate the medical staff with the hospital's management hierarchy. The separation of the clinical enterprise and administrative enterprise has been disappearing (Birk 2013). There is much variety, and if you've seen one hospital organization chart . . . you've seen one hospital organization chart.

A hospital has a bureaucratic structure designed by managers using the organizing principles explained in this chapter. It also has a medical staff structure comprising physicians (and, if hospital bylaws allow, dentists and other clinical professionals). Together, these structures are sometimes referred to as a dual structure. The medical staff is organized into departments and divisions for medical specialties (e.g., oncology) and subspecialties (e.g., dermatologic oncology). **The hospital board of directors delegates to the medical staff the authority and responsibility for medical care in the hospital. The board of directors also dictates that physicians and the medical staff must comply with hospital bylaws, policies, and standards.** These bylaws, policies, and standards are generally based on laws, regulations, accreditation requirements, national or state guidelines, professional norms, and other external standards. Then physicians design their medical staff structure and expect some degree of autonomy as in a professional bureaucracy.

The organized medical staff is essential to fulfill the hospital's goals and mission. Yet, the medical staff structure might—or might not—be shown in detail on a hospital organization chart. The structure might be depicted by a medical staff box connected to a board of directors box or a CEO box at the top. In a large academic medical center, the medical staff will likely be the medical faculty organized as a separate entity that contracts with the hospital—shown on the main organization chart as a box to the side. Sometimes the two structures are separate and appear this way on the organization chart. In other hospitals, the two structures are partly or almost completely blended together into one structure. For example, physicians and the medical staff hierarchy and committees may be shown reporting to a VP of medical affairs who reports to the hospital CEO. Another approach is to use the matrix structure for service line management but to appoint a physician as a clinical comanager and a nonphysician as an administrative comanager for each service line (e.g., neurology, cardiology, pediatrics). This approach is used at Presbyterian Healthcare Services in Albuquerque, New Mexico (Birk 2013). There are many structural variations.

In recent years, the trend has been to more tightly combine the medical and management structures for better organizational responsibility and accountability. This combination enables physicians and hospitals to improve patient care, strengthen finances, manage population health, and adapt to demands of stakeholders and the external environment (Buell 2014). The medical staff and the management team appoint liaisons to each other's committees, councils, and departments to help coordinate their work. The chief of the medical staff and a few other physicians sit on the board of directors. One or more administrative representatives attend meetings of the medical staff and its departments and committees. In the administrative structure, some departments have an administrative manager and a physician as codirectors. A hospital might assign codirectors to specific problems that involve both medicine and administration, such as patient safety or quality of patient care (Calayag 2014). Disagreements are inevitable, so leaders of the medical staff and management (sometimes with the board of directors) must be ready to resolve conflicts. **These two structures—the traditional organization hierarchy and the medical staff hierarchy—coexist and together form the total hospital organization.**

Within the medical staff are physicians with different relationships to the hospital, as mentioned in Chapter 4. Some physicians are based in the hospital, such as radiologists, emergency physicians, and hospitalists. Others are based in the community in their physician office practices. They all must obtain hospital privileges to perform medical work in a hospital. Some physicians work in the hospital's administrative organization structure and are employed and paid by the hospital.

Confused? If so, you are not alone! Even managers who work in hospitals sometimes feel confused. That is because

1.   there are different kinds of hospitals,

2.   there are different kinds of jobs and positions filled by physicians, and

3.   there are different kinds of relationships between hospitals and physicians.

To make things even more interesting, these relationships are evolving to adapt to the trends and issues discussed in Chapter 1.

This discussion of physicians and the medical staff in an HCO has revealed several general points. First, physicians may fit into a hospital organizational structure in a variety of ways. Managers should not assume all physician–hospital relationships are alike. They must examine and understand each one individually.

Second, physicians have authority and responsibility for medical care, whereas managers have authority and responsibility for administrative matters. However, the boundary between medicine and administration is blurred, which creates conflicts between managers and physicians. Hospital patient care employees may be directed by both physicians and managers, so unity of command can be violated.

Third, hospitals have an administrative hierarchy (shown in the hospital organization chart) and a medical staff hierarchy (not always shown in the hospital organization chart). These hierarchies have been merging in recent years. Several organization structures are used to coordinate the medical staff with administration, including medical–management committees, physician and administrator codirectors, appointment of managers to medical staff committees, and liaisons between the medical staff and administration. Medical staff representation on the hospital board of directors is an organization structure for coordinating the governing board and medical staff.

Recall also from Chapter 4 that physicians have power and influence based on their medical expertise, which confers high status that affects their relationships with others.

Managers, of course, have their own expertise—management—and the authority of their positions. Yet, they should be careful about when and how to assert managerial authority when working with physicians who expect autonomy based on professional expertise. Ongoing collegial discussion often can resolve problems, though managers must sometimes assert authority—for example, to obtain physicians' compliance with accreditation standards and licensure requirements. Ultimately, hospital managers combine traditional bureaucracy with professional bureaucracy.

CONTRACT DEPARTMENTS

Do you remember learning in Chapter 4 about contract workers who fill positions in HCOs? In some cases, these workers are not limited to just a few temps from a nursing agency.

Even more interesting and potentially complicated is when an HCO contracts with an outside company to operate an entire department, such as food service or housekeeping. This type of contracting is similar to the modular outsourcing approach of a service, although here the external company puts its own employee in the HCO's department manager position (e.g., food service manager). In some arrangements, the outside company will install its own workers in other positions (e.g., dietician, lead cook). People in these positions work inside the HCO with HCO workers but work for (and are paid by) the outside company. Here, too, the unity of command can be violated. The HCO's top managers must decide how much authority to delegate to the food service manager if the position is held by an outside person who is not on the HCO payroll. Coordination with other parts of the HCO may be awkward if other employees question the food service manager's loyalties. These arrangements do work in many HCOs, but they can cause problems and confusion if not organized well.

Top managers must devote care and attention to formally stating how the contract workers (and department) fit in the hierarchy and what their authorities, coordination, and responsibilities are.

HERE'S WHAT HAPPENED

Tallia and colleagues (2003) studied the organization designs of 18 primary care medical groups. These medical groups varied in environment, size, mission and goals, and other contingencies. The researchers found much variation in how the groups were organized. Some followed a traditional model, such as functional or matrix, while others developed their own form. The 18 medical practices varied in standardization, departmentalization, decentralization of authority, vertical hierarchy, job specialization, and coordination. Some were clearly more mechanistic or organic than others, and some reflected a traditional bureaucracy more than a professional bureaucracy. Groups with more autonomy responded better to changes in their environments and had better performance.

Evolving forces and factors will continue to influence how HCOs organize in the future. Some of these factors were noted earlier in this chapter and in others. Think back to the trends and issues discussed in Chapter 1. How do you think they will affect the organization structure of medical groups, nursing homes, diagnostic clinics, outpatient surgery centers, hospitals, pharmaceutical companies, and other types of HCOs?

ONE MORE TIME

Managers must decide how to organize and coordinate work to accomplish goals and adapt to the environment. Thus, organizing is closely tied to planning. Lower-level managers organize tasks into positions and departments; higher-level managers organize departments into an entire organization. They decide which departments to group with others for close interaction, and they arrange coordination of departments vertically and horizontally in the organization. Because it is an open system, the organization must be linked to other organizations and people in its environment. Managers use hierarchy, span of control, delegation of authority, centralization, line and staff positions, and departmentalization to create the whole organization.

Managers can organize their HCO to generally follow one of several organizational forms:

- *Functional form* organizes departments and positions according to the functions workers perform and the abilities they use.
- *Divisional form* organizes departments and positions to focus on particular groups of customers or services.
- *Matrix form* combines the functional and divisional forms to obtain advantages of both.
- *Parallel form* starts with a functional structure to produce the routine work and then adds a parallel structure to organize for multidepartmental problem solving.
- *Modular (or virtual network) form* outsources much work to other organizations and connects them with contracts and electronic information systems.

Each of these five forms has pros and cons. Managers often combine elements of more than one organizational form to create a mixed form. Thus, much variation exists as HCOs organize according to their unique combination of environment, mission, goals, size, work, technology, and culture. Within an HCO, managers coordinate departments vertically, horizontally, and diagonally using supervision, mutual adjustment, groups, standardized work process, standardized worker skills, standardized work output, and jobs with responsibility for coordination. Managers link their organization to other organizations using specific tasks, jobs, and interorganizational structures. Most HCOs have a governing body (or board) at the top of the organization structure to act on behalf of the owners and bear ultimate responsibility for the organization.

   When physicians are the main type of labor or are largely responsible for producing an HCO's outputs (services), they expect to work in a structure that respects professional expertise and autonomy. In a hospital, physicians organize into a medical staff structure that operates as part of the hospital but to some extent is outside of the management structure. This structure complicates how hospitals are organized—and how managers manage them.

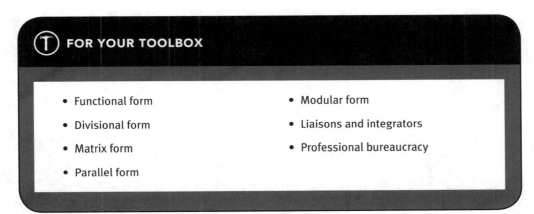

FOR YOUR TOOLBOX

- Functional form
- Divisional form
- Matrix form
- Parallel form

- Modular form
- Liaisons and integrators
- Professional bureaucracy

FOR DISCUSSION

1. Discuss the pros and cons of the functional form versus the divisional form.

2. Explain the matrix form. What are pros and cons of the matrix form?

3. Discuss what you believe are the most important responsibilities of a governing board.

4. How can managers coordinate work among different departments within an HCO?

5. Some HCOs do not design their organization structure exactly like one of the five forms discussed in this chapter. Instead, they begin with one of those structures and then modify it—sometimes creating a unique organization structure. Why might that be a good idea?

6. In a hospital, how does the medical staff complicate the traditional organization hierarchy?

CASE STUDY QUESTIONS

These questions refer to the Integrative Case Studies at the back of this book.

1. I Can't Do It All case: Based on the information in this case, draw a functional organization chart for Healthdyne. Assume Healthdyne grows and Mr. Brice wants to reorganize Healthdyne with a West Region and an East Region. Draw a new organization chart for Healthdyne.

2. Nowhere Job case: Try to draw an organization chart for Jack's company. (Drawing the chart might not be easy.)

3. Nowhere Job case: Which coordination mechanisms (described in Chapters 4 and 5) is Jack supposed to use to coordinate with other people in his company? Does Jack think his coordination with others is sufficient? If not, which coordination mechanisms should he use to improve it?

→ TRY IT, APPLY IT

Riverbend Orthopedics is a busy group practice with expanded services for orthopedic care. It now has seven physicians and a podiatrist, plus about 50 other employees. At its big, new clinic building, Riverbend provides extensive orthopedic care. Several technicians provide diagnostic medical imaging from basic X-ray to magnetic resonance imaging. The physicians perform surgery in their own outpatient surgery center with Riverbend's own operating nurses and technicians. Therapy is provided by three physical therapists and one part-time contracted occupational therapist. Besides the actual medical care, the clinic has staff for financial management, medical records, human resources, marketing, and information systems/technology. Riverbend is managed by a president. She has asked you (a summer intern) for advice on how to design Riverbend's organization structure. Using information from this chapter, what would you suggest? Be sure to include internal and external coordination linkages. Justify your recommendations.

CHAPTER 6

ORGANIZING: GROUPS AND TEAMS

Coming together is a beginning. Keeping together is progress. Working together is success.

Henry Ford, founder of the Ford Motor Company and
inventor of the assembly line

LEARNING OBJECTIVES

Studying this chapter will help you to

➤ define *groups* and *teams*;

➤ state the purposes of groups and teams;

➤ explain structural characteristics of groups and teams;

➤ explain process characteristics of groups and teams;

➤ describe helpful and harmful roles played by group members; and

➤ explain how to make group meetings effective.

HERE'S WHAT HAPPENED

Partners HealthCare had established goals. To accomplish these goals effectively, managers organized teams, committees, and other groups of workers. For example, Partners had a strategy implementation group and transition teams. When organizing them, managers likely had to make important decisions about the group and teams or else they would not succeed. For example, for the strategy group, key decisions may have included: the purpose of the group, whom to appoint to the group, how much authority it should have, and to whom it would be accountable. Managers, or the group members themselves, had to decide who should chair (lead) the group, how often it should meet, with whom it would communicate, and how it would make its decisions. Managers probably had to orient new members to their roles on the committee. Potential conflict among group members (perhaps because of differences in professional viewpoints) could have deterred them from working together, so managers had to avoid creating conflict. If managers succeeded, then the strategy implementation group likely would be prepared to achieve its purpose and help Partners achieve its organizational goals.

This chapter, the third about organizing, helps us understand why and how HCOs must organize people into groups such as teams, committees, task forces, and councils. As we learned in Chapters 4 and 5, organizing is a form of coordination that HCOs use to achieve goals. We saw that Partners HealthCare used these types of groups. It would be hard to imagine how even a small HCO—much less a large, complex one—could succeed without organized groups and teams. This aspect of organization matters because patients' health and lives are at stake. Good teamwork and effective groups matter to employees too. After all, would you want to work in an HCO where people did not work well in groups, committees, or teams?

Managers at all levels of an HCO must be ready to create and participate in groups. Top managers must support groups and promote teamwork throughout medical practices, health insurance companies, pharmaceutical firms, assisted living centers, mental health clinics, and other HCOs. Managers at lower levels must do the same within their own departments and work sections. For career advancement, new managers can volunteer for teams and committees to become more widely known in the HCO. Working with others in groups outside your department or work unit will give you wonderful opportunities to grow professionally and develop rewarding work relationships with others. This chapter will help you to function well on teams, which is important to succeed in healthcare management jobs.

Think of some clubs, teams, groups, and committees that you have belonged to. You might have belonged to some that you felt were effective and fun to be part of. Perhaps you have been in other groups that you dreaded. Why are some groups effective and fun whereas others are not? Good groups and teams are not automatically good; they are good because managers created them properly. How can managers do that? In this chapter we learn how, beginning with basic ideas about groups and teams and their purposes. Next, we study how managers create the structure and the process of groups—both of which influence the groups' success or failure. Additionally, we examine several roles that group members perform and see which roles help and harm a group. All these things matter for a group—whether it is a board of directors, a children's health task force, or an employee softball team.

This chapter focuses on formal groups and teams—the ones that appear in the organization's official written documents and are created by top managers. We know from Chapter 4 that an informal organization exists, which includes informal groups that influence employees. However, those groups are not created by managers and thus are beyond the scope of this book. Here, we will focus on what managers can do to create and manage their organization's formal groups.

REASONS FOR GROUPS AND TEAMS

A **group** involves the social interaction between two or more people in a stable arrangement who have common goals or interests and who perceive themselves as a group (Borkowski 2011). A **team** is a special kind of group with specific complementary abilities, strong commitment to common goals, and shared accountability for goal achievement (Borkowski 2011). Although teams may differ from groups in general, we can study them together. A **committee** is a formal group that is established with an official purpose, charge, or mandate; is linked and reports to the organization hierarchy; and is held accountable to accomplish its mandate (Dunn 2010). Consider these other characteristics of committees:

◆ Some have line authority to make decisions; others lack authority and only recommend.

◆ Some exist within a single department, but many have members from multiple departments (i.e., are interdepartmental) or multiple disciplines (i.e., are interdisciplinary).

◆ They exist at all levels of hierarchy, from the board of directors on down.

◆ They may be permanent (standing) for ongoing work, or they may be temporary (ad hoc) for specific one-time work.

◆ Some exist in a building with members physically interacting face-to-face, whereas others exist in cyberspace with members electronically interacting keyboard-to-keyboard (or keypad-to-keypad).

Why do you think HCOs have groups? What are their purposes? Here are several, although not all groups have all of these purposes:

Group
Social interaction between two or more people in a stable arrangement who have common goals or interests and who perceive themselves as a group.

Team
A group with specific complementary abilities, strong commitment to common goals, and shared accountability for goal achievement.

Committee
A formal group that is established with an official mandate, is linked to the organizational hierarchy, and is accountable for its mandate.

◆ Combine and coordinate work that is fragmented because of division of work and specialized expertise

◆ Enable workers to grow, try new roles, and develop professionally

◆ Expand workers' knowledge of the HCO beyond their own departments

◆ Enable workers to exchange skills, knowledge, and organizational learning with others

◆ Build commitment (through participation) to solutions, changes, and new plans

◆ Improve problem solving and decision making by bringing in diverse and necessary input, points of view, experience, and expertise

◆ Obtain input, representation, and support of stakeholders, interest groups, and constituents

In addition to these positive purposes, committees may sometimes be used for the purpose of delaying or avoiding something (Liebler and McConnell 2004). A committee might even be known as "the graveyard" if proposals are sent there and never heard of again. Although this fortunately does not happen in all HCOs, you should realize it does occur in some.

GROUPS IN HEALTHCARE ORGANIZATIONS

HCOs have many groups, teams, committees, councils, and task forces. The following examples show the variety of groups in HCOs:

◆ Population Health Coordination Council

◆ Board of Directors Strategic Planning Committee

◆ Telehealth Network Installation Task Force

◆ Medical Staff Interdisciplinary Practice Committee

◆ Accountable Care Organization Team

◆ Cross-Functional Readmissions Committee

◆ Self-Managed Rehabilitation Team

◆ Consumer Engagement Advisory Council

◆ Virtual ICU Design Task Force

◆ Cut Carbon Footprint Committee

While groups form in all businesses, they seem to be especially common in HCOs. Why? Healthcare is multidisciplinary, involving disciplines of medicine, nursing, pharmacy, occupational therapy, social work, and dozens of others. Many disciplines have specialties, such as cardiology, neurology, surgery, and many others in medicine. Nurses specialize in pediatric nursing, emergency nursing, psychiatric nursing, and so forth. Besides all the clinical disciplines and professions, there are others such as management, information technology, finance, and marketing. As one commentator put it, healthcare "takes a village" (Scott 2009, 46). These disciplines have sometimes been too focused on their own specialized area such that "silos" have evolved. Groups and teams can overcome the silos. Perhaps at your college you have heard of interprofessional healthcare education, which combines students of several health professions in the same class (group) to learn together. The Affordable Care Act also reflects this idea. This healthcare reform law calls for and rewards more healthcare teams, interdisciplinary teams, and team models of healthcare delivery (Kaiser Family Foundation 2013). **Managers create groups to coordinate work among the many different professions, disciplines, departments, shifts, and days of an HCO.**

As noted earlier—and worth repeating—groups are not automatically good. **Groups become good because managers create them properly and then lead them properly.** How can managers do that? First, managers properly create the purpose and *structures* of a group. Second, managers properly create the *processes* of a group. You can learn how to do these tasks in the next two sections.

PURPOSE AND STRUCTURES OF GROUPS

When you form a group, think carefully about these seven structural characteristics: purpose, size, membership, relation to the organization hierarchy, authority, leader, and culture. The characteristics are interrelated and affect each other. Get them right so that your group can succeed. This section presents seven aspects of group structure that affect group performance (Borkowski 2009; Costa 2009; Fried, Topping, and Edmondson 2012).

PURPOSE

What is the purpose of the group? Each group must have a clear purpose, which is sometimes called the *charge* or *mandate*. This charge will guide the group in many ways, such as outlining who should be part of the group, how often it will meet, which resources it will need, and if it is temporary or ongoing. When group members have a clear purpose, they can stay focused rather than drift aimlessly or shift from one direction to another. A group can also more easily measure progress and achievement when it has a targeted purpose. The purpose of a group is usually stated (at least in rough-draft form) when people first decide that a group is needed. A written statement of purpose often comes from the manager who formally creates the group and holds it accountable for achieving the work stated in the group's purpose.

Managers should devote careful thought and effort to writing the purpose. That effort will pay off later by giving clear guidance to the group and its members. Groups should periodically update the purpose, if needed, to reflect changing situations.

SIZE

The size of a group strongly influences how well it performs. Managers at Partners had to decide how big the strategy implementation group ought to be. Pop quiz: What size would be best? If you said, "It all depends," you are correct! Bonus question: What does it depend on?

Several factors are relevant when managers decide the size of a group, team, or committee. A manager who forms a group must weigh the advantages of a big group against the advantages of a small one. The best size depends on the group's purpose. For example, the purpose might require certain departments, stakeholders, or others to be represented and able to participate. If the group's purpose is to coordinate the work of seven departments, then the group size should at least be seven people so that each department participates.

Sometimes the purpose requires certain expertise, such as marketing and finance. In that case, the group's size must be big enough to include members with the needed expertise. When the purpose of a group is to advise and offer input to others who will then make a decision, a large size would bring in a wider range of views and relevant information. If the purpose is to build support for a strategic plan, a large size would allow more people to participate so that they would be more likely to support the final plan. If the purpose requires lots of work to accomplish, then a large group would enable tasks to be spread among more members so that no one is overloaded.

While big groups have advantages, they also have disadvantages. See Exhibit 6.1 for the respective advantages of big and small groups. Bigger groups are harder to manage because of less cohesiveness and cooperation among members. Smaller "splinter" groups and informal groups often emerge within large groups. If this happens, it may signal a need to subdivide a large group into several smaller subgroups, each focused on a part of the full group's purpose. More time and effort are needed for large groups to meet, discuss, gather input, resolve differences, and reach decisions. Costs rapidly increase in big groups as the salary meter runs. Costs for food, supplies, and other resources also increase. When HCOs must control costs and decide quickly, small groups of five to seven members are better than larger groups.

MEMBERSHIP

The members greatly affect group performance. Managers might decide (or recommend) who should be on a committee, team, or council. Alternatively, people might elect or choose a member to be in a group, such as the social services department choosing

Advantages of Big Group Size	Advantages of Small Group Size	
More opportunity for diverse views, ideas, expertise, and input	Less cost per meeting due to fewer participants	
More people become committed to the group's purpose and work	Less time needed for members to get acquainted and be comfortable with each other	
More stakeholders feel they have a say and are represented	More group cohesiveness and cooperation	
Tasks and work can be spread among more people	Easier to manage	
Better for solving complex problems	Easier to reach agreement	

EXHIBIT 6.1
Group Sizes and Advantages

SOURCES: Borkowski (2009); Fried, Topping, and Edmondson (2012).

someone to represent that department on the consumer engagement advisory council. When choosing or electing members to serve on teams, committees, and groups, managers should consider these questions:

◆ Who can provide the knowledge, skills, and attitudes the group needs?

◆ Who can perform helpful task and maintenance roles, and who would not harm the group?

◆ Who works well with people and in groups (or could after training and coaching)?

◆ Who has sufficient time for this group while still doing his regular job?

◆ Who might grow professionally from group membership?

◆ Who can represent certain stakeholders, constituents, and work groups?

Managers should realize that members' similarities (e.g., gender, age, culture, education, professional status) increase group cohesiveness, but they also decrease the breadth of views and ideas. Too much similarity among members promotes **groupthink**, which means members quickly agree (politely and superficially) in order to maintain group harmony. Unfortunately, they avoid critical thinking, discussion, and thoughtful analysis, which would improve problem solving and decisions. Diversity of members creates diversity of ideas, viewpoints, attitudes, and values and often leads to innovative solutions to complex problems. However, diversity of members reduces (at least initially) trust and

Groupthink
Group members quickly, politely, and superficially reach agreement without considering diverse ideas; usually done to maintain group harmony.

cooperation. Diversity of team members' ages, education levels, and statuses may impede communication, participation, cohesiveness, and decision making. Thus, managers who appoint committee members of diverse backgrounds should provide time, training, and activities to strengthen trust and communication. (Chapters 7 and 8 on staffing and Chapter 15 on professionalism offer ideas for such activities.) Related to diversity is the duration of membership in a group. If members serve only for one year and meet only six times per year, they might not have enough time to develop enough trust and cohesiveness. Managers should then appoint members for longer durations.

HERE'S WHAT HAPPENED

Virginia Mason Medical Center in Seattle, Washington, was concerned about how much it was spending on thousands of different supplies. A Product Review Team was analyzing physicians' requests for new clinical supplies, implants, and devices, and a vice president made the decisions. This process took too long (six to seven weeks for each decision), and in the end the team rarely denied a request even if less expensive options existed. Managers realized the team lacked clinical expertise to properly challenge a request or discuss it with a requesting physician. A part-time physician advisor was added to help analyze clinical supply requests and talk with physicians about less costly options. Now, with better membership, the team is progressing toward a goal of about two weeks for reaching decisions, and it is saving the HCO thousands of dollars (HFMA 2009).

Exhibit 6.2 shows three types of roles that group members may perform (in much the same way people perform roles in a school play or movie). When group members perform task roles, they help their group achieve its purpose and get its work done. When they perform maintenance roles, they help group members work together and support each other, which is necessary for the group to succeed. When group members perform personal roles, they are trying to achieve their personal desires and may harm the group in doing so. Which of these roles have you seen group members perform? Which ones were helpful?

When managers pick people to serve in groups, they should think not only about people's technical knowledge or skills but also about task and maintenance roles people could contribute to the group. As a new manager who wants to succeed, be sure you perform task and maintenance roles, not personal roles.

RELATION TO THE ORGANIZATION HIERARCHY

Another structural feature of a group is the way it relates to the HCO's overall organization hierarchy. This relationship also affects how the group performs and how effective it can be. A committee that ties into the formal organization at a high level is perceived as more

EXHIBIT 6.2
Roles of Group Members

Task roles help the group achieve its tasks.

Role/Function	Actions and Behaviors
Initiator	Suggests new tasks, directions, problems, solutions, procedures
Information seeker	Requests relevant facts, opinions, information, data
Information giver	Provides relevant facts, opinions, information, data
Clarifier	Clarifies and explains terms, ideas, issues, opinions, information, data
Elaborator	Explains in depth giving examples, details, interpretations, implications
Evaluator	Judges ideas, information, progress, results
Agreement tester	States possible agreement, asks if members agree
Energizer	Keeps members going, stimulates members, urges progress
Orienter	Keeps discussion on track, redirects group to stay on task
Recorder	Takes notes, prepares records

Maintenance roles help group members maintain good feelings about the group and about working with group members.

Role/Function	Actions and Behaviors
Encourager	Praises others, affirms contributions of others, recognizes others
Harmonizer	Smooths over conflict, reconciles disagreements, reduces stress, eases tension
Compromiser	Offers or accepts compromises, admits own mistakes, changes opinion to maintain cohesion
Facilitator	Invites participation of members, suggests procedures for discussions, keeps communication open for all
Observer	Monitors and comments on feelings of the group and how well it functions
Follower	Accepts ideas, goes along with the group, passive

Personal roles do not help the group; rather, they help members fulfill personal needs.

Role/Function	Actions and Behaviors
Aggressor	Attacks others, attacks group, harshly disagrees
Blocker	Opposes group's ideas, impedes progress, is excessively negative
Dominator	Tries to dominate and control group, asserts authority
Help seeker	Seeks help with personal problems, seeks sympathy and support
Recognition seeker	Calls attention to self, seeks praise and recognition
Special interest seeker	Speaks up for a different group

SOURCES: Adapted from Benne and Sheats (1948); Fried, Rundall, and Topping (2000); and Myers and Anderson (2008).

important and powerful than a committee that is accountable to a lower level of the HCO. The high-level association will provide more political clout and resources, which could help the group succeed. This point is important because a group cannot perform well if it does not have sufficient resources from higher-level managers. Group members' main jobs also create linkages to the HCO's organizational structure.

When a manager creates a committee, task force, or team, he must decide to whom it will be accountable. For Partners HealthCare, the top managers had to decide to whom the strategy implementation group would be accountable (perhaps the chief strategy officer) and to whom it would report its work (perhaps the senior management team).

AUTHORITY

When creating a task force, a committee, or another group in an HCO, managers must decide what (if any) authority the group will have. Will a patient safety committee have the authority to set policy requiring nurses to repeat verbal orders from a physician to ensure that the verbal orders were heard correctly? Or will the committee lack that authority and only be able to advise nurses to repeat back verbal orders? Or perhaps the committee will only make recommendations to the nursing manager who first created the committee. How about an HCO's employee picnic task force—how much authority will it have to spend funds? At a healthcare consulting firm, the picnic task force wanted unlimited authority, but the chief executive officer (CEO) authorized it to spend only up to $1,000, after which it would need to get further approval from the CEO. Authority might vary over time or because of other factors. For example, a new task force might initially have little authority but later be given more authority after it becomes more proficient.

LEADER OR CHAIRPERSON

Another important structural feature for a group is its leader position and the person who serves in that position. Suppose the president of a large medical group practice in Boca Raton, Florida, creates an employee advisory council to advise managers about employees' concerns. Will the president appoint the leader of the council, or will the council members elect their own leader? For standing committees that continue for years, how long should someone be allowed to serve as chairperson? What duties and authority will the leader have? The more clearly these details are stated at the beginning, the better the group will perform. Depending on the size and purpose of a group, there may be more than one leader. Larger formal committees and councils might have a chair, a vice chair, and a secretary.

Another consideration is who will serve in the formal leadership position. For example, a nursing council has a chairperson position with designated responsibilities. Who should be the chairperson? Earlier, we learned about task roles, maintenance roles, and personal roles in groups. How well a group leader performs task and maintenance roles will strongly affect the group's success. Ideally, the formal leader position of a group will be filled by someone with the right knowledge, skills, abilities, and role behaviors. If you have been in a group led by an incapable chairperson, then you know how the group leader affects the group's performance.

 TRY IT, APPLY IT

> When you read through the roles in Exhibit 6.2, did you think of people you know who tend to take on those roles? Do you know someone who is a natural initiator, clarifier, energizer, harmonizer, or observer? (Perhaps you also know a blocker or dominator.) Try to list people you know who could perform task and maintenance roles without performing personal roles. Those are people to have in a group or on a team!

CULTURE

A final feature of a group, team, or committee is its culture—the values, attitudes, and norms (behaviors) that reflect and guide a group's members. A group might value risk taking and thinking outside the box—or it might not. A committee should establish its expected behaviors, such as "no side conversations during meetings" and "make new members feel welcome." The culture of the group strongly influences its effectiveness. Culture may include sensitive issues such as trust, conflict, civility, group loyalty, and ownership of group outcomes.

The culture should fit the purpose of the group and should not strongly conflict with the HCO's overall culture. For example, if a strategic planning committee is to brainstorm new ideas, its culture must not be rigid and stifling. Group members must have the attitude that it is OK to ask "stupid" questions and suggest "crazy" ideas. A group's culture will affect how members feel about being part of the group and whether they continue to actively participate. If a patient safety committee's culture allows physicians to behave in an arrogant manner toward other members, then nonphysicians will not fully support the committee. A culture that supports and even encourages disagreement and debate will have less groupthink and enable people to safely express different points of view.

Managers and group members must decide what the culture or personality of the group should be and take steps to establish it. More information is provided in the section on group developing (and in Chapter 11 on culture in HCOs.)

PROCESSES OF GROUPS AND TEAMS

Besides structure, groups in HCOs must have processes to do their work. Structure only creates a committee. The processes make the committee come to life with activity. Listen closely to a group and you will hear the hum of activity; with some groups, you might also hear shouting, cheering, arguing, and other sounds! When you are on a team or committee, think about five processes: developing, leading, communicating and interacting, decision making, and learning. Group leaders and members together create these processes, which all affect group performance. Additionally, these processes may affect structure, such as by shaping the group's culture. This section explains the five group processes (Costa 2009; Fried, Topping, and Edmondson 2012; Ivanitskaya, Glazer, and Erofeev 2009).

DEVELOPING

As Henry Ford's quote at the beginning of this chapter implies, groups of workers go through stages. Before actually working together, they begin by coming together and then progress toward staying together. Bruce Tuckman (1965) created those ideas in a Team Development Model that he later expanded (Tuckman and Jensen 1977). The Team Development Model is frequently used today, and it suggests that groups go through five stages of development: forming, storming, norming, performing, and adjourning. The model provides a broad understanding of groups. Although it does not portray every group exactly, the model does provide a useful guide for understanding how to manage and participate in groups. Following are the five stages of the Team Development Model (Costa 2009; Fried, Topping, and Edmondson 2012):

1. Forming Stage
   - Members get acquainted, act polite, and try to figure out what is OK and not OK.

   - Members learn the group's purpose and "why we are here."

   - Members reduce barriers with icebreakers (e.g., self-introductions, interviewing and then introducing other members, scavenger hunt, team-building exercises).

   - The leader should set a positive tone and stimulate new thinking and motivation.

2. Storming Stage
   - Members argue and disagree about the group's methods, rules, and tasks; conflicts arise.

   –   Some members strive for control and leadership, creating conflict.

   –   The leader should demonstrate cooperation and teamwork; the leader should emphasize teamwork and team purpose.

3.   Norming Stage
   –   Members figure out how to work together and agree on ground rules, expected norms (behaviors), a code of conduct, and methods for deciding, cooperating, and communicating in the group.

   –   Cooperation increases, conflict decreases, and the group feels more cohesive.

   –   The leader should emphasize the group's goals and purpose.

4.   Performing Stage
   –   Members have figured out how to work together and now focus on achieving the group's purpose and goals.

   –   Members plan how to accomplish goals, divide work, and make assignments.

   –   Members perform their tasks.

   –   The leader should guide progress toward goals and motivate members.

5.   Adjourning Stage
   –   Temporary groups finish their goals and disband.

   –   Members acknowledge and celebrate what they have achieved.

   –   If members worked well together, they may mourn, feel sadness, and express farewells.

   –   The leader should help members reach closure.

   Managers use this model to understand group behavior, realizing that some groups may not go through all stages or develop in a linear way. For example, maintenance workers at a personal care home who already know each other could be appointed to a departmental task force to develop a new preventive maintenance schedule. Because they know each other, they will not have to go through the forming stage. Members may quickly progress to the performing stage. Alternatively, if an ongoing community advisory board expands its purpose and increases its size from 7 to 15 members, it should back up and redo the earlier forming stage.

   Managers who lead or serve on virtual teams in cyberspace should be sensitive to where members are in these stages of development. Some group members—particularly those who have not been in a virtual group before—may need extra time and support to work through the stages. The forming stage will take more time and patience. Members will have a harder time meeting and becoming comfortable with each other because they will not be able to watch body language and facial expressions to judge how others feel. Members may argue about rules for communicating and norms for interacting. A virtual team needs time, careful leadership, and perhaps training to work through the stages of developing. Otherwise, the team will struggle for group success (Khan 2011). Local, regional, national, and global HCOs use virtual teams with carefully managed trust, intra-group communication, cohesiveness, teamwork, and group dynamics. Regional, national, and global HCOs that use virtual teams include nursing home chains, hospital management companies, and pharmaceutical firms. When team members come from countries with different cultures, the challenges of team development are even more evident. Challenges can arise even with team members from different regional cultures of the same country (e.g., the cultures of the Northeast, the South, and the West Coast in the United States).

LEADING

In a group, leading motivates and influences group members to work toward a purpose. We learned earlier that managers create a group's leadership structure (e.g., a team captain, committee chair, task force director). These are structural positions—they are not the same as the process behaviors and actions expected from someone in a leader position. Perhaps you have been in a club in which the formal leadership position was filled by someone who later left. Did the next leader (in the same position) exhibit the same behaviors and perform the same actions as the first person? Probably not. Leaders vary in how they lead. Leading greatly affects a group's performance. As a manager or group member, pay attention to who is leading and how. **The leader should explain the group's vision and goals, divide the work, arrange assignments, resolve conflicts, and motivate everyone to help the group succeed. The leader should perform many task and maintenance roles (shown in Exhibit 6.2) and should interact effectively with each member.** The person in the leadership position will (ideally) lead the group to achieve its purpose.

For a group's formal leader, the process of leading sometimes includes stepping back and letting a different group member lead. The formal leader lets a member with specific expertise (e.g., social media expertise) lead the group when it must handle a specific matter (e.g., a social media problem) pertaining to that person's expertise. This approach strengthens the group by actively involving more members, using group members' expertise, and enabling more people to develop leadership skills for the future.

One or more group members might act as unofficial informal leaders and form subgroups of followers. People with high energy who like to socialize may become informal leaders in a committee. Or, a more experienced person might take on this role. Suppose a patient care council has 20 members, including 4 nurses. The nurses might sit together at council meetings, text each other between meetings, and be led by the most experienced nurse who becomes their informal leader. Sometimes informal leaders are helpful and support the official leader. However, if they strongly disagree with the leader, they might do the opposite. As we learned in Chapter 4, the formal leader must identify informal leaders and try to work effectively with them.

COMMUNICATING AND INTERACTING

Group members must communicate with people inside and outside their group, so communication processes are important for the group's success. Chapter 15 teaches the subject of communication. For now, realize that group members and leaders must work to create effective communication processes for the group.

First, **effective communication processes (e.g., speaking, listening, persuading) are needed inside the group.** Ideally, all members would easily communicate with all other members in meetings and in one-to-one conversations. However, we know that does not always happen. Cultural diversity among members can impede communication, because of language barriers and feelings about communicating with others. People who are younger or who have less status may defer to older or higher-level group members and not interact with them. If members are not comfortable interacting, communication will be limited as shown in Exhibit 6.3.

In other groups, some members may share information with one or two other members but not the entire group, which also restricts the communication processes.

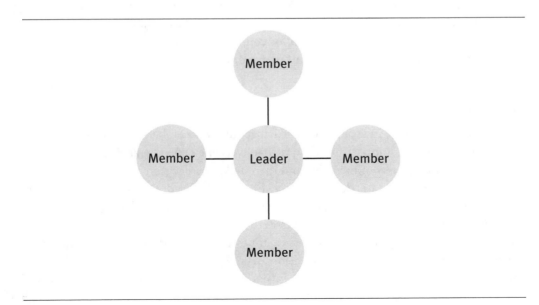

EXHIBIT 6.3
Limited Communication Among Group Members

Leaders should help groups create effective communication and interaction processes so that group members—and the group—can be effective. A group leader should ensure that members interact and communicate with others as needed, but not more than is needed. Too much unnecessary interaction or information could overload group members and cause them to back away from the group. However, closed or restricted communication among members will reduce trust, cohesiveness, and effectiveness. A group leader must manage these issues carefully.

Task, maintenance, and personal roles (shown in Exhibit 6.2) all shape the communication processes of a group. When group members together perform the task and maintenance roles, they create effective communication processes. However, members who strive to satisfy personal needs (e.g., recognition, sympathy) by acting out personal roles in groups may impede communication.

Second, **effective communication processes with people outside the group are also needed.** Recall from previous chapters that an HCO must be open to its environment. Similarly, a group in an HCO must be open to factors outside the group. Groups in an HCO must communicate with departments, people, and other groups inside the HCO. In addition, they might have to communicate with people outside the HCO. Why? To obtain inputs (e.g., resources, information, political support, expertise) from outsiders and to coordinate its work with, form relationships with, and distribute its outputs to other parts of the HCO.

Communication processes must be created by groups, which may require training and coaching. These processes can by enhanced by several methods and technologies, including meetings, conference calls, documents, e-mail, social media, intranets, and blogs. Group members' communication and interaction strongly affect the group's performance. For example, when Vladlena became chairwoman of a community health council, she expanded the number and frequency of communication processes so that members would get to know each other sooner and then work together better.

Decision Making

How are decisions made in groups you participate in? Do members vote? Does the leader try to build consensus support for an idea that everyone generally agrees with? Or does the leader obtain input from members and then make the decision alone? Decision making can range from autocratic decisions made by the group leader to democratic decisions made by all the members. This subject is more fully addressed in Chapter 13. For now, remember that groups can use many processes to make decisions. A single committee may use different decision processes at different times because of different leadership, time urgency, members, and training in decision making. Members must develop decision-making processes that best fit the group given its goals, time, resources, and members' ability to make decisions. Group members can become better at making decisions through training, coaching, and experience.

Group members and leaders should watch for two possible problems. The first occurs when responsibility for a group decision is spread among group members so that no one individual is accountable for the decision. This situation is reflected in the saying "When it is everybody's decision, it is nobody's decision." Knowing they will not be held individually responsible, members might take group decision making less seriously than they would individual decision making. Thus, group leaders must create and reinforce individual as well as group accountability by using words, norms, incentives, and actions such as calling on each person to participate.

Second, groups should strive to avoid groupthink. This occurs when leaders and group norms (developed in the norming stage) support harmony more than critical thinking. Members feel strongly that "we must all get along"—thus, they will not disagree with each other. Yet, some disagreement is good for organizations to prevent quick, superficial, and ineffective decisions. When groups have people who perform the task and maintenance roles (and do not allow the personal roles), they will avoid groupthink and reach better decisions. Groups potentially can make better decisions than individuals because groups can bring a wider range of information, experiences, perspectives, and insights to the decision. However, groupthink will block these potential benefits of groups for decisions. Group leaders should create team norms that support critical thinking to get beyond quick, superficial statements. They should not only allow but also encourage disagreement early in the decision-making process, which is explained further in Chapter 13.

LEARNING

A final important group process is team or group learning, as explained by Fried, Topping, and Edmondson (2012). The group must learn as a group. That is not the same as individual learning by individual group members. The group must reflect on its structure and its processes (described earlier in this chapter) to learn how it is doing as a group. Based on what it learns about itself, the group then can improve its structures and processes.

For example, suppose a safety-net primary care clinic in Chicago, Illinois, appoints a new fundraising committee to obtain $50,000 in donations. The group comprises thirteen members, some of whom do not know the others. The group will have to develop itself, lead itself, communicate within and beyond itself, and make decisions. How well does the group perform all these duties? Kiera feels there is not enough communication between the leader and herself. Travis thinks the group members have been wishfully guessing how much local businesses will donate rather than carefully analyzing data. Colleen and Taylor feel the group is struggling and might not reach its goal. Group learning is needed. The group's members can candidly discuss its processes and how it is doing. The leader, in open discussion or in confidential surveys, can ask group members for feedback about the group's processes and outcomes and seek suggestions. (The following Check It Out offers a group self-assessment survey to help guide group learning.) To overcome weak processes, the group can engage in team-building exercises

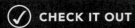

CHECK IT OUT

If you are part of a team or group at college, you may perform a self-assessment of your group. At the Mind Tools website (www.mindtools.com/pages/article/newTMM_84.htm), you will find a Team Effectiveness Assessment with 15 questions. After answering these questions, you can click the Calculate My Total button to learn the results. Then check the brief guide that explains how to interpret your results to better understand how your team functions and performs. This assessment can be used to guide team learning and improvement.

and training in group processes (e.g., communicating, decision making). The group can reaffirm its norms and, if necessary, return to the norming stage to develop new norms. It might have to change its structures, such as reducing group size or strengthening leadership authority. As a manager and as a group member, realize that people do not automatically work well as a group. They must learn how to work together as a group. **The group learning process enables a group to learn about itself and then adjust structures and processes to improve group performance.** Group learning is essential—especially for new groups!

EFFECTIVE GROUPS AND TEAMS

Some groups and teams are more effective than others in achieving their intended purposes and satisfying members. Managers can help groups do well by creating effective group structures and processes. While developing the structure and processes, managers should also ensure that group members have the skills needed to work in groups. Training, coaching, and mentoring might be necessary. Many employees have excellent knowledge and skills for their task-oriented jobs yet lack skills for group decision making, communicating, interpersonal relations, and discussions. Role playing, mini-cases, practice exercises, and other forms of hands-on learning can help. Providing time, funds, and other resources for training is one way top managers demonstrate support and commitment to a group. Executives at Peninsula Regional Health System in Salisbury, Maryland, provide thousands of hours of training to the system's 4,000 employees to help them communicate better with each other and improve group performance (Scott 2009).

This chapter has provided tools and techniques that managers can use to create effective teams. Managers can change and control these factors. They can "turn the dials" to adjust group size, membership, leaders, processes, culture, and so forth. Yet managers must realize that external factors also affect how well groups perform and achieve their purposes. Each of the prior five chapters made the point that external factors affect an HCO. The same lesson applies to groups: External factors (i.e., factors outside a group) affect a group. Thus, factors in the external environment (recall Chapter 1), such as laws, customers' preferences, competitors, and new scientific discoveries, can affect groups. In addition, a group can be affected by factors that are inside an HCO yet external to a group that is inside that HCO. For example, suppose Medical Diagnostics, Inc. is a business that provides outpatient testing including lab tests, medical imaging, and cardiology tests.

Within this business, an equipment committee decides which equipment to buy each year. The committee will be influenced by factors outside of the equipment committee yet inside other parts of Medical Diagnostics, Inc. The business's managers, financial situation, political relationships, workload, and competing priorities will all affect how well the equipment committee performs and achieves its purpose.

MANAGERS' GUIDELINES FOR EFFECTIVE MEETINGS

What would groups (and HCOs) do without meetings? Because groups meet often (sometimes too often), managers should do their best to ensure that meetings are worthwhile. Employees gripe about meetings that are pointless, unproductive, and a waste of time. Managers who know how to make meetings worthwhile are rewarded with better results and happier employees. Managers should consider doing the following (Costa 2009; Liebler and McConnell 2004):

◆ Before calling a meeting, ensure a meeting is really needed.

◆ Plan the meeting: who, what, where, when, why, and how.

◆ Send participants the agenda and necessary reading materials early enough so that they can read them and prepare.

◆ Orient new members before the meeting.

◆ Arrange for someone to record the minutes (and distribute them later).

◆ Respect people's time—begin on time, stay on time, and end on time.

◆ Set the tone and state ground rules (e.g., be on time, turn off cell phones, maintain confidentiality, avoid blaming, no slacking or free riding, no side conversations, everyone participates, support each other).

◆ State the purpose of the meeting.

◆ Lead the meeting, stay on agenda, and use time wisely to cover all agenda items.

◆ Respect everyone by leading a balanced discussion, seeking input from everyone, and performing task and maintenance roles.

◆ Don't spend meeting time on issues that are better discussed by smaller subcommittees or one-to-one.

◆ Use time-outs, mediation, and separate conflict resolution meetings if necessary.

◆ End on a positive note, summarize the meeting, review assignments, and thank participants.

◆ Follow through on decisions, assignments, and arrangements for the next meeting.

ONE MORE TIME

A group involves the social interaction between two or more people in a stable arrangement who have common goals or interests and who perceive themselves as a group. Groups such as teams, committees, task forces, and councils coordinate work in an HCO. At all levels of an HCO, managers must create and participate in groups. Top managers must support groups and promote teamwork. Managers of departments and work sections must do the same within their own areas.

Group success requires proper group structure and process. Group success also depends on group members performing task and maintenance roles. When forming a group, think carefully about seven structural characteristics (purpose, size, membership, relation to the organization hierarchy, authority, leader, culture) and five processes (developing, leading, communicating and interacting, decision making, and learning). Group development includes five stages—forming, storming, norming, performing, and adjourning. When group members perform task roles, they help their group achieve its purpose and get its work done. When they perform maintenance roles, they help their group members work together and support each other. Managers should nurture these roles in groups and discourage members from performing personal roles for their own needs. Managers should follow practical tips to make meetings worthwhile. Two final ingredients for group success are visible active support from top management and training of employees for work in groups. Group members should periodically evaluate their groups to identify and resolve possible problems.

(T) FOR YOUR TOOLBOX

- Group structures
- Group processes
- Roles of group members
- Team development model
- Guidelines for effective meetings

FOR DISCUSSION

1.   Why are teams, committees, and other groups needed in HCOs?

2.   Identify structural factors that affect the performance of groups and teams. Give examples.

3.   Identify process factors that affect the performance of groups and teams. Give examples.

4.   Name a group you were in that was fun and effective. Which structure characteristics and process characteristics do you think made the group fun and effective?

5.   Discuss how groupthink can harm a group. How can a group leader avoid groupthink?

6.   Explain the difference between task, maintenance, and personal roles in groups. Which roles would come easily to you? Which roles would you like to develop in the future?

7.   Discuss your top three "Managers' Guidelines for Effective Meetings."

CASE STUDY QUESTIONS

These questions refer to the Integrative Case Studies at the back of this book.

1.   Decisions, Decisions case: Using this chapter, advise Mr. Martin on how to create the subcommittee. How many people and which people and positions would you appoint? What should the purpose and goal of the subcommittee be? What would you do to ensure the subcommittee fulfills its purpose?

2.   Disparities in Care at Southern Regional Health System case: Suppose Tim Hank wants to appoint a healthcare disparities council to advise him on how to reduce healthcare disparities. Use this chapter to help Mr. Hank create the council. How many people and which stakeholders would you appoint? What would the purpose and goal of the council be? What would you do to ensure the council fulfills its purpose?

3.   Taking Care of Business at Graceland Memorial Hospital case: Think about the two-hour meeting at the end of the case. Explain which task roles and maintenance roles would help during that meeting. Describe which personal roles might have interfered with reaching agreement.

TRY IT, APPLY IT

Suppose a local hospital established the goal of reducing its carbon footprint by 25 percent in three years. As an intern there, you are asked to help create a new Cut Carbon committee. Write a short statement of purpose for the committee. What would you suggest for its membership? To whom should it be accountable? What authority would you recommend this committee have? After you write your answers, share them with colleagues and ask for their feedback.

CHAPTER 7

STAFFING: OBTAINING EMPLOYEES

Our employees are our greatest asset.

Business slogan

LEARNING OBJECTIVES

Studying this chapter will help you to

➤ define the staffing function of management;

➤ describe how human resource specialists can help managers obtain employees;

➤ realize how laws, regulations, and court decisions affect staffing;

➤ explain how managers plan staffing;

➤ describe how managers design jobs; and

➤ understand how managers recruit, select, and hire staff.

HERE'S WHAT HAPPENED

Partners HealthCare revised its mission and developed ambitious goals to improve the quality and cost-effectiveness of patient care. More specifically, managers intended to use technology to improve priority health conditions: diabetes, heart attack, stroke, and colorectal cancer. To achieve their goals, managers had to staff the organization. They planned which jobs were required (e.g., telemonitoring nurse) and how many positions were needed for each. They organized jobs by identifying the tasks, responsibilities, authority, and qualifications of each job. For example, the telemonitoring nurse job was responsible for monitoring remote patients' vital signs via telehealth technology, responding when the telehealth system signaled vitals were abnormal, and guiding patients through biweekly heart education. Managers had to recruit applicants for the positions and evaluate the applicants using selection criteria. Careful selection of telemonitoring nurses was needed because some nurses prefer working with patients by standing at the bedside rather than by sitting at a monitor. After managers decided whom to hire for each position, they likely prepared job offers with compensation, starting dates, and other essential information. By performing this staffing function, managers were progressing toward their goals.

A s we see in the opening Here's What Happened, healthcare organization (HCO) managers must get people—and keep them—to do the work to achieve the HCO's mission and goals. This function is staffing—the third fundamental management function we learned in Chapter 2. We can think of **staffing** as obtaining and retaining people to fill jobs and do the work. Previous chapters on planning (the first management function) and organizing (the second management function) often referred to workers, employees, jobs, positions, and staff. Building on that, this chapter and Chapter 8 teach us how managers perform the staffing function. Staffing requires managers to perform several management roles we studied in Chapter 2: monitor, entrepreneur, disturbance handler, resource allocator, and negotiator.

Staffing
Obtaining and retaining people to fill jobs and do work.

As we learned in Chapter 4, healthcare is usually a service, and services are performed by people (rather than manufactured by machines). Most HCOs are labor intensive and depend on many people to perform the services. These people may be called staff, workers, employees, personnel, human resources, or talent. Even though we might be impressed by the amazing medical equipment used in HCOs, we must remember that people (human resources) are needed to operate the equipment (physical resources). Further, some medical work and much nonmedical work (e.g., management itself) often does not use fancy gadgets and equipment. **Always remember that healthcare is a service provided by people, so managers must excel at staffing.**

Many organizations, including HCOs, proclaim, "Employees are our greatest asset." What should managers do to make employees great (e.g., empathetic, innovative, honest, flexible, industrious, cooperative, patient centered)? How can managers obtain their "greatest

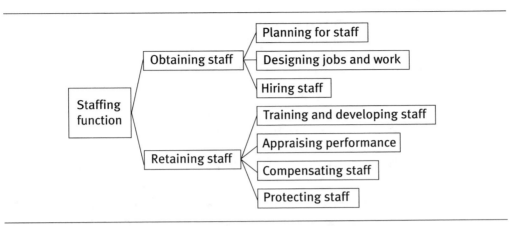

Exhibit 7.1
Staffing Processes

asset"? How can managers then retain their "greatest asset" to avoid the time, expense, effort, and lost revenue of replacing workers (and also avoid negative comments on employer rating websites such as Glassdoor)? Chapters 7 and 8 answer these questions. First, we learn how managers staff their HCOs by using seven staffing processes. Then we examine how specialized experts and departments may assist managers in staffing their HCOs. Staffing is done in a legal environment that regulates how the function must—and must not—be done. After considering this background, we study in more depth the seven processes used to staff an HCO. The first three are discussed in this chapter and focus on *obtaining* workers. The other four processes are explored in the next chapter and focus on *retaining* workers.

When you become a manager, you will soon become involved in staffing. This chapter and the next one will help you prepare for that work.

Staffing Processes

The management staffing function can be explained by breaking it into seven processes that managers should do. These processes are shown in Exhibit 7.1 and defined as follows (Fallon and McConnell 2014; Fottler 2008a; French 2007; Fried and Gates 2008):

1. **Planning for staff:** Forecasting the organization's future staffing requirements and deciding how to ensure the needed workers are available

2. **Designing jobs and work:** Determining work tasks to be done by a job, along with working conditions, rules, schedules, supervision, and qualifications

3. **Hiring staff:** Recruiting and selecting workers for jobs, which may include reassigning existing workers by promotion or transfer

4. **Training and developing staff:** Enabling employees to acquire new knowledge, skills, attitudes, and behaviors for current and future jobs

Planning for staff
Forecasting the organization's future staffing requirements and deciding how to ensure the needed workers are available.

Designing jobs and work
Determining work tasks to be done by a job, along with working conditions, rules, schedules, supervision, and qualifications.

Hiring staff
Recruiting and selecting workers for jobs, which may include reassigning existing workers by promotion or transfer.

Training and developing staff
Enabling employees to acquire new knowledge, skills, attitudes, and behaviors for current and future jobs.

**Appraising
performance**
Evaluating the job
performance of
workers and discussing
those evaluations with
the workers.

Compensating staff
Determining and
giving wages, salaries,
incentives, and
benefits to workers.

Protecting staff
Ensuring that workers
have proper work
conditions and
that their opinions
are considered by
managers.

Compensation
Wages, salaries,
incentives, and
benefits for employees.

5. **Appraising performance:** Evaluating the job performance of workers and discussing those evaluations with the workers

6. **Compensating staff:** Determining and giving wages, salaries, incentives, and benefits to workers

7. **Protecting staff:** Ensuring that workers have proper work conditions and that their opinions are considered by managers.

Which of these processes have you experienced in a summer job or part-time job during college?

This chapter studies the first three processes, which get people in the door to start working. Chapter 8 explains the other four processes, which keep people so they do not walk out the door. **These seven staffing processes interact and affect each other.** For example, a respiratory therapist's expanded *job design* may lead to new *training*, which might later lead to higher *compensation*. Also, these processes can contribute to both obtaining and retaining staff. For example, **compensation** must start high enough to hire people, and it must later increase to keep people.

Managers in HCOs should ensure that all seven staffing processes are done well to help their HCOs survive and thrive. Managers are likely to do much of the staffing function themselves but also rely on internal or external staffing experts to help. A small HCO, such as a new home care business in Ithaca, New York, may have only an owner-manager, a few nurses, and a clerical assistant. This owner-manager will likely do much of the staffing with help from a business consultant. Larger HCOs have specialized human resources (HR) employees to assist managers with the seven processes. When HCOs become even larger, the HR staff expands and becomes an HR department. In recent years, many HCOs have been merging, affiliating, networking, and in other ways combining to gain size and power. With this trend, smaller HCOs have become part of bigger HCOs that have HR departments. Then the small HCO does not have to outsource as much routine staffing work to consultants.

Recall from Chapter 5 the discussion of the modular approach to organizing, in which some work is outsourced to other businesses. HCOs outsource some staffing work to firms that specialize in, for example, developing compensation packages, implementing workforce reductions, or training employees for patient engagement. Outsourcing may be important for strategic purposes (Brown and Fink 2012), when in-depth expertise is required, or for temporary or unusual staffing requirements. As a manager, you will have to decide how much of the staffing function to do internally and how much to outsource.

MANAGERS AND THE HUMAN RESOURCES DEPARTMENT

Staffing processes are performed by managers who are responsible for their subordinates. As mentioned earlier, managers often receive help from HR departments and from staff such as human resource specialists, talent recruiters, and compensation analysts. If your HCO has an HR department, you as a manager should not view your role as merely helping the HR department with staffing. Rather, you will be responsible for staffing your work unit in cooperation with higher-level managers and HR staff.

An HR department creates staffing programs, policies, and procedures for managers to use in their departments with their employees. The HR staffing specialists may prepare an orientation program for new employees, create a procedure for announcing job opportunities via social media, and design an employee performance evaluation form. These programs, policies, and procedures help create consistency and fairness when individual managers use them throughout the HCO. Yet, the manager of a department is still the person responsible for using those programs, policies, and procedures to staff her department.

HR staff and departments also should have current information systems, computer programs, communications technology, and mobile apps to support the staffing processes, employees, and managers. HR software can be used to manage databases for many aspects of staffing and for thousands of applicants, employees, and former employees. For example, HCO managers can keep track of all approved jobs and positions, track applicants, manage recruitment and selection for jobs, measure diversity and inclusion, manage employees' benefits and compensation, identify which employees are due for annual performance appraisals in a given month, and track employee safety problems. In this way, HR staff help managers with many staffing duties.

New supervisors, experienced managers, and senior executives can all benefit—and avoid serious legal problems—by working with HR staff and experts. Although managers *should* work closely with the expert HR staff, they sometimes do not. Why would managers turn down free, expert help?

In HCOs, conflict can arise between managers of departments (e.g., admissions, infomatics, radiology, marketing, supply chain, health education) and the HR staff. Some managers view the HR staff as bureaucratic—for example, requiring many forms, following numerous rules, and creating delays when hiring staff (Fallon and McConnell 2014). Suppose Amanda, the office manager of a large, busy multispecialty medical group, wants to hire someone quickly to fill an unexpected vacancy. To ensure fairness and prevent a lawsuit, the HR staff carefully checks that all laws are followed when advertising the opening, interviewing applicants, and making a hiring decision. (Grrrr, delay.) Amanda then wants to raise the starting salary to fill the vacancy quickly. The HR staff advises that doing so would not be fair to current employees and would upset them if they found out. (Grrrr, an obstacle.) The HR staff also wants to check each applicant's references, which could take several days. (Grrrr, more delay.) Thus, conflict arises between Amanda and the HR staff.

Most managers realize that HR policies, procedures, rules, and forms are for the good of the HCO and its employees and managers. These processes help prevent lawsuits, bad press, and a revolving door of workers who leave soon after starting. If a manager ignores HR staff advice and makes a foolish or illegal hiring decision, that mistake will reflect badly on him. As a manager, you must work cooperatively with the staffing experts.

LAWS AND REGULATIONS

It would be hard to exaggerate how much staffing is influenced (controlled, really) by laws, court decisions, and regulations. Laws affect how managers recruit staff, interview applicants, compensate workers, promote or discharge employees, and perform most aspects of staffing. If you have had a job, you probably already know that laws require workplace safety and forbid discrimination in hiring. Here are a few of the laws that affect staffing in HCOs:

◆ National Labor Relations Act of 1935

◆ Civil Rights Act of 1964

◆ Occupational Safety and Health Act of 1970

◆ Equal Employment Opportunity Act of 1972

◆ Americans with Disabilities Act of 1990

◆ Family and Medical Leave Act of 1993

◆ Fair Minimum Wage Act of 2007

◆ Patient Protection and Affordable Care Act of 2010

◆ Veterans Opportunity to Work (VOW) to Hire Heroes Act of 2011

Some of these laws are studied in health law or business law classes.

To comply with labor laws, managers and supervisors should confer with HR experts. Labor law is so complex that many HCOs regularly consult with labor attorneys; some large HCOs hire their own labor attorneys. **In addition to acting fairly and consistently, managers and supervisors should also carefully document all staffing processes, decisions, and actions.** Job applicants and employees might file lawsuits if they feel unfairly turned down for a job, promotion, pay raise, or even a preferred work schedule. The saying "If it isn't documented, it didn't happen" means you need documentation of your actions in case a legal challenge arises.

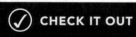

CHECK IT OUT

The US Department of Labor has a practical online resource for employment laws (www.dol.gov/elaws/). It explains many laws and regulations affecting small businesses and workers. The guide is especially useful to people who need hands-on information on topics such as wages, benefits, safety, health, and nondiscrimination. This valuable resource can help you learn more about staffing laws now and during your career.

PLANNING FOR STAFF

In Chapter 3, we learned that HCOs create their mission and goals along with implementation plans to achieve the mission and goals. This work often requires planning for staff, which includes planning changes in staff positions and workers, and planning for changes in staff programs and policies (Noe et al. 2015). Changes to positions and workers might include

- three new nurses,

- two fewer supply clerks,

- a new social media coordinator,

- two new data analysts, and

- a new population health coordinator.

Changes to staffing programs and policies might include

- a different merit pay system that will reward innovation,

- a training program to help staff work with other employees for whom English is a second language, or

- a new hiring policy for returning military veterans.

This type of planning can become complex, given the trends of HCOs merging, forming accountable care organizations, or affiliating with others. Merging HCOs leads to merging (and perhaps reducing) staff as well as merging programs and policies. Think about combining two different policies for compensation, two different methods for writing job descriptions, and two different hiring policies. The staff planning process is a good place to begin this work.

To plan jobs, positions, and workers, the HCO's managers must forecast several factors on the basis of input from supervisors and managers. These factors include the following:

- Expected turnover, retirements, resignations, and other departures, as well as promotions, transfers, and other transitions—all based on historical data, future plans, and good judgment

- Numbers and types of positions needed to achieve intended goals for the coming year

- The HCO's strengths, weaknesses, and internal situation, such as its financial situation, support for a diverse workforce, use of temporary workers, and reputation as a place to work

- External threats and opportunities, such as emerging health problems, new employment laws, changing availability of workers, customers' demands for patient-centered care, plans of local colleges and vocational schools, workforce diversity, and emerging technology

Given these factors, managers must anticipate and plan staff accordingly. How many retirees will have to be replaced next year? How many therapists will be needed to staff the new chronic pain clinic? How will the Affordable Care Act affect staffing needs? To deal with the nursing shortage, should we contract with a nursing agency and freelance workers?

Managers also must plan the HR programs, policies, procedures, systems, methods, and tools that will be used for all the other staffing processes. They help ensure workers are available and perform well. Here are examples of planning for the other staffing processes:

◆ *Job designing:* During the coming year, we plan to develop standard job description formats, rules for who can change a job description, and policy for who must approve new job descriptions for the HCO.

◆ *Hiring:* During the coming year, we plan to create standard procedures for hiring, including placing employment ads online, checking references from previous employers, and approving a starting salary.

◆ *Training:* During the coming year, we plan to prepare training programs to improve employees' care of disabled clients.

◆ *Appraising:* During the coming year, we plan to revise performance appraisal methods to require each employee to do a self-evaluation.

◆ *Compensating:* During the coming year, we plan to revise the policy for using vacation days so that it better meets the needs of employees with young children.

◆ *Protecting:* During the coming year, we plan to create a workforce diversity celebration to recognize and celebrate the diversity of our staff.

DESIGNING JOBS AND WORK

Recall from Chapter 4 that the terms *job* and *position* are similar but not the same. "A job consists of a group of activities and duties that entail natural units of work that are similar and related" (Fottler 2008a, 163). Some jobs, such as president, are performed by just one person. Other jobs, such as nurse, are performed by more than one person if the amount of work is too much for one person. There are multiple nurse positions, and each is filled by a person who performs the nurse job. "A position consists of different duties and responsibilities that are performed by only one employee" (Fottler 2008a, 163). Thus, five people may fill five nurse positions that all perform one nurse job.

JOB ANALYSIS

Job analysis is used to design jobs. In Chapter 4, we studied how work and jobs are designed as part of organizing work in an HCO. This function is linked with staffing. Job and work design involves determining which tasks and activities must be done and how they should be grouped into jobs, positions, teams, and work units. For example, in the Here's What Happened at the beginning of this chapter, Partners HealthCare designed the telemonitoring nurse job to include monitoring patients' vital signs along with other tasks. Job analysis dissects jobs to identify specific tasks, activities, and behaviors of each job and their relative frequencies. Job analysis historically assumed jobs were stable and constant. Today, however, managers view jobs as more flexible and even adaptable to fit particular people and situations (Noe et al. 2015).

Managers and HR staff analyze jobs using several methods, including observation, written surveys, and interviews. This information is used to create **job descriptions** (also called **position descriptions**), which were explained in Chapter 4. HCOs use different formats for job descriptions, but all state the job title and work to be done based on job analysis. Most job descriptions also include the authority, reporting relationships, and minimum qualifications (e.g., knowledge, skills, competencies, licensures) to perform the job. More detailed job descriptions include the equipment and materials used, working conditions, usual work schedule, mental and physical demands, interactions with others, and salary range (Fallon and McConnell 2014).

Line managers, including lower-level beginning supervisors, work closely with HR staff and top managers to do job analysis. Accuracy matters because job analyses are used to guide other staffing processes and to manage employees. The seven staffing processes are interrelated. Managers use job analyses and descriptions to explain jobs to applicants, to decide which applicants could best perform jobs, to evaluate employees' job performance, to determine the pay for a job, and so forth. Incorrect or sloppy job analysis can lead to bad hiring choices, employee lawsuits, poor organizational performance, and an HCO's inability to achieve its goals. For example, in 2012 the Medicare program began reimbursing hospitals based partly on patient satisfaction. A related trend is patients' increased participation in their healthcare and engagement in the healthcare decision-making process. Given these developments, HCO managers have had to redesign jobs to achieve better customer satisfaction and to allow more patient participation in healthcare.

Job description (also position description) States the job title and work to be done; usually includes the authority, reporting relationships, and minimum qualifications to perform the job; may include the equipment and materials used, working conditions, work schedule, mental and physical demands, interactions with others, and salary range.

WORK RULES AND SCHEDULES

Besides job descriptions (written from job analyses), designing jobs and work involves creating work rules, schedules, and standards of behavior. Managers are responsible for this work, but sometimes workers participate in the process. Although many of us feel that rules are confining, most employees desire the structure, predictability, and civility in their work setting that rules can provide. Managers must balance the needs of the HCO with the needs of employees. For example, rules may limit socializing at work to ensure patient care is not delayed while employees discuss sports scores or weekend parties. Rules continually evolve to address new issues, such as limiting what employees may view online during work hours or tweet on Twitter after work. If two employees do not like each other, can one bully the other on Facebook? Managers may have to create work rules for such situations.

As a manager, you will have to ensure fair work schedules as part of job design. Scheduling can be challenging for any organization, especially for HCOs that operate around the clock. Is it Jose's turn to work weekends? Did Zainab work nights last month? Could Brittany work on New Year's Day? Managers must balance the needs of the HCO and patients with employees' schedules. Trends in scheduling now permit more flexibility to let employees arrive (and depart) at different times. Some staff members may work five eight-hour days per week, whereas others may work four ten-hour days. Some jobs allow telecommuting and working from home to increase the job satisfaction of workers with small children. Scheduling must consider full-time and part-time jobs and how they fit in a schedule. Complications arise when an employee is on vacation or out sick. Here, too, managers should work closely with the HR department to ensure their department schedules adhere to labor laws and are consistent with the HCO's overall staffing policies.

HIRING STAFF

After designing jobs and positions, managers hire people to fill them. Some HCOs refer to this function as *talent acquisition*. Perhaps you have been a job applicant and participated in this process. It includes

◆ recruiting applicants,

◆ selecting from among applicants,

◆ making a job offer, and

◆ sometimes reassigning a worker (e.g., promotion, transfer).

To begin recruitment, managers should ensure that a current, accurate job description is available to guide recruitment and later selection. Then, upper management must authorize filling a vacant position; authority for filling positions may be delegated to HR staff. Vacant positions are not always filled right away, and a decision must be made about each vacancy. For example, in 2009 the economic recession reduced demand for services, and fewer workers were needed in some HCOs. Some vacant positions were kept vacant. Later, when the economy improved and more customers demanded services, managers gave approval to hire workers for those vacant positions.

RECRUITING

Managers recruit applicants for each position. Can you suggest ways to recruit people? How did you find out about jobs you have applied for? **Internal recruitment** (inside the HCO) uses the HCO's bulletin boards, newsletters, and intranet; networking among staff; and managers' conversations with current employees about job openings. Managers also use **external recruitment** by going to job fairs and professional conferences; networking beyond the HCO; posting job openings on job search websites such as Monster and CareerBuilder; talking with representatives of schools and colleges; contacting former employees; and placing ads in newspapers, professional newsletters, and trade magazines. Social media—such as Facebook and LinkedIn—provide a newer way to "e-cruit" externally that can easily reach many potential applicants. Recruiting with social media creates a connection that goes beyond the one-way methods (Baldwin 2011). Employee-generated content helps employee recruitment (Miller and Tucker 2013). Many applicants respond well to recruiting via social media and mobile devices. Managers should be sure to use methods and sources that will reach people of diverse cultures. For example, an HCO could advertise jobs in media that appeal to diverse ethnic groups and state its support for workers of diverse cultures.

What are the pros and cons of internal and external recruiting? Take a minute to jot down some ideas, and then read Exhibit 7.2.

Here are several other ideas to keep in mind when recruiting:

◆ Offer incentives, such as sign-on bonuses to attract applicants or bonuses to your employees for referring an applicant.

◆ While recruiting, subtly sell the HCO as a place to work by honestly identifying things an applicant might appreciate.

◆ Focus the recruiting process on applicants. Design the application process from their perspective. Make it easy to apply for a job. Do not mislead applicants with exaggerated promises.

Internal recruitment
Seeking job applicants from inside the organization.

External recruitment
Seeking job applicants from outside the organization.

⊙ TRY IT, APPLY IT

Suppose you work at a hospital in a large urban area such as New York City, Houston, or Los Angeles. The lead cook is going to retire in three months, and a replacement must be hired. How could you recruit a culturally diverse pool of applicants for this job? Use what you have learned in this chapter to outline a recruitment plan.

Advantages of Recruiting Internally	Disadvantages of Recruiting Internally
Applicant already familiar with HCO and thus is more likely to fit in	Employee may apply for promotion and then be upset if not promoted
Applicant already known by the HCO	Employee may become the boss of former coworkers, which can create problems
Employees see opportunities to grow, which strengthens employee morale and retention	Fewer new ideas, methods, innovations brought into the HCO from outside; inbreeding
Inexpensive	Small pool of potential applicants
Helps retain good employees	Internal promotion creates a new vacancy
Fast	

Advantages of Recruiting Externally	Disadvantages of Recruiting Externally
New ideas, methods, innovations brought into the HCO	Can be expensive for some methods
Large pool of potential applicants	Time and effort required to onboard and acculturate new employee
Applicant comes without political baggage or problems with coworkers	Applicant not known by HCO, so more time and effort needed to select and hire
Creates awareness of the HCO	

SOURCES: Adapted from Fried and Gates (2008) and Noe et al. (2015).

SELECTING

Managers use a selection process to choose the person to whom they will offer the job. A hiring decision has big consequences for the HCO, so managers should invest time and effort to make the right choice. The manager of the department with the vacancy must work with HR staff and agree on a hiring process that complies with laws and the HCO's policies. The process varies depending on the organization and the job and is longer and more complex for higher-level jobs. The HR staff and manager responsible for the job must be involved in the process, and it has become common for a team to make the hiring decision (Fottler 2008b). This team might include future coworkers (of the person to be hired) from both inside and outside the department.

After the HCO receives applications, HR staff screens them using preset criteria to select applications for further consideration. Pop quiz: What did we already learn in this chapter that would provide useful standards to screen applications? You should have answered "job descriptions." Job descriptions indicate the basic qualifications, skills, and competencies applicants should have. They can be used to eliminate unqualified applicants and identify good applicants for further consideration. Managers, HR staff, or automated systems read each application (or resume) and compare it to the job description. Applicants who do not meet a basic requirement (e.g., having a nursing license) can be eliminated; their applications go in the C pile. Managers can keep these applications until the hiring process is complete and any follow-up inquiries by these applicants have been answered. From the applicants who do possess the required qualifications, managers select the applicants who (at least on paper or online) seem best for the job; their applications go in the A pile for immediate consideration. Other applications are set aside in a B pile as backups in case none of the A applicants are offered and accept the job. This is a general approach with many variations.

Next, depending on the job, selected applicants may be asked to perform tests. One-third of organizations in the United States test for personality traits—for example, conscientiousness (Noe et al. 2015). A hiring manager might also test applicants to measure and learn about their knowledge, aptitude, mental ability, and physical ability. Managers should use tests that are valid, reliable, and not culturally biased.

Managers then interview candidates—perhaps three to five—selected from the A list of top candidates (who also passed any necessary tests). If applicants live far away, a telephone interview may be done first. If that call goes well, an on-site, face-to-face interview, which is more expensive and time consuming, is arranged. Guidance from the HR staff is essential regarding questions that may (and may not) be asked during interviews. **Laws forbid most questions about applicants' race, religion, age, culture of origin, gender, marital status, family, health, disabilities, and personal lives;** the few exceptions must be narrowly and carefully worded (Fallon and McConnell 2014, 248–49). Interviewers may ask if someone is at least 18 years old, is a US citizen, or has an impairment or obligation that would prevent full performance of the job.

Interviews are essential for understanding applicants well enough to select the right one. HCOs often hire based on applicants' personality traits (e.g., cooperativeness, initiative) rather than only technical skills (e.g., calculating cash flow, writing software code) (Fottler 2008b). How well a new employee would fit in with the HCO's values and other workers is more important than it was in the past. Interviews (rather than applications and resumes) enable managers to judge personality traits and fit.

Managers in many HCOs use behavioral interviewing (also called competency-based interviewing) to predict how an applicant might fit in the organization and perform in a certain situation or role (Broscio 2013). This approach helps managers better understand who has a necessary competency. For example, during an interview, an HCO manager in Jackson, Mississippi, might say, "Craig, describe a situation in which you had to work on a team with people you did not know" or "Deb, please tell me about a time when you handled a complaint." The manager judges the applicant based on the applicant's reported behavior in the situations. Recall from earlier in this chapter that Medicare reimbursement is now linked to patient satisfaction. Managers could use behavioral interviewing to hire employees who interact well with patients!

Effective interviews take time and effort. The following tips can improve interviews and help managers make good choices (Fallon and McConnell 2014; French 2007; Noe et al. 2015):

◆ Decide who (e.g., the manager, coworkers in the department) will do the interview and if they will meet with the applicant together or separately.

◆ Prepare by reviewing a current job description, the applicant's file, and other information.

◆ Arrange a suitable time (without interruptions) and a comfortable place for everyone involved.

◆ Ensure the work site will leave a good impression on the applicant.

◆ Put the applicant at ease with initial chitchat for a minute or two.

◆ Ask questions that require more than a few words to answer.

◆ Ask questions that require answers that will reflect how well the applicant *could do* the job (is capable), *would do* the job (is willing), and *would fit in* at the HCO.

◆ Ask situational questions for which the applicant must explain how she would handle a situation (e.g., What would you do if you felt a coworker was posting confidential information on Facebook?).

◆ Allow time for the applicant to think before speaking, and wait for the applicant to answer.

◆ Listen closely for content and feeling; pay attention to the applicant's body language, voice, emotions, and responses.

◆ Be respectful, friendly, genuine, and professional toward the applicant.

◆ Ask questions related to how well an applicant could perform the job; avoid questions that are inappropriate, illegal, biased, or culturally insensitive.

◆ Gather information about the applicant's abilities, personality traits (e.g., dependability, initiative), and expectations.

◆ Softly sell the job and the HCO, but do not overdo it or misrepresent anything.

◆ Be sure the applicant understands the job, expectations, schedule, pay and benefits, and what it would be like to work at the HCO.

◆ Ask for and fully answer the applicant's questions.

◆ Avoid writing many notes during the interview, but do write detailed notes soon afterward.

As a manager, you might interview applicants whose native language and culture differ from yours. You might participate in selection decisions that consider culturally diverse applicants. Such situations require careful communication, sensitivity, and emotional intelligence. The preceding guidelines can help ensure a fair, useful interview. Chapter 15, on professionalism, gives more advice on how to handle potential language and cultural barriers when interviewing and selecting people for jobs.

After each interview, the manager should gather feedback from everyone who interacted with (or even observed) the interviewee. These people include HR staff, everyone who interviewed the applicant, and perhaps a receptionist who observed how the applicant behaved while waiting outside the manager's office.

Depending on the HCO's hiring process, the manager or a committee might make the final decision. Sometimes the final choice is easy and straightforward. Sometimes it is difficult; all candidates have strengths and weaknesses and perhaps no candidate stands out as the best. Some applicants might "look good on paper" but not in a live interview. Managers should openly involve others in making the final selection to obtain different perspectives.

If necessary, a second interview can be arranged to further evaluate an applicant. Although another interview will take more time, it can lead to better hiring decisions. Even when trying their best, managers might make a hiring decision they later regret, but they must strive to avoid poor decisions by being thorough. A bad choice will not only haunt the manager but also hurt the HCO. Chapter 13 offers good advice on making decisions. As we will see, some managers use intuition in making decisions—including hiring decisions—and to rethink a preliminary decision if it does not feel right the next day.

At some point during the selection process, managers or HR staff will perform reference checks to confirm some applicant information (e.g., the applicant's college degree) and try to obtain new information (e.g., the applicant's empathy toward patients). The timing of reference checks varies depending on the situation. Confirmation of a college degree may be done early in the process by contacting the applicant's college. Talking to an applicant's current boss by phone may be done after obtaining the applicant's permission. If the applicant does not want her boss to know she is looking for a new job, this reference check might be done after the job offer has been made subject to satisfactory reference checks.

While it seems like a good idea to check references (and most managers do), this step is not a strong predictor of how well someone will perform in a new job (Noe et al. 2015). Why is that? When asked to provide a list of references, applicants of course list people who will give favorable references. Also, references often are vague and rarely identify an applicant's weaknesses or past problems. Many HR policies do not allow much information for reference checks of former employees (other than dates of employment and job title) for fear of being sued by someone who does not get a job. Some organizations have a culture of silence and are reluctant to share negative information (Malvey, Fottler, and Sumner 2013, 225).

Because official references often are too vague or minimal to be useful, some employers look online and at social media to learn about applicants. This check might occur in the initial screening process to verify applicants' prior employment and to gather information that may help decide which applicants to interview. Later, an HR manager might informally contact an unofficial reference on LinkedIn whom the applicant and manager both know. The manager might obtain more information from that person than from an official reference. Members of a search committee might look at an applicant's information and photos on Facebook. Managers who want to hire people to provide compassionate, sensitive healthcare to sick people might decide not to hire someone because of information obtained from or seen on social media (Roberts and Roach 2009). This situation presents potential ethical and legal issues related to privacy, justice, and the employer's obligation to avoid hiring incompetent or dangerous workers who could abuse patients or employees (Slovensky and Ross 2012).

Once the manager or selection committee decides whom to hire, it must make a firm job offer with a starting date and salary. The offer may be made subject to background checks and tests, such as for criminal background or prior drug abuse. After a candidate accepts the job offer and clears all background verifications, the HR staff contacts other interviewed applicants to thank them for their interest and inform them someone else was chosen.

After working in a job, employees are sometimes promoted, transferred to other jobs, laid off, or discharged. The selection methods explained in this section may help a manager decide whether to promote or transfer an employee to an open position as part of internal recruiting, or whether an external applicant should be hired instead.

ONE MORE TIME

The management function of staffing involves obtaining and retaining employees (human resources) to do the work required to achieve the HCO's goals and mission. Healthcare is a service and thus depends on people. Staffing may be understood by studying seven interrelated processes, and this chapter presented three of them. First, managers plan for staff—forecasting the organization's future staffing requirements and deciding how to ensure the needed workers are available. Next, they design jobs and work—determining work tasks to be done by a job, along with working conditions, rules, schedules, supervision, and qualifications. Then managers hire staff—recruiting and selecting workers for jobs, which may include reassigning existing workers by promotion or transfer.

Managers must use careful, legal, and effective interviewing to select people who will fit in the organization and work well with others. HR staff and departments (or consultants) often assist managers with staffing. The HR staff is usually responsible for creating staffing programs, policies, procedures, methods, and tools that managers throughout the organization use to staff their individual departments. This approach helps create consistency and ensure fairness throughout the HCO. It also helps managers comply with the many laws, court decisions, and regulations that affect how managers staff their HCOs.

 FOR YOUR TOOLBOX

- Internal and external recruiting
- Job interview methods

FOR DISCUSSION

1. Briefly describe the seven processes that managers use to staff an HCO.

2. Which staffing processes do you think are most important? Why?

3. Discuss the purpose of a job description. What information is often included in a job description?

4. Discuss several methods that managers can use to recruit new employees for an HCO.

5. Discuss the advantages and disadvantages of internal and external recruiting for the following jobs at a large metropolitan hospital:
    - Plumber
    - Website manager
    - Chief financial officer
    - Nurse

6. Compare and contrast the information that may be obtained from a resume and the information from an interview. Which do you think is most important? Why?

7. Give examples of questions that are appropriate and not appropriate for a manager to ask an applicant during a job interview. Why are some questions inappropriate?

CASE STUDY QUESTIONS

These questions refer to the Integrative Case Studies at the back of this book.

1. Disparities in Care at Southern Regional Health System case: Suppose SRHS sets a goal of reducing disparities by 50 percent during the next three years. Using this chapter and the case information, what would you suggest that SRHS include in staff planning to achieve the goal? Consider new positions and new policies or programs.

2. Nowhere Job case: Write a job description for Jack's job. Use case information, and make inferences to further develop the job description.

3. I Can't Do It All case: Healthdyne had to recruit a new CEO to replace Ms. Huggins. Use Exhibit 7.2 to explain the pros and cons of Healthdyne recruiting internally and externally.

 TRY IT, APPLY IT

The recruitment plan you prepared (see the Try It, Apply It in the middle of this chapter) was a huge success. Many good applicants applied for the lead cook job, and three have been chosen for interviews. Use what you have learned in this chapter and think about who, where, when, and what for the three interviews. Write an interview plan stating, at a minimum, who will be involved, where and when interviews will be held, what will be done during interviews, and ten questions to ask. How would you ensure your questions are legal? How would you make the interview convenient and appealing for the applicants?

CHAPTER 8

STAFFING: RETAINING EMPLOYEES

A company is only as good as the people it keeps.

Mary Kay Ash, entrepreneur and businesswoman

LEARNING OBJECTIVES

Studying this chapter will help you to

➤ explain how managers train and develop staff;

➤ understand how managers appraise staff performance;

➤ describe how managers compensate staff;

➤ explain how managers protect staff; and

➤ describe how onboarding helps improve staff retention.

HERE'S WHAT HAPPENED

When implementing their new strategic goals, managers at Partners HealthCare performed the staffing function. This function enabled Partners to obtain new workers and retain existing ones. An essential part of staffing was to decide financial compensation for each position and employee. Compensation included base pay, incentives, and bonuses as well as benefits such as paid vacation days, health insurance, and retirement plan contributions. In making compensation decisions, managers had to figure out what compensation would be needed to obtain and then retain the people Partners wanted. Managers also had to understand and comply with dozens of laws regulating compensation and other aspects of employment. Another part of staffing was to decide how to evaluate staff job performance and how performance evaluations would affect future compensation. Partners HealthCare's strategic goals were going to require innovation and change, so managers also knew they would have to provide training to prepare employees for changes in their jobs. By doing all these tasks well, managers were able to achieve ambitious goals and the Partners HealthCare mission.

As we see in the opening Here's What Happened, staffing a healthcare organization (HCO) is complex and requires much thought by managers. It is another way managers make a difference and add value to their HCO. Chapter 7 identified seven staffing processes and explained in depth the first three, which are used to obtain staff. This chapter builds on that discussion and studies the other four staffing processes, which are used to retain workers: developing staff, appraising staff, compensating staff, and protecting staff. The processes overlap to some extent because they are interconnected and because some processes support both obtaining and retaining workers. This chapter concludes with the topic of onboarding, which combines several staffing processes to improve staff retention. If an HCO's managers perform these seven staffing processes well, employees will like working at the HCO. The staff will not wonder, "Should I stay or should I go?" (as the punk rock band The Clash sang in their hit song from the 1980s).

TRAINING AND DEVELOPING STAFF

In Chapter 7, we defined *training and developing staff* to mean enabling employees to acquire new knowledge, skills, attitudes, and behaviors for current and future jobs. Employees will need training to continually perform their jobs well; most employees will need it the day they begin work! Employees need training and development to motivate them, help them feel competent, enable them to succeed in their jobs, and give them opportunities to grow (Fallon and McConnell 2014). Can you see how training contributes to staff retention? Training also enables HCOs and their workers to adapt to changes in the external environment (e.g., the changes we saw in Chapter 1). If an HCO does not train workers for those changes, it will fall behind. Despite these reasons for training and development, some HCOs have cut training budgets and spend little time developing employees. Managers in HCOs should strive to avoid skimping on training—even when faced with financial difficulties.

We will next study orientation of newly hired employees to help them successfully begin working. Then we will consider how to train and develop all employees so they can improve their performance and prepare for growth and promotion.

ORIENTATION FOR NEW EMPLOYEES

After a manager hires a new employee to work in her department, she then must orient the new employee to the department and the HCO. **Orientation of new staff should focus on both the technical aspects of work (how to do the job well) and the social aspects of work (how to fit in and get along with coworkers).** The manager must orient new workers to help them succeed—which then helps the manager succeed. How the manager orients new staff varies among HCOs. Some orientation may start online after workers have accepted a job but before they begin their first day of work. Compared to big HCOs, smaller HCOs usually provide a shorter, more casual, and less organized orientation. New, start-up HCOs may not yet have a planned orientation, and new workers will become oriented day by day. In larger HCOs, orientation might be part of a comprehensive, year-long onboarding process (described at the end of this chapter). Top managers orient all new employees to the HCO. Middle- and lower-level managers orient their new employees to their specific work departments. They use media and materials that include videos, handbooks, manuals, meetings, and checklists.

Managers are likely to divide new-employee orientation into several sessions spread over several days (or weeks) so that new workers are not overloaded with information. For example, suppose Juan (the reimbursement manager at a healthcare system in Miami) hires Erin as a Medicare reimbursement specialist. Juan and the human resources (HR) department arrange for Erin to complete her payroll forms, enroll in the health insurance plan, and buy a company parking permit online, all before her first day of work. Juan then schedules time to orient Erin to the reimbursement department when she arrives for her first day at work. This departmental orientation includes

◆ a welcome to the healthcare system and the department;

◆ introductions to coworkers;

◆ a tour of the work area and department;

◆ specifics of the Medicare reimbursement specialist job—what, why, when, where, and how to do it the way Juan expects it to be done (which might differ from how Erin has done similar work elsewhere);

- information about work schedules, breaks, meals, and overtime;

- information about workstation, equipment, and supplies;

- explanation of essential policies, procedures, rules, and standards of behavior—especially those that pertain to the department (rather than to the entire healthcare system); and

- helpful, supportive answers to Erin's questions.

Juan and Erin then meet with Carla (an experienced reimbursement specialist), who will be Erin's mentor/buddy. Carla and Juan have already discussed this arrangement, and Carla has agreed to offer on-the-job guidance to Erin and help Erin socialize with others. Juan will talk with Erin at the end of her first day and during her first week to ensure she is starting well.

After orientation to the department, a new employee will be oriented to the organization. Whereas departmental orientation should be done the day an employee begins, organizational orientation can be done later. Organizational orientation includes new employees from all departments of the HCO—they will all attend organizational orientation that might take place once a month. Returning to the example in Miami, the healthcare system's top managers and HR staff welcome Erin and 16 other new employees from 9 different departments. They explain the healthcare system's

- history, mission, vision, values, and goals;

- organization chart and management team;

- essential policies, procedures, rules, and standards of behavior that pertain to all employees; and

- employee benefits that pertain to all workers.

After an hour of organizational orientation, new employees should be better informed, but often they are restless. Break time! Snacks are provided, and people chat informally. Then the orientation continues. After covering all topics, a top manager walks the new employees around the organization's campus to provide a guided tour and answer their questions along the way.

In the real world, managers sometimes struggle for weeks to keep a department going while a job is vacant. People work extra hours (or days) to cover the job's tasks until a new employee begins. When a new employee finally arrives, everyone wants her to jump right in and get to work! The manager should resist a quick "Here's what I want you to do" orientation. A new employee will have questions and feel anxious about a new job, new place, new people, and so forth. She will feel supported—or not—depending on how her first day goes. The first day, first week, and first month will greatly affect how well the new employee does her job and how she feels about her job and the organization. Without an adequate, supportive orientation, she may soon be wondering, "Should I stay or should I go?" If she goes, then the manager, department, and HCO have to redo the hiring process. As a manager, remember: **Employee orientation improves employee satisfaction—which then improves employee performance and retention.** For the employee, manager, department, and organization it's a win-win-win-win!

TRAINING

Although employees might have graduated with the latest knowledge and skills or might have years of experience, that knowledge will not be "best practice" forever. In fact, it can become outdated within months because of rapid changes in the external environment of HCOs. A manager must train and develop employees so that they can adapt to those changes. Recall from Chapter 7 that Medicare began reimbursing hospitals based (partly) on patients' satisfaction scores. Should hospitals give employees more training in how to satisfy patients? Sure, and many hospitals are doing that. New medical procedures, as well as use of social media and mobile apps, keep evolving. Employees must receive training and continuing education to stay current.

When you are a manager, you will have to ensure that your workers are trained for their jobs—the equipment, methods, processes, and so forth. Training specifically for your department may be handled by you, someone else in the department, or an expert from another department. You could train your staff how to perform certain procedures in your department. Experts from other departments—such as information technology or infection control—could provide training for their areas of expertise. Large HCOs are likely to have a department for education, training, and development. People in that department could help you plan and implement training workshops for your staff. Some organizations bring in consultants with specific expertise to train staff. One trend, for example, is for more healthcare—and more work in general—to be done in teams. Because many HCO workers are not adequately prepared to work in teams, HCOs are using consultants to conduct workshops on effective teamwork.

Training (a kind of education) is a complex subject, and many books are dedicated to it. Good training that has a lasting effect usually is not simple. Sometimes an HCO is in such a hurry to train staff that it does not take time to effectively train. When workers (with the hourly pay meter running) go to long training sessions that use ineffective methods, what is the result? Much time and money is spent for results that fade away, and workers end up doing things the old way.

How can managers prepare and provide effective training? They can use the training methods shown in Exhibit 8.1. These methods can improve training so that it has a lasting effect. (To really stick, training must be supported by other organizational factors, such as leadership and organization culture, that will be studied in later chapters of this book.)

Exhibit 8.1

Training Checklist:
What Managers
Should Do

✔ Determine what training is needed, based on surveys, employees' job performance appraisals, on-the-job safety reports, customer satisfaction data, employees' input, future goals, the changing external environment, job redesign, and other information.

✔ Clearly write the specific purpose, objectives, and desired outcomes for the training. As a result of the training, which new knowledge, skills, attitudes, and behaviors should employees have?

✔ Identify the individual workers who should be trained. Use employees' names—not just "everybody in Pediatrics" or "all second-shift workers." Names will be useful for planning the training, executing it, and following up afterward.

✔ Gain support for the training from supervisors whose staff will be involved (i.e., pulled from their jobs to attend training sessions). If these supervisors are not committed to the training, they may not let the staff go because of other priorities. The supervisors can help motivate their staff about the training so that employees understand why they need the training. After training, supervisors can support employees who try to apply the training to their jobs.

✔ Decide appropriate content, curriculum, learning methods, and desired outcomes for the people to be trained. Keep it simple, practical, and job related. Include plenty of hands-on application.

✔ Calculate a budget based on number of trainees, training time per person, supplies, materials, equipment, facility space, and other resources. Ensure sufficient funds and resources.

✔ Schedule training as conveniently as possible for the trainees. Find out which days and times would avoid disrupting their work and service to customers.

✔ Plan, prepare, and practice the training beforehand. Be sure the trainers can easily and smoothly deliver the training so that trainees do not lose interest while someone leaves to get supplies or the trainer struggles to explain a procedure.

✔ Ensure that trainees (employees) are ready to be trained. They need to feel motivated and capable ("OK, I can do this"). For some kinds of training, they may need basic skills before trying more advanced skills.

✔ After the training, evaluate all aspects of training and monitor (initially and later on) how well it achieved its purpose. Make notes on how to improve the training next time.

SOURCES: Information from Fallon and McConnell (2014), French (2007), and Noe et al. (2015).

There are many possible training methods and approaches (Noe et al. 2015). Some training is done alone with self-study modules and online apps, some is done one-on-one with a supervisor, and some is done in groups. Team members that work together should be trained together (if work schedules allow). Classroom teaching methods may be used along with hands-on learning (e.g., case studies, simulations, behavior modeling, role play) and feedback from trainers. Training can be done with teleconferencing, webcasting, and mobile apps. Job shadowing, apprenticeships, and mentoring are other useful methods. Managers may combine methods, such as individual online video tutorials followed by live hands-on practice and feedback from the manager.

Managers should also help their staff develop for career growth and promotions. This function goes beyond training for an existing job and develops workers for other jobs in the HCO. Educational programs for workers, which are longer and more comprehensive than short-term training sessions, can be planned by managers using the methods listed in Exhibit 8.1. Managers can also arrange for carefully chosen mentors to help workers grow and develop for higher-level jobs and promotions. Without development and career growth opportunities in an HCO, it will be hard to retain younger workers (Haeberle, Herzberg, and Hobbs 2009) and clinical professionals, such as physical therapists.

Often in HCOs, the "best" worker is promoted to supervisor when that position becomes vacant. If not given preparation for the job, a new supervisor is likely to make mistakes when supervising former coworkers. He might maintain peer-to-peer relationships rather than shift to superior–subordinate relationships. He might hesitate to delegate tasks to other workers and will instead try to do all the work to ensure tasks are done his way. A new supervisor might avoid giving necessary, critical feedback to her staff. Job development programs can help good workers prepare for a promotion to a supervisory or management job. For example, Main Line Health in Pennsylvania created a Peer to Boss class (White 2005). An interesting example of clinical job development is described in the next Here's What Happened.

HERE'S WHAT HAPPENED

Banner Health operates hospitals in seven states and strives to provide excellent patient care. To help ensure quality care, it set up a nurse training and development program with career growth opportunities. Banner Health organized five levels of clinical nurse jobs—from novice to expert. These positions enable nurses to grow in nursing work rather than move into management work (e.g., head nurse, nursing supervisor). Training and development comes from preceptors, clinical academies, certifications, and other methods. This example of staff development has helped employees grow in their careers and helped Banner Health achieve its mission of excellent patient care (Banner Health 2009).

As noted earlier, in the real world, employees and their managers sometimes resent having to participate in training. While they understand the value of training, they view it as less urgent than the daily workload in the department. Some managers may say staff is needed in the department to do "the real work" rather than sit in a half-day workshop. Training can create conflicts over priorities, and managers have to make choices among competing needs. Chapter 13 on making decisions and problem solving will help you learn how to make these choices.

APPRAISING PERFORMANCE

In Chapter 7, we defined *appraising performance* to mean evaluating the job performance of workers and discussing those evaluations with the workers. Managers might formally appraise each employee once a year. However, managers should often informally appraise and talk with employees about their performance throughout the year.

Top managers and HR staff usually design performance appraisal methods, schedules, and forms for the entire HCO. Supervisors and department managers use those methods and forms to appraise the workers for whom they are responsible. This process achieves several purposes (Fallon and McConnell 2014; Fried 2008):

- lets employees know what is expected and how well they are meeting expectations;

- guides and urges employees to improve their performance;

- plans future training and development programs for each worker and for the HCO as a whole;

- guides and supports managers' decisions about pay, promotion, transfer, discipline, and termination;

- enables discussion between manager and employee; and

- complies with accreditation and legal requirements.

Unfortunately, appraisals are not always done well (Fallon and McConnell 2014). In fact, they may be dreaded by both the appraiser (manager) and the appraisee (employee). Perhaps you have dreaded a performance appraisal at your job. What are the barriers to good appraisals? First, the appraisal process, forms, and methods must be designed well and based on clear, up-to-date job descriptions—which takes time. Even when processes and forms are done well, they are used by managers who are only human (Fried 2008). Managers may be (consciously or unconsciously) influenced by emotions, biases, favoritism, personalities, organizational politics, time pressures, and non-job factors (Noe et al. 2015). Managers might inflate or deflate an appraisal for reasons unrelated to performance, such as wanting to get along with everyone or wanting to treat everyone equally. Some people are uncomfortable judging or being judged by other people; that makes performance appraisals awkward and difficult. This discomfort may cause managers to avoid an appraisal or hurry through it in a superficial way. When not done well, an appraisal can create employee resentment and distrust, which makes the next appraisal even harder for both manager and employee. Fortunately, managers can avoid some of these problems by using the methods explained next.

Who provides input for an employee's appraisal? The manager always does. The employee can do a self-appraisal. Coworkers who interact with (and perhaps depend on) an employee may be invited to give input. **Today, many HCOs use a 360-degree evaluation in which selected workers above, below, and at the same level as the employee all provide input into that employee's appraisal.** Feedback and data from bosses, peers, subordinates, and team members reflect an employee's performance from multiple perspectives. Depending on the employee's interactions, input may also be obtained from nonemployees, such as patients, vendors, and people in other organizations. They provide input via several methods including checklists, questionnaires, and surveys that involve marking choices from among prepared statements and factors.

Some managers use a less focused approach and ask people to write essays or answer open-ended questions about an employee. In all cases, managers should plan ahead and give people several weeks to provide the information. The manager uses all the input to prepare a performance appraisal. Usually this information is recorded on the HCO's standard forms, although some HCOs are flexible about using other forms. A common approach in HCOs is to use forms with rating scales. These scales should measure how well a worker performs—what he actually does—in relation to his job description and job standards. Some scales measure employees' skills, knowledge, behaviors, or traits. A better approach is to measure employees' results. Here is a sample rating scale:

	(Low)				(High)
1. Rate the employee's results on the job.	1	2	3	4	5
2. Rate the employee's work quality.	1	2	3	4	5
3. Rate the employee's quantity of work.	1	2	3	4	5

Unfortunately, these scales leave room for manager opinion and bias. Thus, HCOs often use more specific rating forms that define what each number rating means. For example, a 1 might be defined as "results are often late and less than assigned." Yet, different managers still might interpret the rating scale differently. What does "often late" and "less than assigned" really mean? Managers should strive to use measureable standards and benchmarks for what ratings 1, 2, 3, 4, and 5 mean. Here are some examples:

✔ Number of patients treated per day

✔ Average cost of supplies per week

✔ Numerical patient satisfaction scores in Medicare's Hospital Consumer Assessment of Healthcare Providers and Systems (HCAHPS) surveys

Another useful approach is to design the rating scales with only three ratings to indicate that performance was below, met, or exceeded job standards (Fallon and McConnell 2014).

Rate the employee's quantity of work:

1 = performance was below standards

2 = performance met standards

3 = performance exceeded standards

For each numerical rating, the manager should give specific examples to support the rating, especially for a low rating that the employee may challenge. A manager could keep track of and then identify specific examples of late work, such as "the monthly budget analysis was late in April, June, July, and October during the past year."

After rating performance of each essential job expectation, a manager should then write about the worker's strengths and weaknesses and give recommendations for the coming year. This aspect of the appraisal takes careful thought and work because managers must pay attention to their employees throughout the year! The manager writes a performance appraisal to steer an employee's future efforts toward the HCO's future goals and strategies. The next appraisal should then consider how well the previous recommendations were achieved.

While the rating method is common, a manager can use other appraisal methods. She may apply the comparative approach to all employees (or groups of employees) and rank them from best to worst. Or, he may use the forced distribution method that assigns (distributes) all employees among categories such as the top 20 percent, middle 60 percent, and bottom 20 percent.

In the final part of performance appraisal, the manager must arrange and conduct a review meeting with the employee. This discussion may create anxiety for both of them, especially if performance was inadequate, they do not have a good working relationship, or the past review meeting was unpleasant. To make the review meeting effective, a manager can use the methods shown in Exhibit 8.2.

Think about all the work that is involved! A good appraisal takes a lot of time, thought, and effort—for every employee. Suppose Rebecca supervises seven employees

Exhibit 8.2
Performance
Appraisal Meeting
Checklist

✔ Ensure that top management supports the performance appraisal process. Give feedback to the employee during the year to continually guide performance as needed and to avoid (unpleasant) surprises at the review meeting.

✔ Allow one month of lead time to schedule the review meeting, gather information from multiple sources, review the job description, and write the appraisal.

✔ Give performance feedback and recommendations; reinforce good aspects of performance; be specific and objective.

✔ Collaboratively plan future goals and expected outcomes; discuss the future more than the past.

✔ Anticipate how the employee may react, then plan how to respond.

✔ Arrange the review meeting to take place in a comfortable, private place at a convenient, uninterrupted time.

✔ Lead a collaborative discussion that seems supportive rather than punitive; when the employee talks, listen for content and feeling.

✔ Focus on the employee's performance, behavior, and results (not personality).

✔ Document the appraisal review, sign it, and have the employee sign it.

✔ Give copies of the appraisal to the employee and HR department; keep a copy to use for periodic follow-up. The appraisal is confidential, so do not share it with other employees.

SOURCES: Information from Fallon and McConnell (2014), Fried (2008), and Noe et al. (2015).

at a medical company in Edmonton. She does the math and realizes she must set aside a lot of time to do seven performance appraisals well. Formal appraisals have tended to be an annual event, along with appraising new workers after a 90-day probation period. However, trends show that some managers do more frequent (though less comprehensive) appraisals on a real-time basis using performance management software and information technology (Biro 2013). Attentive and engaged managers also make rounds in their HCOs and their departments to informally assess workers and give them feedback throughout the year. Many workers like this more frequent feedback.

The appraisal methods listed in Exhibit 8.2 are useful for middle managers and supervisors who must evaluate their frontline workers. These methods can also be used by top managers to appraise middle managers and to some extent by a chief executive officer (CEO) to appraise other C-suite managers and executives. Appraisals of managers should be done as a narrative explaining how well the manager has fulfilled the position's responsibilities, accomplished preset goals, and achieved outcome targets (White and Griffith 2010). These factors pertain to finances, customer satisfaction, clinical outcomes, human resources, legal compliance, population health, and key organization-level outcomes under an executive's control. As much as possible, objective data—such as from a balanced scorecard—should be used to measure goal achievement and outcomes (White and Griffith

2010). If an executive has an employment contract with the HCO, the appraiser must consider and comply with it.

COMPENSATING STAFF

In Chapter 7, we defined *compensating staff* to mean determining and giving wages, salaries, incentives, and benefits to workers. Compensation includes cash compensation (e.g., wages, salaries, merit increases, bonuses, incentives) and benefits (e.g., paid vacation, health insurance, child care, retirement contribution) to workers (Noe et al. 2015). Partners HealthCare, for example, must compensate its many workers and also decide how to compensate people hired into new positions. Compensation strongly affects how well an HCO obtains and retains employees. In other words, it strongly affects an HCO's survival.

Besides receiving compensation as financial reward, employees may also receive nonfinancial rewards as part of a total rewards approach. Nonfinancial compensation includes

1. praise, recognition, and awards;

2. promotion and advancement; and

3. an organizational culture and policies that enable workers to balance work lives and personal lives (McSweeney-Feld and Rubin 2014).

Together, these nonfinancial rewards and financial rewards make up a total rewards approach to compensate employees for their work. This chapter focuses on financial compensation, while nonmonetary rewards are discussed in Chapters 7, 9, 10, and 11.

Compensation is complex for several reasons:

1. It is an important and sensitive matter for each employee. Today's management tip: Do not make a mistake with someone's paycheck!

2. Dozens of laws and court decisions affect how HCOs compensate workers.

3. When it comes to pay and benefits, one size does not fit all. Many compensation differences among employees in an HCO arise because of differences in the value of jobs, laws that regulate how workers must be compensated, individual human motivations, and other factors. Workers come from four unique generations that differ in what they value and want. Some employees do not want benefits and say, "Just give me cash!"

4. Differences in pay must occur, yet employees may question differences (real or perceived).

Top managers and HR staff develop their HCO's compensation system. In large HCOs, someone in the HR department will have compensation expertise to help managers. Some HCOs contract with compensation and benefit consultants to design effective, legal plans for compensation.

The compensation system includes pay scales and opportunities for additional pay through bonuses, incentives, overtime, and other means. The compensation system also includes employee benefits, which vary according to several factors including full-time or part-time status, salaried or nonsalaried status, and number of years worked at the HCO. Before developing the compensation details, top executives make broad decisions about how competitive their HCO will be in their labor market. Will it pay above-average, average, or below-average wages? How will the wages affect spending on other forms of compensation (e.g., employee benefits) and spending on other needs (e.g., medical equipment)? How will it affect staffing recruitment and retention?

Managers have important roles in compensating employees (Fallon and McConnell 2014). First, they must work with HR and payroll staff to apply the HCO's overall compensation program to their own department. For example, Nina, the director of business development at a health insurance company in Austin, decides merit pay or bonuses for her employees. Second, managers must be familiar with the compensation methods and benefits so they can answer questions from their employees. A worker may ask Nina how many vacation days he gets or when he is eligible for a pay increase. Nina should be able to answer these questions (perhaps after referring to HR manuals or records). Detailed questions may be referred to HR and payroll staff. Third, managers must be attentive to employees' complaints about pay and compensation and strive to resolve issues with help from HR staff and higher managers when necessary. Nina can give those managers feedback from her staff who feel the company should offer profit-sharing as a financial incentive.

HOW IS PAY DETERMINED?

Pay, wages, and salaries are the income employees earn. How much income does an employee earn? It depends on several factors, especially the worth of the job performed. Large HCOs may have hundreds of unique jobs. Managers assign each job a value to determine how much it is worth. In doing so, they must strive to ensure fair pay for each job in relation to all other jobs. This valuation is not easy, especially for an HCO with hundreds of jobs that competes with other HCOs for workers. When managers determine the worth of a job, they depend on accurate position descriptions to analyze jobs and assign points that determine pay levels.

A common approach to figuring job values is the **point-factor method** (Noe et al. 2015). This method assigns points to each job based on how it rates on a common set of factors. Thus, each job (e.g., strategic planner, medical utilization analyst, computer

Point-factor method
Assigns points to a job based on how that job rates on a common set of factors used to rate all jobs; points are used to determine pay for a job.

programmer, groundskeeper, sales representative, health educator) may be assigned points (e.g., 0 to 10) based on how it rates for the same factors (e.g., supervising others, difficulty of working conditions, independent judgment, responsibility, experience, particular skills) (Smith et al. 2008). For each job, points for each factor are summed to reflect the total value of that job. This calculation is done for all jobs. Then jobs are ranked or grouped based on their points. This method helps create **internal equity** so that jobs in the HCO are paid fairly relative to each other.

Dollar pay rates are set for each job based on (1) the points or values of each job; (2) what the HCO can afford; and (3) what seems to be the going rate in the community for key jobs, such as a computer programmer. The assigned pay rate for a job is a base rate. Let's consider the computer programmer job. Managers evaluate it and assign points for all factors. Here are examples for just three of those factors:

◆ Education = 45 points

◆ Difficulty of working conditions = 20 points

◆ Independent judgment = 50 points

Suppose the points for *all* factors equal 200. As a result of the points, the HCO's available funds, and local pay rates for programmers, the HCO's managers set the programmer's base pay at $42,000 per year. Each point is worth $210 pay. After the groundskeeper's job was assigned 90 total points, managers set its base pay at $18,900.

Sometimes compensation becomes more complicated. Suppose a manager later finds that the base pay rate is no longer high enough to obtain and retain workers because of higher base pay in the community. If the average local base pay for a programmer is now $45,000, the HCO may have to set its own base pay close to that amount (or else offer a much richer benefit package). Raising programmer pay to meet the prevailing pay in the community helps create **external equity** of the HCO's programmer's pay compared to programmers' pay outside of the HCO. However, this raise means the programmer job is paid more than the internal job point value ($210 per point). It upsets the internal equity of the programmer pay compared to pay for other jobs inside the HCO. Sometimes managers face a dilemma and will have to balance between internal and external equity.

After the *base pay for a job* is set, the *pay for a specific person in that job* might be increased because that person has extra education or years of experience beyond the minimum required. Suppose Samantha is a programmer with five more years of experience than the minimum required. Managers may decide to pay her $3000 more because of her extra years.

The base pay rate of all jobs in an HCO will usually increase each year. If funds are not available, base pay might have to be held constant. If an HCO is struggling financially, base pay might even be reduced. Managers make these compensation decisions each year. Sometimes they make further adjustments mid-year to adapt to internal and external changes.

Workers in lower-valued jobs receive hourly wages generally based on *how many hours they work* times their *hourly rate of pay*. Workers in higher-level jobs, such as managers and professional staff, receive a salary regardless of how many hours they work. Beyond their base pay, some workers may be eligible for additional pay such as

◆   individual incentive pay or team incentive pay;

◆   overtime pay for nonsalaried workers;

◆   pay-for-performance bonuses for reaching performance targets;

◆   extra pay for working second shift, third shift, weekends, and holidays; and

◆   profit sharing in for-profit HCOs.

HOW ARE BENEFITS DETERMINED?

Besides paying workers, managers must compensate them with benefits. Some benefits are required by law, such as the HCO contributing to employees' social security (for retirement) and workers' compensation (for on-the-job injuries). Other benefits are voluntary but are expected by most workers and thus essential for staffing an HCO. For example, workers expect health insurance and want to know how much is paid by the employer and how much by the employee, what the insurance will and will not cover, what restrictions exist, and so forth. There are dozens of possible benefits, and employees differ in which ones they prefer. Many younger employees want day care for children, whereas middle-aged workers want contributions to a retirement plan. Therapists like payment for continuing education, whereas housekeepers would rather have another paid day off. Thus, managers often create flexible cafeteria benefits plans, which allow each employee to choose from a variety of benefits up to a certain dollar value. Although this approach is harder to manage, it increases employees' satisfaction because they have more control and can pick benefits they really want.

 TRY IT, APPLY IT

Suppose you and one of your parents began working this year at a large for-profit medical supply business. The company offers a flexible cafeteria approach to employee benefits. List the top ten benefits you would choose. Then list the top ten benefits you think your parent would choose. How are the lists similar? Different? (Discuss this exercise with your parent if possible.)

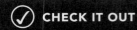

CHECK IT OUT

The US Department of Labor has much information about federal laws for pay and benefits. Its wages website (www.dol.gov/dol/topic/wages/index.htm) provides information for employees and employers. As a future employee and manager, you should be interested in both perspectives (employee and employer).

The value of employees' benefit packages often exceeds one-third of their base pay. **Employees usually underestimate the value of their benefits, so managers should periodically inform them and provide data showing the value of their benefits.** In addition, managers should be prepared to answer their employees' basic questions about benefits and can refer them to HR staff for more detailed or unusual questions.

As noted earlier, compensation is influenced by several factors. Laws, some of which were identified earlier, are important. To properly manage benefits and compensation, managers must obtain clear advice from experts, such as labor attorneys or compensation consultants. Managers may check the US Department of Labor website to learn more about these laws. Benefits (and all compensation) are affected by how much an HCO can afford, so managers must plan benefits with the HCO's overall strategic plan and financial plan in mind.

PROTECTING STAFF

Imagine how hard it would be for an HCO to achieve its mission and goals if employees stayed home because of on-the-job accidents, uncontrolled infections, job stress, low morale, an abusive coworker, or an uncaring supervisor. In Chapter 7, we defined *protecting staff* to mean ensuring that workers have proper work conditions and that their opinions are considered by managers. When staffing an HCO, a manager must protect staff, which is the last of the seven staffing processes. Similar to the other staffing processes, protecting staff helps an HCO maintain the workforce needed to achieve its mission and goals. The importance of this process is reflected in the shift toward protecting *employees* rather than *employers* (Fottler 2008b). Employee protection is good for several reasons. It is required by the Occupational Safety and Health Act and other laws, and it helps an HCO avoid being known as an unsafe place to work. In the long run, safety and health violations are costly because of lost business, lawsuits, overtime wages to cover absent staff, employee resignations, higher insurance costs for liability and employee health, and other reasons.

Managers must protect their employees against many potential dangers in HCOs. Pause and think of some of these dangers. There are physical hazards, such as radiation, biological waste, possible fires, infectious diseases, noise, dangerous equipment, repetitive motions, slippery floors, and workplace violence. There are mental and emotional hazards, such as stress, verbal abuse, privacy violation, burnout, and harassment (which can be based on race, gender, religion, age, disability, and other characteristics). When a manager helps protect her workers, she helps retain her workers.

Managers are responsible for safety in their own departments and work areas. They should frequently inspect work conditions; advocate for proper lighting, ventilation, and comfort; arrange repair of defective equipment; report workplace accidents and injuries; arrange training for workplace safety; orient employees to policies needed for safety and protection; and include safety as part of the annual performance appraisal. (Notice how the protection process ties in with other staffing processes.) Managers can protect employees by enforcing safety and health policies, procedures, standards, and rules. Managers should learn about their HCO's employee health services and employee assistance programs and then refer employees to them when needed.

Managers should also strive to protect employees' basic rights at work. Basic rights include speech, privacy, justice, nondiscrimination, and due process. While employees' rights are not absolute in the workplace, they are not absent either. **Managers (and employees) must strike a balance between the rights of employees and the rights of others, including patients, visitors, suppliers, and the HCO.**

Workers should be able to present problems and grievances about their rights, jobs, and work to managers and then receive managers' response to those concerns. How can managers enable this communication? **Managers and the HR staff should establish multiple ways that workers can be heard and can see their concerns addressed** (French 2007; Fallon and McConnell 2014), including

- policies supporting employees' rights;
- communication via open-door policies, suggestion boxes, and town hall meetings;
- formal written grievance procedures with prompt follow-up and resolution;
- top managers' visits to all departments, including on weekends and on second and third shifts at HCOs operating around the clock;
- a disciplinary review board by which an employee may seek a review of disciplinary action;
- HR staff who present employees' views and concerns at management staff meetings and help managers consider how their potential decisions would affect the workforce;
- HR staff who assist employees in voicing individual concerns to management;
- sensitivity to and respect for people of diverse cultures and backgrounds;

◆   an employee ombudsman;

◆   an employee advisory council that meets regularly with managers; and

◆   supervisors and managers who genuinely care about their workers and manage that way.

Labor union
An outside organization that represents specific groups of employees and negotiates on their behalf with managers for workers' schedules, work conditions, compensation, and terms of employment.

What happens when employees' rights and concerns are *not* presented to top managers or taken seriously? Employees might elect a **labor union** to represent them. A labor union is an outside organization that represents specific groups of employees and negotiates on their behalf with managers for compensation, schedules, work conditions, and terms of employment (French 2007). When employees feel mistreated by managers and think their rights are violated and their concerns are ignored, they may choose this route. A union enables workers to join together and gain power as a group to present their concerns to managers. Here too, relevant laws and court decisions apply. Some people think workers join unions to gain better compensation. That is only part of the story. Workers also join unions for protection against perceived unfairness, humiliation, harassment, anxiety, insecurity, dangers, and managers who do not seem to care.

Protection is especially important for a diverse workforce in which employees have beliefs, cultures, and behaviors that differ from those of the managers. Thus, managers must clearly set the policy and model the behavior to establish protection for culturally diverse workers. The methods described in this chapter, and in later chapters on leadership and communication, can help managers protect workers.

HERE'S WHAT HAPPENED

On May 19, 2010, a jury found that drug company Novartis had been violating labor laws since 2002 by discriminating against its female workers. Novartis had paid women less than men, promoted fewer women, and allowed a hostile workplace. The jury awarded $250 million in punitive damages against the company, after awarding $3.3 million in compensation to 12 women. The company admitted it might have been slow to investigate the women's complaints (Neumeister 2010).

Onboarding
The process of helping new hires adjust to social and performance aspects of their new jobs quickly and smoothly.

ONBOARDING

"**Onboarding** is the process of helping new hires adjust to social and performance aspects of their new jobs quickly and smoothly" (Bauer 2010, 1). Methods already discussed in this chapter are used to onboard staff, so a discussion of onboarding is a nice way to conclude this chapter. Recall what you learned earlier about orientation of new employees, mentoring, training, feedback and performance appraisals, HR support, and management support. Managers do all these tasks to onboard new employees.

To make onboarding effective, managers should do it proactively and systematically in a deliberate way. They should intentionally address four levels of onboarding (Bauer 2010, 2) from basic to complex:

1. *Compliance* is the most basic level and teaches employees basic rules and regulations.

2. *Clarification* ensures that employees understand their new job and all expectations.

3. *Culture* helps employees understand the history, mission, values, and expected behaviors (formal and informal) of the organization.

4. *Connection* helps employees develop their interpersonal relationships and information networks.

Notice that these four levels of onboarding, combined, help new employees adjust to their new job and organization so that they can perform their job well and fit in socially with coworkers. When done well, onboarding improves staffing outcomes: better employee satisfaction, better employee job performance, and better employee retention. Achieving that will surely help you feel good about your work and advance in your career!

ONE MORE TIME

Managers must staff their HCOs to perform the HCO's work and achieve its mission and goals. They must obtain and retain people to perform jobs. While managers are responsible for these tasks, HR specialists often assist in staffing the HCO. Four staffing processes were studied in this chapter: training and developing staff, appraising performance, compensating staff, and protecting staff.

Training and developing staff enables employees to acquire new knowledge, skills, attitudes, and behaviors for current and future jobs. All employees in a manager's department will need training at some time. To achieve lasting results, managers should follow a structured approach to training with appropriate learning methods.

Appraising performance evaluates the job performance of workers and discusses those evaluations with the workers. For this, a manager should obtain input from multiple sources by using valid reliable questionnaires, checklists, interviews, and other sources of information. The appraisal must be discussed with the employee to share results and plan future goals. This discussion should focus on performance (not personality) and on future performance (more than past performance). Managers and employees may feel uncomfortable about appraisals, so managers should prepare properly to make them more effective.

Compensating staff determines and gives wages, salaries, incentives, and benefits to workers. Managers decide compensation, and payroll and HR staff help managers administer pay and benefits. Pay is largely based on the value of a job, which may be judged using the point-factor method. Many HCOs offer flexible benefit plans so that individual employees may choose preferred benefits up to a preset dollar value. Managers and staff must carefully decide pay and benefits to achieve internal and external equity.

Protecting staff ensures that workers have proper work conditions and that their opinions are considered by managers. Workers should have fair and safe work conditions, and their rights should be protected. Without that, and without all the other staffing processes, managers will be unable to obtain and then retain the different kinds of workers that an HCO needs.

Onboarding combines many elements of training, appraising, and protecting workers to improve their satisfaction, performance, and retention. Other factors also affect retention, such as organization structure, which we studied in prior chapters. Leadership also affects staff retention—that is the focus of the next three chapters.

(T) FOR YOUR TOOLBOX

- Training checklist
- Performance rating scales
- Performance appraisal meeting checklist
- Point-factor method
- Methods to hear employees' concerns

FOR DISCUSSION

1. Discuss reasons that employees' training might not have lasting effects. How can managers ensure that training lasts?

2. Using Exhibit 8.2, describe how a manager can effectively and fairly evaluate employees.

3. Explain the pros and cons of 360-degree appraisals of employees.

4. Discuss how managers can determine pay for a job.

5. Compare internal versus external equity in determining compensation.

6. Why might a cafeteria benefit plan be useful for workers whose ages range from 18 to 65?

7. Discuss some of the rights employees have at work. What can managers do to ensure that employees' rights are not ignored?

CASE STUDY QUESTIONS

These questions refer to the Integrative Case Studies at the back of this book.

1. Nowhere Job case: Suppose the point-factor method will be used to determine Jack's base pay. List the factors you would use to rate his job and assign points to it. Besides base pay, which other kinds of pay mentioned in this chapter would you offer to Jack?

2. I Can't Do It All case: Explain how Mr. Brice could use the training, performance appraisal, and compensation processes to help his subordinates make decisions.

3. Ergonomics in Practice case: Explain how Riverlea Rehab's administrators could use the four staffing processes discussed in this chapter to reduce staff injuries.

4. Taking Care of Business at Graceland Memorial Hospital case: Explain how Graceland Memorial Hospital's administrators could use the four staffing processes in this chapter to prevent staff injuries.

→ TRY IT, APPLY IT

Suppose you are an administrative intern in a personal care home. Many of these facilities have excessive turnover of nurse aides, who have minimal education and perform low-skilled tasks. Personal care home administrators often struggle with continual rehiring as aides resign or are discharged—often after working for less than a year. You must help develop a retention plan to reduce turnover of nurse aides. Use what you learned in this chapter to identify possible staffing-related causes of turnover, and then write recommendations to reduce turnover. Justify your approach. Discuss your ideas with classmates.

CHAPTER 9

LEADING: THEORIES AND MODELS

"Born to Lead or Learned to Lead . . . The Leadership of Bruce Springsteen"

Title of academic paper by Dr. Steven Ronik, CEO,
Henderson Mental Health Center, Fort Lauderdale, Florida

LEARNING OBJECTIVES

Studying this chapter will help you to

➤ define leadership and explain its relation to management;

➤ explain how leadership is related to planning, organizing, and staffing;

➤ identify, compare, and contrast leadership theories; and

➤ describe methods for leading physicians in professional bureaucracies.

HERE'S WHAT HAPPENED

The Partners HealthCare board of directors hired a chief executive officer (CEO) to lead the organization. The board looked for someone with the necessary leadership traits, skills, and behaviors. The CEO then led thousands of employees to achieve the organization's vision and mission. Yet he was not the only manager who led. People in other top management jobs, such as executive vice president and chief information officer, also were leaders who used leadership traits, skills, and behaviors to lead employees. So, too, did managers in middle and lower levels of the organization who led their own departments and workers. Throughout the organization—at all levels—managers led. They influenced people to accomplish work, tasks, projects, goals, mission, and vision. For example, implementation of one goal required staff to use telehealth technology to monitor discharged hospital patients at home. Telehealth would help patients stay healthy and not have to be readmitted to the hospital. But some nurses resisted the "high-tech" approach because they favored their "high-touch" approach to patient care. Managers used appropriate leadership to influence the nurses, overcome resistance, and gain support for the telehealth approach.

The opening Here's What Happened presents leadership in a healthcare organization (HCO). You know there are leaders at the top of an HCO, such as the Partners HealthCare CEO. But did you also know there are leaders in middle and lower levels of an HCO? As we learned in Chapter 2, this book views leading as one of the five main management functions; leading is something that managers at all levels of the organization do. We can even think of nonmanagers as leaders. For example, a consultant who chairs the consulting firm's employee suggestion committee leads seven committee members through consideration of five new suggestions. An occupational therapist leads a nervous client in trying adaptive equipment after an accident. A health administration student leads her team of students to complete a group project.

This chapter is the first of three chapters on leading. It focuses on leading as part of management. Leadership is defined and related to other management functions. We examine several perspectives of leadership—trait theory; skill theory; behavior theory; contingencies; and theories X, Y, and Z—plus the transactional, transformational, servant, and collaborative approaches to leadership. Each perspective should deepen our understanding of what leadership is and how it is done. Because we are studying leadership in HCOs, this chapter also teaches how leading physicians is different from leading many other types of workers. In Chapter 10, we will study how to motivate and influence people, which is a big part of leadership. Then, in Chapter 11, we will examine organizational culture and ethics that are essential for effective leadership.

How does leading connect to what we have already learned in this book? To sum up the book so far in 50 words or less: **First, managers *plan* the HCO's mission and goals.**

Second, they *organize* the HCO's tasks, jobs, and resources to achieve the plans. Third, they *staff* the HCO with people to do the jobs to achieve the plans. Fourth, they *lead* the people who do the jobs to achieve the plans. We see how the fourth management function—leading—connects to three other management functions. (Stay tuned, because in Chapter 12 we will get to the fifth and final management function.)

What Is Leadership?

What do you think of when you read the word *leader* or *leadership*? Perhaps you think of people who are considered leaders. Maybe you think of a time when you were a leader. We can assume that leaders and leadership have been around for as long as people have been around. Aristotle and Confucius wrote about leadership, and scholars have studied it for centuries. So what is it?

Well, for one thing, it is hard to define! If we look at definitions, we often see several concepts, such as influencing and motivating people and followers as well as setting direction and goals. "Leadership is among the most valued management abilities," according to Dennis Pointer (2006, 128), who then defines it: "Leadership is a process through which an individual attempts to intentionally influence human systems in order to accomplish a goal." We can slightly modify this definition and say that leadership is a process through which an individual attempts to intentionally influence *people* to accomplish a goal. Pointer dissects his definition to identify the main points:

◆ Leadership is a process, not a one-time event.

◆ Only individuals (not organizations) lead.

◆ Leadership is intentional, not accidental.

◆ Leadership is influencing.

◆ The focus of leadership is other people—the followers.

◆ The purpose of leadership is goal accomplishment.

Recall from Chapter 2 the definition of *management*: the process of getting things done through and with people. Leading people is part of the process by which managers get things done through and with people. Also recall from Chapter 2 the ten roles performed by managers (Mintzberg 1990). One of the roles is the role of leader, in which the manager creates a vision and motivates others to work toward it. Being a leader is part of being a manager. **Leadership is not the same as management, nor is it separate from management. Rather, it is part of management.** All managers lead—that is the view taken in this book.

However, there are other points of view. Writers, managers, and leaders have long debated what leadership and management mean, how they are related, and who does them (Ledlow and Coppola 2009). To further complicate things, these words may be used differently in everyday language than in professional and scholarly books. This book's definition of leadership, and its relation to management, is consistent with those of writers cited earlier and with others cited later. (However, we will not stay up all night debating definitions with someone who has a different view.)

This book defines **leadership** as a process through which an individual attempts to intentionally influence people to accomplish a goal. This definition implies that leadership can occur at all levels of an organization—and in fact it must for complete success. Leadership is not done only by people at the top. **For an HCO to succeed, leadership must be done by people at all levels of the HCO.** A top manager in an HCO leads (influences) the HCO's workers to accomplish the HCO's goals. A middle-level department manager leads (influences) the department's workers to accomplish the department's goals. A lower-level office manager leads (influences) the office's workers to accomplish the office's goals. Although not all health administration students will become CEOs in HCOs, many will become leaders at multiple levels throughout HCOs (Glandon 2014).

Glenn Bodinson, a quality consultant, has worked with more than 300 organizations (including HCOs) and helped some of them earn the prestigious Malcolm Baldrige National Quality Award. For an HCO to become great, Bodinson believes that leaders are needed at all levels throughout an organization. This idea is reflected in statements from his leadership assessment tool (Bodinson 2005, 25):

◆ "Leaders at all levels are accessible to patients, physicians, and staff, building relationships that foster trust, confidence, and loyalty."

◆ "Leaders at all levels have the necessary leadership skills and technical knowledge to achieve our organization's top goals."

> *Leadership*
> A process through which an individual attempts to intentionally influence people to accomplish a goal.

LEADERSHIP THEORIES AND MODELS

Scholars have developed theories of leadership over many years of study. These theories help us to better understand, explain, and predict leadership and leaders. No single theory fully explains all aspects of leadership or all success factors in leaders. Consider some leaders throughout world history, such as Alexander the Great, Abraham Lincoln, Indira Gandhi, Martin Luther King Jr., Queen Elizabeth I, and Nelson Mandela. It would be difficult to fully explain these leaders and their leadership success using only one theoretical perspective. By using several theories, we can more fully understand these leaders and what enabled them to succeed.

 CHECK IT OUT

Many ideas exist about what leadership is. Try Googling "leadership definition" and you'll get more than 86,000,000 results! You can find leadership definitions from leaders, famous people, and scholars.

Perhaps you have heard someone say, "He is a born leader!" Are people really *born* leaders? Or do they *learn* to lead? Or maybe both? These questions are reflected in the quote about Bruce Springsteen at the beginning of the chapter. He suffered a difficult childhood and in his youth became "a loner and something of a social leper" (Alterman 2001, 10). Yet, during his career of more than 40 years as a songwriter and musician, he grew into a charismatic leader. His lyrical songs and stories about people, their relationships, their emotions, and their ups and downs in life—and his legendary high-energy concerts—have led, influenced, motivated, and inspired millions of people worldwide. The good news for students is that leadership can be developed during one's career. You do not have to be "born to lead." You can learn to lead! "Effective leadership can be learned," according to Carson F. Dye (2010, xii), who has spent decades in healthcare, human resources, leadership development, leadership education, and executive search consulting. Today, many college academic programs and professional organizations (e.g., the American College of Healthcare Executives and the Healthcare Leadership Alliance) are helping people to learn and develop their leadership.

TRAIT THEORY

Trait theory of leadership examines traits and characteristics of leaders and how they contribute to leadership effectiveness. Think about some good leaders you know from a job, club, sports team, or other activities. Which personal traits do you think enabled these leaders to succeed?

According to Gerald R. Ledlow and M. Nicholas Coppola (2009), early studies of effective leadership suggested that it was associated with traits such as intelligence, extroversion, confidence, and initiative. Later research found effective leaders (as compared to ineffective leaders and to followers) were more likely to be ambitious, adaptable, persistent, cooperative, assertive, decisive, energetic, social, and responsible. These ideas generally make sense; an effective leader—for example, in a health insurance company—would likely have some of these traits. Perhaps you can think of leaders who have these traits. However, we should not assume that all effective leaders would have all these traits.

Some of these traits (e.g., Justine is decisive) can also be viewed from a skills perspective (e.g., Justine has good decision-making skills). Thus, the skill theory emerged.

SKILL THEORY

The **skill theory** of leadership examines skills and abilities of leaders and how they influence leadership effectiveness. Take a minute to brainstorm skills you think leaders would need to succeed. Write down at least five leadership skills.

Some writers emphasize that leadership effectiveness depends on three core skills or broad skill categories (Pointer 2006). These skills were first found in research by Robert Katz (1955) and are still useful today:

1. Technical skills for working with things (e.g., making health products and services)

2. Conceptual skills for working with ideas (e.g., thinking of new goals)

3. Human skills for working with people (e.g., coaching employees).

The skills leaders need can generally be grouped into these three skills categories.

Do some leaders rely on one kind of skill more than another? Leading in high-level management positions requires conceptual skills more than technical skills (Katz 1955; Pointer 2006). The opposite is true for leaders in low-level positions. For leading in mid-level management jobs, both technical and conceptual skills are moderately important. Human skills are important for leaders at all levels of management.

In the Partners HealthCare case, conceptual skills would be especially important for the new CEO to conceive mission, vision, values, and long-range goals for the system. Technical hands-on skills are especially important for lower-level leaders, such as a pharmacy shift supervisor, to ensure that technical tasks are properly done. Leaders lead people, so human skills would be important for leaders throughout Partners.

BEHAVIOR THEORY

Researchers also looked beyond traits and skills to behaviors, actions, and conduct. The **behavior theory** examines leadership behavior (sometimes called *leadership styles*) and how it influences leadership effectiveness. Rather than study the traits and skills a leader *has*, this theory looks at what a leader *does*—how she behaves or how he conducts himself. When you are a leader in healthcare, which behaviors will you use? How will you conduct yourself? Suppose you are a mid-level manager at an information technology (IT) company in Jacksonville, Florida, that provides IT support to medical businesses. Your management team decides it must relocate to a bigger office building. Which behaviors would you use to lead (influence) your employees to support relocation?

The Ohio State University's leadership studies directed by Ralph Stogdill in 1947 helped develop behavior theory. This research examined two dimensions of leader behavior (Ledlow and Coppola 2009):

1. *Consideration:* The leader considers followers (workers) and their concerns.

2. *Initiating structure:* The leader initiates action, work, and tasks to complete jobs and achieve goals.

Leaders were rated as "high" or "low" in each of these dimensions, which created four types of leaders:

Behavior theory
Leadership theory that considers what a leader actually does and how a leader behaves.

◆   Low initiating structure / Low consideration

◆   Low initiating structure / High consideration

◆   High initiating structure / Low consideration

◆   High initiating structure / High consideration

Behavior theory was further developed by Rensis Likert (1961) at the University of Michigan. Leaders were rated low or high on *job-centered behavior (behavior that was concerned about work, jobs, goals)*. They were also rated low or high on *employee-centered behavior (behavior that was concerned about employees)*. Again, four leadership styles emerged based on low or high ratings for the two kinds of behavior. This kind of research was done by other scholars in the 1950s and 1960s to further investigate which leadership behaviors led to the best employee satisfaction, job performance, goal achievement, and other outcomes (Pointer 2006).

Pop quiz: In the leadership behavior studies discussed, which leadership style do you think was most effective?

a.   Low initiating structure / Low consideration

b.   Low initiating structure / High consideration

c.   High initiating structure / Low consideration

d.   High initiating structure / High consideration

e.   It depends.

Hmmm, seems like *High initiating structure / High consideration* would be a good answer. But try again. In Chapter 2, we learned contingency theory. So maybe the answer is *It depends*. Yes, that is correct!

The best leadership style depends on the situation. *High initiating structure / High consideration* is not always a good approach. Research has shown that a leader who initiated structure (i.e., initiated action to complete jobs and goals) when structure was already sufficient *decreased* employee satisfaction. In that situation, it would have been better to use a low initiating style. The bottom line is: "It was more important for a leader to strike a balance between what is appropriate for the situation rather than consistently displaying high consideration and high structure at all times" (Ledlow and Coppola 2009, 175).

Managers today often use a managerial grid that is based on leadership behavior theory and research (Blake and Mouton 1964). Like the prior studies, this grid uses two dimensions: *production orientation* and *people orientation*. Leaders were rated from 1 (low) to 9 (high) for each dimension. These orientations (leadership styles) are shown in Exhibit 9.1.

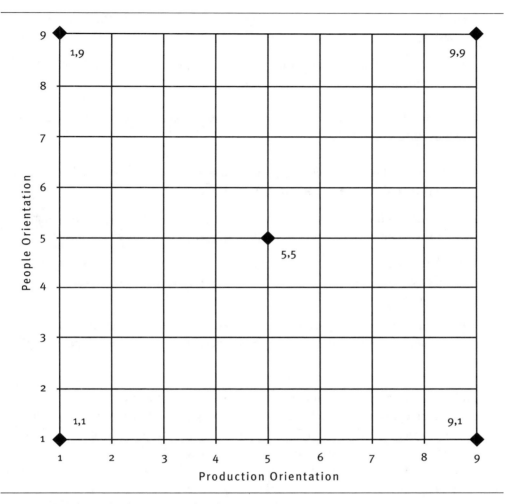

SOURCE: Adapted from Blake and Mouton (1964).

EXHIBIT 9.1
The Managerial Grid

The researchers who developed the managerial grid conceived the same four leadership styles as the Ohio and Michigan studies and added a fifth style in the middle:

◆ Low production orientation / Low people orientation (1,1): Impoverished style

◆ Low production orientation / High people orientation (1,9): Country club style

◆ High production orientation / Low people orientation (9,1): Authoritarian style

◆ High production orientation / High people orientation (9,9): Team leader style

◆ Middle production orientation / Middle people orientation (5,5): Middle-of-the-road style

Leaders who use one of the four corner styles in Exhibit 9.1 would lead as follows (Esparza and Rubino 2014, 10).

◆ Impoverished style: detached, uncommitted to work or workers, let workers do whatever, "delegate and disappear"

◆ Country club style: use rewards and recognition to encourage workers, avoid authority and discipline, maintain positive relationships with workers

◆ Authoritarian style: tough on workers, expects workers to get work done no matter what, not interested in workers' input, doesn't want dissent, expects loyalty

◆ Team leader style: leads by example, helps workers achieve their highest potential, promotes goal achievement, develops close relationships among workers

The middle-of-the-road style is in between these styles—a little of each.

The managerial grid model was developed long ago, and managers today still use it to guide organization leaders' behavior. Many managers seem to like it and think it works well. The team leader style is often best. However, leaders should not assume it is always best. Pointer (2006) notes that little research supports the belief that a team leader style (high production / high people style) is best regardless of the situation. As the Ohio State studies found, no single style always leads to the best productivity and satisfaction results. Apparently, something else affects the results. What could it be? Read on.

CONTINGENCIES

By the early 1960s, scholars and leaders realized that the trait, skill, and behavior theories of leadership did not fully explain leadership effectiveness. Furthermore, they realized there was no universal best way to lead. Organizations and people are too complicated for that.

The best leadership approach seemed to vary from situation to situation and from person to person. The best approach was **contingent**, which meant that it depended on something. Further studies and theorizing led to deeper understanding of how effective leadership depended on three contingencies (Deckard 2011b; Pointer 2006):

Contingent
Dependent on something.

1. Characteristics of the leader (e.g., skills, traits, behaviors)

2. Characteristics of the followers (e.g., skills, traits, behaviors, relationship with leader)

3. Characteristics of the situation (e.g., clarity of goals, urgency, work to be done)

When leading employees who are assertive self-starters in a medical research institute, a hands-on, task-oriented leadership style might stifle and annoy the employees. With those people, the leader should back off and try a looser style with less day-to-day oversight of tasks and production. As another example, consider an extroverted leader in a health insurance company who likes to chitchat with subordinates. Sounds like a good idea; after all, leaders should get to know their followers. However, such a style might not work equally well with all employees. Why? Because the best style is contingent on characteristics of the followers. An extroverted style would likely work well with extroverted followers. It would not work as well with introverted followers; with them, the leader should adjust to a less chatty style.

How about a contingency example based on the situation? A personal care home leader might prefer to have long group discussions to lead staff to collaboratively make team decisions. However, if the building is on fire and the fire alarm goes off, the leader will quickly assess the urgency of the situation and use a more direct, take-charge style.

A manager must develop a mix of leadership styles (e.g., those in the managerial grid) and then figure out when to use which style. This skill cannot be developed in a semester of study or a year of work. Experience and trial-and-error are necessary. Everyone makes mistakes, and we can learn from them. Good role models and mentors can help too, so choose role models and find mentors to help you develop your leadership styles. Developing your emotional intelligence and your cultural competency can also help—we will learn about these in Chapter 15 on managing with professionalism. Besides developing a mix of leadership styles, you will also develop the ability to assess yourself, your followers, and situations. Based on those assessments, you can decide which style to use in leadership situations. Returning to the managerial grid, perhaps leaders like this tool because it helps them stop and deliberately ask themselves: For the leadership situation I now face, where should I be on the grid? How much should I use a people orientation and how much should I use a production orientation?

 CHECK IT OUT

Employers sometimes use personality tests to learn more about their employees. One commonly used assessment is the DiSC, which measures a person's levels of dominance, influence, steadiness, and conscientiousness. Another popular test is the Myers-Briggs Type Indicator, which measures attitudes, functions, and lifestyles. You can learn more at www.discprofile.com and www.myersbriggs.org.

THEORY X, THEORY Y, AND THEORY Z

Research in the 1960s led to the belief that leaders hold one of two different views of people and workers. These two views came to be known as **Theory X** and **Theory Y** (McGregor 1960; Borkowski 2011; Ledlow and Coppola 2009).

Theory X assumes people	Theory Y assumes people
◆ dislike work,	◆ like meaningful work,
◆ are lazy and stupid,	◆ are creative and capable,
◆ are motivated extrinsically (by rewards from other people),	◆ are motivated intrinsically (by rewards from within themselves),
◆ lack self-discipline and must be directed,	◆ have self-control and can direct themselves,
◆ want security, and	◆ want to contribute and participate, and
◆ do not want responsibility.	◆ want responsibility.

These two views are important for contingencies and leadership. A city health department's manager (leader) who views the world from a Theory X perspective would lead employees (followers) with an autocratic style of close oversight, distrust, coercion, monetary rewards, minimal communication, and solo decision making. In the same health department (situation) with the same employees (followers), a manager (leader) with a Theory Y perspective would lead with a participative style of trust, open communication, shared decisions, freedom, self-direction, and personal development rewards. The leadership style depends on the leaders' different views: Theory X or Theory Y.

In the 1970s, **Theory Z** emerged. This approach emphasizes concern for workers and strives to develop long-term cooperative relationships among workers, peers, and the organization (Ouchi 1981; Dunn 2010). Growth opportunities for workers are important but are developed more slowly and deeply in Theory Z than in Theory Y. Individual responsibility is important, and so is collective responsibility for coworkers and the organization. Theory Z seeks lasting employment and relationships with workers, discouraging the short-term job hopping common among some workers and in some organizations. Thus, Theory Z could help in HCOs where employee turnover is a costly problem, as explained in Chapters 7 and 8.

TRANSACTIONAL AND TRANSFORMATIONAL LEADERSHIP

Leadership has often been viewed from a transactional perspective, in which the leader transacts a deal with the followers: You perform tasks to help achieve the organization's

Theory X
Leader assumes people dislike work, are lazy and stupid, are motivated by rewards from others, lack self-discipline, want security, and do not want responsibility.

Theory Y
Leader assumes people like meaningful work, are creative and capable, are motivated by rewards from within oneself, have self-control, can direct themselves, and want responsibility.

Theory Z
Leader emphasizes concern for workers, develops long-term cooperative relationships, gradually provides growth opportunities for workers, and promotes individual and collective responsibility.

goals, and I will reward you with pay, benefits, and other rewards. That's the deal, and it can be a win–win situation for everyone. But the deal tends to maintain the rules and the status quo. Many organizations have **transactional leadership**, and followers go along with it.

An alternative is the **transformational leadership** approach (Burns 1978). Leaders who use this approach do not focus on transacting deals with followers (employees). Instead, they strive to do the following (Deckard 2011a):

◆ Inspire others by appealing to higher-level human needs of self-actualization and fulfillment, rather than lower-level basic survival and economic needs

◆ Appeal to the greater good for everyone, so people think less about "what's in it for me?"

◆ Challenge how things are done, and innovate with new ideas

◆ Revitalize the organization with change—sometimes radical change

Transformational leaders transform work and the workplace so that employees become excited about their work (Elkins, Melton, and Hall 2014). These leaders are guided by their organization's mission and values, and they communicate those often to workers. The leaders know their employees, interact with them in the employees' work setting, and look for ways to enable them to become more self-fulfilled and satisfied. With so much support from leaders, the workers develop loyalty and respect for the transformational leaders and organization. Workers want to help their organization succeed. They feel they are contributing to something important! All of this motivates employees to work hard for the organization's mission and values, which in turn leads them to feel more fulfilled.

Earlier, we learned about the trait, skill, and behavior theories of leadership. Which traits, skills, and behaviors do you think are needed for transformational leadership? What would it take to inspire others, challenge the status quo, and create radical change? Take a few minutes to brainstorm and jot down your ideas. Perhaps you thought of characteristics such as being flexible, creative, open minded, and trusting—all good ideas. Here are more characteristics that transformational leaders possess (Deckard 2011a):

◆ *Charisma:* provides a vision and purpose, develops pride, and earns respect and trust

◆ *Inspiration:* clearly and simply communicates purpose and expectations and focuses efforts

◆ *Intelligence:* promotes rational thinking, careful problem solving, and use of intellect

◆ *Individual consideration:* coaches, advises, and gives personal attention to each employee

Transactional leadership
Leadership based on transactions in which workers perform tasks to achieve goals and then the leader gives workers pay and other rewards.

Transformational leadership
Leadership based on inspiration, the greater good for everyone, people's need for fulfillment, innovation, and revitalizing the organization with change.

Transformational leadership has the potential to help each employee and an entire HCO grow and achieve great performance (rather than merely good performance). But it does not happen easily and takes much hard work.

A leader is not all transactional or all transformational. Each leader is likely to have some elements of each style. However, some leaders may be mostly transactional whereas others may be mostly transformational.

SERVANT LEADERSHIP

Servant leadership
Leadership that emphasizes that a leader should serve the followers by listening, mentoring, teaching, and helping.

A leadership style with some similarity to transformational leadership is the **servant leadership** approach (Dye 2010). This approach emerged in the 1970s and is similar to transformational leadership because they both are concerned with followers. However, the servant leadership approach emphasizes that a leader should serve the followers (not just be concerned about them). A servant leader unselfishly listens, mentors, teaches, helps, and has an interest in people. The servant leader serves followers by providing them with necessary resources, meeting their needs, understanding and respecting their views, and helping them grow (Dolan 2013). Servant leaders allow a bottoms-up approach that delegates more power and control to followers than top-down leaders would delegate. This approach is expected to improve workers' morale and goal achievement as well as develop future managers for the HCO.

COLLABORATIVE LEADERSHIP

Collaborative leadership
Leadership used to form alliances, partnerships, and other forms of interorganizational relationships.

Collaborative leadership is used to form alliances, partnerships, and other forms of interorganizational relationships. This type of leadership has become—and will continue to be—essential for future healthcare managers. Recall from Chapter 1 the trend of hospitals, medical groups, insurers, ambulatory clinics, long-term care companies, community agencies, and other HCOs forming more mergers, alliances, networks, integrated delivery systems, accountable care organizations, patient-centered medical homes, and other collaborative structures.

This leadership style is complex because it involves leading people from other organizations toward a common purpose (Borkowski and Deppman 2014). But the leader does not have direct control or authority over these people. The leader must influence people from other organizations who are likely to have different goals, cultures, management styles, attitudes, assumptions, knowledge, constraints, awareness of problems, and commitments. To make this task even more challenging, some of the organizations may be competing—trying to take resources, customers, market share, and revenue away from each other. Do those organizations trust each other? Can somebody lead this group toward a common purpose? Yes, it can be done by using the collaborative leadership style. A leader will need specific skills, traits, and competencies for collaborative leadership. The transformational leadership and servant leadership styles are often equated with collaborative leadership style because they use similar skills and behaviors. Additional competencies are also important for collaborative leadership (Borkowski and Deppman 2014). These leaders must be able to manage conflict, coordinate teams, create trust, share power, share credit, work with people while not having authority over them, apply political skills, and use emotional intelligence. Patience is a virtue because life in the collaboration lane is usually slow. Some of these competencies were explained in prior chapters; others will be addressed in future chapters.

 TRY IT, APPLY IT

Use what you have learned in this chapter to describe your usual leadership style (although it might sometimes change because of contingencies). Apply the leadership theories and models to yourself while you reflect on your past leadership experiences. Think about how you did—and how you would—lead a club, team, or group of students. Which skills, traits, and behaviors do you possess? After some thought, write a page to describe your usual leadership style.

LEADING IN A PROFESSIONAL BUREAUCRACY

Do you remember (from Chapter 5) what a professional bureaucracy is? We learned it is an organization in which authority is based on highly specialized education, training, and expertise of professional workers. Some HCOs are, at least partly, professional bureaucracies with many professional workers providing patient care. Examples include hospitals and medical office practices, where the main products and services require workers with extensive education and training—such as physicians. Other HCOs, such as a medical supply business, do not rely on physicians to produce the work and are not professional bureaucracies.

In a professional bureaucracy, performance is guided and controlled by professional norms and culture that come from outside the organization and its leaders. Internal bureaucratic authority and rules are less important. Professional workers (e.g., physicians, other healthcare professionals) expect autonomy without much managerial oversight as long as they work within their professional training. Physicians in particular expect managerial authority to defer to professional expertise.

This expectation is one of the main ways physicians (and some other patient-care professionals) think and behave differently from managers. These different thoughts and behaviors result from differences in education, professional norms, job purpose, and perhaps even personality among people who choose these kinds of jobs. Exhibit 9.2 contrasts managers and physicians in relation to several interesting factors. These comparisons are broad generalities that will vary depending on the level of management and type of HCO. However, they do offer useful insights for managers.

As Exhibit 9.2 shows, physicians think and behave differently than managers do. Yet, managers sometimes incorrectly assume the opposite. **As a manager, realize that**

EXHIBIT 9.2
Comparison of Managers and Physicians

Factor	Managers	Physicians
Authority	Bureaucratic, individual, and shared	Professional, individual
Responsibility	Individual and group	Individual
Work relationships	Hierarchical, bureaucratic	Peer, collegial
Allegiance, loyalty	To the organization	To patients, clients
Decisions	Deliberative, uses input from others, based on consensus	Quick, based on own judgment
Resources	Viewed as limited, must be used wisely	Assume resources will be available for patient care
Patient focus	Groups and populations of patients	Usually one patient at a time
Time frame	Ranges from now to years in the future	Now, today, this week, short-term
Dealing with uncertainty	Accepted as part of the job	Expects more certainty
Feedback	Sporadic, vague	Specific, frequent
Responsiveness	To patients, families, physicians, board members, employees, accreditors, other stakeholders	To patients, families, other physicians
Whom they help to survive	Organization	Patients
Compensation	Salary	Usually payment per patient or procedure

SOURCES: Information from Gill (1987), Pointer (2006), and Welch (2010).

physicians think and behave differently than managers do. Some managers have created problems (and even derailed their careers) by trying to lead physicians the same way they lead other workers. With proper leadership of physicians, problems can be reduced and shared purpose developed. Understanding this concept is essential for managers because in today's healthcare environment, physicians and HCOs are interdependent and interconnected (Birk 2014). Contingency thinking tells us that the best style depends on the leader, followers, and situation. When the followers are physicians, leaders should adjust their style to what works well with physicians. Here are suggestions for what to do when you are managing physicians (and other professional patient-care workers) in HCOs that are professional bureaucracies:

- Realize how your view of the world differs from that of physicians.

- When possible, show how your ideas will help a physician and her patients, but avoid trying to spin everything as "good for patient care."

- Develop trusting relationships with a few key physicians who can help you interpret other physicians' actions, can explain your ideas to other physicians, and can give you advice on working with specific physicians.

- Use collegial physician–physician (i.e., peer-to-peer) competitiveness, such as showing a physician his performance scores compared to those of his peers.

- Use data that can be easily understood and easily judged as valid and reliable.

- Acknowledge physicians' medical expertise in medical matters; point out your managerial expertise in management matters.

- Minimize use of authority, bureaucratic rules, and organization hierarchy.

- Explain yourself to physicians who may misinterpret your ideas and actions.

- Respect physicians' time, and avoid long or unnecessary meetings.

- Allow data, ideas, and opinions to sink in and take root; do not try to change physicians' views overnight.

ONE MORE TIME

Leadership is a process through which an individual attempts to intentionally influence people to accomplish a goal. It is one of the five management functions, and thus it is performed at all management levels in an HCO.

Leadership has been studied for more than a century by examining traits, skills, and behaviors of leaders. Leaders need human skills at all managerial levels. Technical skills matter more at lower levels, and conceptual skills matter more at higher levels. One behavioral approach looks at how much leaders focus on getting the *tasks and goals* done and how much they focus on *employees and their needs*. Managers can use the managerial grid to think about how much to focus on each of them. The proper focus is contingent on the leader, followers, and situation. Leadership may also be viewed in relation to two contrasting styles — Theory X and Theory Y. Managers may decide how much to use Theory X versus Theory Y based on the same contingencies (leader, followers, situation). Another behavioral approach is transactional versus transformational. Transactional behavior tends to maintain the status quo. But today, with the external environment changing so much, HCOs themselves must change (sometimes a lot). The transformational style is better for adapting to change, although the style is hard to implement. Managers should also use servant leadership and collaborative leadership when appropriate.

Finally, when the followers are physicians, HCO leaders must remember that they think differently than physicians do. Physicians expect managers to allow physicians much professional autonomy based on their extensive medical education and training.

People can learn, develop, and improve their leadership. During their careers, leaders should develop a mix of leadership styles and be flexible. Then they can assess contingencies and use the style that is best for themselves, their followers, and the situation. These abilities will enable leaders to better understand, interact with, and lead other people.

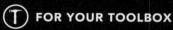

ⓣ FOR YOUR TOOLBOX

- Trait theory
- Skills theory
- Behavior theory
- Managerial grid
- Theory X, Theory Y, and Theory Z

- Transformational leadership
- Servant leadership
- Collaborative leadership
- Differences between managers and physicians

FOR DISCUSSION

1. How did your understanding of leadership change while reading this chapter?

2. Do you think there are born leaders? Discuss why or why not.

3. Discuss which leadership perspective—traits, skills, or behaviors—you think is most important for an HCO leader.

4. How do contingencies affect leadership? Give examples to illustrate your answer.

5. Explain the differences between transactional and transformational leadership.

CASE STUDY QUESTIONS

These questions refer to the Integrative Case Studies at the back of this book.

1. I Can't Do It All case: Use leadership theories, concepts, and models from this chapter to compare and contrast the leadership styles of Ms. Huggins and Mr. Brice.

2. Taking Care of Business at Graceland Memorial Hospital case: Assume that you are Mr. Prestwood trying to lead Ms. Thompson in this case. Refer to the managerial grid in Exhibit 9.1. Where on the grid (i.e., how much people orientation and how much production orientation) would you be with Ms. Thompson?

3. Disparities in Care at Southern Regional Health System case: Using the information in this chapter, describe the kind of leadership approach you would use if you were Tim Hank. Justify your answer using information from the case and chapter.

→ TRY IT, APPLY IT

Suppose you are the top manager of an outpatient surgery center that is owned and used by dozens of surgeons. You report to the board of directors, which consists of nine surgeons. Insurance companies are cutting payments for surgery, so you must reduce expenses by 5 percent next year. Using what you learned in this chapter, explain how you would lead surgeons to accomplish this goal.

CHAPTER 10

LEADING: MOTIVATING AND INFLUENCING

Pleasure in the job puts perfection in the work.

Aristotle

LEARNING OBJECTIVES

Studying this chapter will help you to

➤ define motivation;

➤ explain eight approaches to motivation;

➤ compare and contrast different approaches for motivating employees;

➤ define and describe power used by leaders in organizations;

➤ identify the different types of power leaders may have; and

➤ explain when power is likely to be used—and abused.

HERE'S WHAT HAPPENED

In Boston (and the entire nation), external forces were changing the way health-care would be organized, delivered, and paid for in the future. Stakeholders were demanding patient-centered care, fewer hospital readmissions, and more affordable services. Implementation of the healthcare reform law was pushing improved qual-ity, cost-effectiveness, and access to care. Managers at Partners HealthCare planned how to adapt to—and align with—these external changes. They planned new stra-tegic initiatives and goals that, if achieved, would enable Partners to survive and thrive in its changing environment. Then managers had to lead the organization and its thousands of employees to carry out these plans. Leading required influencing and motivating. Managers throughout Partners had to motivate their staff to accept the new goals and change how they did their jobs. Employees are not all motivated by the same "carrots" or "sticks," so managers had to figure out which motivational approaches to use with which employees. For example, managers could use author-ity as power to demand and punish. But, when leading change, that approach might not work well with physicians and others. Other types of power, influence, and moti-vation could be more effective.

As seen in the opening Here's What Happened, managers (as leaders) must lead others to do things to accomplish the healthcare organization (HCO) mission and goals. **Influencing and motivating people is a big part of management and leadership.** Managers at all levels of an HCO influence and motivate others, usually begin-ning at the top and flowing through the organization. The top executives motivate their management team and the organization as a whole. Middle managers motivate staff in their departments. Lower-level managers motivate staff in their work units.

This chapter describes how leaders influence and motivate others to accomplish their goals and desired outcomes. It builds on ideas discussed in Chapter 9 and adds to our managerial toolbox of tools, methods, theories, and techniques for managing HCOs. Chapter 9 defined leadership as a process through which an individual attempts to inten-tionally influence people to accomplish a goal. Well, how do leaders influence people?

This chapter answers that question. Perhaps you already have some answers. You probably have influenced people—a sibling, a roommate, or a coworker—to accomplish things. How did you try to influence them? Did you try the same approach with everyone, or did you try different methods with different people? Which methods worked best?

This chapter explains what motivation is and then presents several approaches to motivation. Each approach has strengths and weaknesses, and each has been used in HCOs. **The best motivation approach depends on the situation and the people involved. Manag-ers must understand their employees well enough to judge which motivation approach to use for which situation and which employees.** Motivation and influence involve the use of power, which is also discussed in this chapter. We learn the kinds of power that leaders use and when power is likely to be used (and, unfortunately, sometimes abused).

MOTIVATION THEORY AND MODELS

Motivation is "the desire and willingness of a person to expend effort to reach a particular goal or outcome" (French 2007, 89). Reading this definition carefully, we realize that motivation is not the act of doing something; it is the desire and willingness to do something. Desire to do something is different from actually doing it. For example, Matt may be motivated to shampoo the waiting room carpet at an outpatient surgery facility in Flint, Michigan. He has the desire and willingness. But if the carpet-cleaning equipment is broken, Matt will be unable to do that task despite his motivation to do it. The same would happen if his boss reassigned him to some other tasks for the day.

We will examine eight motivation theories. (These theories are sometimes referred to as motivation approaches or perspectives. Some might not technically fulfill all requirements of a true "theory," so that word is used loosely.) Motivation theories can generally be grouped into two categories (Fottler et al. 2006). **Content theories focus on human needs and other unmet needs that all people have. Process theories focus on the context in which work is done and how people think and feel about work.**

First we consider four **content theories**:

1. Maslow's hierarchy of needs theory (self-actualization, esteem and recognition, belonging and friendship, safety and security, physiological)

2. Alderfer's ERG theory (existence, relatedness, growth)

3. McClelland's learned needs theory (achievement, affiliation, power)

4. Herzberg's two factors theory (motivators and hygiene)

Then we consider four **process theories**:

1. Vroom's expectancy theory (based on effort, performance, outcome)

2. Adams's equity theory (fairness of outcomes relative to inputs)

3. Locke's goal-setting theory (based on goals)

4. Skinner's reinforcement theory (based on rewards and punishments)

Which of these theories or approaches should a leader use? Like many other aspects of management, it all depends. Some people may be motivated by money, whereas others are motivated by recognition. We know that in HCOs today, workers are diverse, with different values, ages, ethnicities, and cultural norms. These differences cause differences in motivators. For example, the American culture values achievement, and Eastern cultures value harmony (Hellriegel and Slocum 2011). So when it comes to motivation, one size does not fit all. Further, one motivator might not fit a person forever. A person's motivators may change over time. When Adrianna graduates from college with loans to repay, she will be motivated by money. After she repays her loans, she may be more motivated by opportunities for professional growth.

So what should a manager do? First, assess the situation and people. Second, choose appropriate motivation methods to fit the situation and people. Think about the quote at the beginning of the chapter. As a leader, figure out what brings pleasure to each of your employees. If you can provide that through their work, they will be motivated to work. If an employee gains pleasure from being with other people and forming friendships, then be sure the job provides opportunities for that.

Think about this process as you study each motivation theory. To strengthen your understanding of each theory, think about how leaders at Partners HealthCare in the opening Here's What Happened could apply each theory. Think too about how these theories could be used to motivate you—in your college studies, in a volunteer service role, in a part-time job, and in other aspects of your life!

MASLOW'S HIERARCHY OF NEEDS THEORY

Abraham Maslow (1954) theorized that human motivation comes from five basic human needs that have a hierarchical order—from the lowest, most basic need for physiological survival to the highest need for self-fulfillment (Borkowski 2011). People were thought to try to fulfill lower needs before trying to satisfy higher needs. The needs are reflected in Exhibits 10.1 and 10.2.

· Think of what HCOs do to satisfy employees' five needs (as theorized by Maslow). Take a few minutes to jot down your ideas, and then confer with someone.

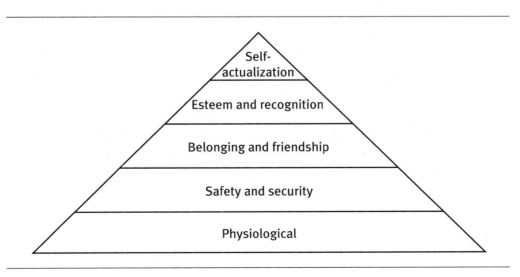

EXHIBIT 10.1
Maslow's Hierarchy of Needs

SOURCE: Information from Maslow (1954).

Maslow's Need	Example from Daily Life	Example for HCO Worker
Self-fulfillment, self-actualization	Accomplishment of personal goals, hobbies	Satisfying job, opportunity for career development
Esteem, respect from others	Praise from friends, status symbols	Recognition for a job well done, job promotion, name in the employee newsletter
Belonging, affiliation, friendship, love	Family, Facebook friends, membership in clubs	Friendly coworkers, a lunch group at work
Safety and security	Shelter, fire alarms, protection from crime	Job security, protection from harassment, safety from bio-hazardous medical waste
Physiological	Food, water, air, shelter	Warm place to work, clean indoor air

Managers should realize several points about Maslow's hierarchy:

1. The five types of needs can overlap (e.g., shelter satisfies the two lowest needs—safety/security and physiological).

2. The hierarchy is culturally biased because it is based on American values (Hellriegel and Slocum 2011).

3. Research has found that people do not always satisfy the lowest need before seeking to satisfy higher needs; Maslow's step-by-step upward progression of needs fulfillment has not been confirmed by research (Fottler et al. 2006). Mother Theresa's pursuit of high-level spiritual calling—rather than low-level material comforts—has been cited to disconfirm Maslow's upward hierarchy of need fulfillment (Borkowski 2011).

4. A manager can motivate employees by enabling them in their jobs to meet their most urgent needs. For example, a manager at a medical clinic in Oshawa, Ontario, Canada, could praise and recognize workers who help implement patient care goals—that would motivate workers who have a need for esteem and respect from others.

ALDERFER'S ERG THEORY

To overcome criticism of Maslow's theory, Clayton Alderfer (1972) theorized that people could be motivated to seek three needs in any order or at the same time (Borkowski 2011).

These needs are shown in Exhibit 10.3. Alderfer's needs are similar to Maslow's although they overlap less and are more distinct:

1.   Existence (equivalent to Maslow's physiological and security needs)

2.   Relatedness (equivalent to Maslow's affiliation and recognition needs)

3.   Growth (equivalent to Maslow's self-esteem and self-actualization needs)

Alderfer believed workers strive to fulfill these needs in any sequence, rather than satisfying existence needs first followed by relatedness needs and then by growth needs. His approach seems more realistic than Maslow's. We can think of our lives and realize we are sometimes motivated by more than one of Alderfer's needs at a time. Further, we do not necessarily fulfill all existence needs before seeking friendships and esteem to satisfy other needs.

Similar to using Maslow's needs, managers can use Alderfer's needs to motivate employees. Consider the medical clinic in Oshawa where managers are trying to motivate workers to improve patient care. For workers with basic existence needs, managers could explain that if the workers help implement the patient care goal, then the clinic will attract patients and earn revenue. As a result, the workers will still have jobs and paychecks to buy things for basic existence needs. Without enough patients and revenue, the clinic might lay off workers, which would threaten the workers' existence needs.

McClelland's Learned Needs Theory

David McClelland (1985) developed another approach to motivation based on learned human needs. McClelland's theory argues that people grow up learning and acquiring

Alderfer's Need	Example from Daily Life	Example for HCO Worker
Existence	Food, water, shelter, protection from crime	Job security, protection from harassment, safety from bio-hazardous medical waste
Relatedness	Family, Facebook friends, membership in clubs, praise from others	Friendly coworkers, a lunch group, recognition from boss
Growth	Accomplishment of personal goals, favorite hobbies	Satisfying job, opportunity for professional growth, job promotion

Exhibit 10.3
Examples of Alderfer's Three Needs

three culturally rooted needs in varying strengths and intensities (Fottler et al. 2006; Hellriegel and Slocum 2011):

1. Achievement: the need to excel and accomplish tasks, responsibilities, meaningful work, high standards, competitive goals, and challenges

2. Affiliation: the need for social interaction, friendships, supportive relationships with other people, and participation

3. Power: the need for control and influence over people and events

An important part of the learned needs theory is that needs are learned and can be learned throughout one's life. People differ in how much they desire to fulfill each need because of differences in their knowledge and life experiences (especially while growing up). In their work lives, people tend to pursue jobs that enable them to fulfill their desired amount of these three needs. For example, many allied health jobs (e.g., therapist, nurse, pharmacist) require much individual work, personal responsibility, and self-sufficiency—all of which enable workers to experience individual achievement. People with a high need for achievement often are found in these jobs, and managers can motivate them by appealing to their need for achievement. Generation Y workers now entering the workforce tend to have a high need for affiliation. Managers can motivate them by creating opportunities at work for participation in groups and interaction with others.

Using McClelland's theory, managers can do two things. First, for each job, consider how much the job would enable someone to experience achievement, affiliation, and power—and then hire someone who has a similar need for achievement, affiliation, and power. As mentioned, jobs vary in how much they enable someone to fulfill each of these three needs. It would not make sense to hire someone with high affiliation needs to fill an isolated job located in a basement cubicle. (As a manager, you can use what you learned about staffing in Chapter 7 to hire people with motivational needs that fit the job.) Second, as someone is working in a job, pay attention to his needs (which may change over time), and adjust the job if possible so that it enables the worker to fulfill unmet needs. Depending on Henrik's needs, his manager might adjust his job to assign more challenging goals, provide more opportunity for affiliation, or give more autonomy and control.

HERZBERG'S TWO FACTORS THEORY

Frederick Herzberg (1966) studied workers' satisfaction and believed that people are motivated by things that increase feelings of satisfaction. His research led him to conclude that satisfaction and dissatisfaction are caused by different factors. One group of factors—which he labeled *hygiene*—is associated with dissatisfaction. The factors are extrinsic—external to the work—and are the context and conditions in which the work is performed.

Hygiene factors include company policies, pay, supervision, coworkers, and other work conditions (Borkowski 2011). If these factors are adequate, they prevent workers from feeling dissatisfied. And if workers are dissatisfied, improving these hygiene factors reduces dissatisfaction. Herzberg argued that better hygiene factors would not make workers feel satisfied but would reduce their dissatisfaction (Fottler et al. 2006).

So what would satisfy workers? A second group of factors—which Herzberg labeled *motivators*—that come from the work itself and include achievement, growth, recognition, challenge, autonomy, and responsibility (Hellriegel and Slocum 2011). Herzberg believed motivators are intrinsic—internal to the work—and arise from the content of the work and how it makes a worker feel. For example, feeling achievement and growth after completing a new, challenging project comes from doing the work. Herzberg argued that more motivators lead to more satisfaction. However, more motivators do not reduce dissatisfaction.

Dissatisfaction and satisfaction are *not* opposite ends of one scale, as shown here:

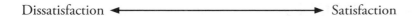

Dissatisfaction ⟵——————————————⟶ Satisfaction

Instead, dissatisfaction and satisfaction are separate concepts. Each may be present in varying degrees, such as on a scale of 0 to 10:

Dissatisfaction   0 _____ 10
Satisfaction   0 _____ 10

HERE'S WHAT HAPPENED

Inova Fairfax Hospital in Virginia was struggling to staff enough nurses amid a nationwide shortage of nurses. The hospital influenced nurses to work there by improving their working conditions. It provided nurses with new equipment, reduced their paperwork, and helped them with work schedules. Better working conditions were influential in helping Inova Fairfax Hospital keep nurses (Haynes 2008). These changes reduced nurses' dissatisfaction at the hospital so that they would not leave to work somewhere else.

Herzberg's theory has limitations (Fottler et al. 2006; Hellriegel and Slocum 2011). Some hygiene factors can affect both dissatisfaction and satisfaction. Both hygiene and motivator factors can motivate workers to higher levels of performance. Workers will perform better because a hygiene factor (e.g., big pay raise) also provides a form of recognition and thus is a motivator. Limitations arise when culturally diverse workers grow up with different feelings about specific hygiene factors (e.g., following rules, interacting with supervisors, accepting on-the-job working conditions) and about motivators (e.g., desire for achievement, challenges, autonomy).

CHECK IT OUT

Have you heard of online leadership style tests? They include short questions, such as "How often do you initiate new ideas in a group?" and "Are you a good listener?" Answer choices are *always*, *sometimes*, or *rarely*. The interactive test immediately interprets and comments on your answers. These tests are fun and easy and give insight into your leadership style. Two examples may be found at http://psychology.about.com/library/quiz/bl-leadershipquiz.htm and www.yourleadershiplegacy.com/assessment/assessment.php. If you Google "leadership style test" you will find others.

Despite its limitations, managers often can and do use the two factors theory. As a manager, pay attention to both dissatisfaction and satisfaction and realize that different factors might be needed to reduce dissatisfaction and to increase satisfaction.

Managers should periodically survey employees as a group and also ask them individually about their job satisfaction and dissatisfaction. The responses will help managers plan what to do. Leaders have to understand their employees well enough to know how to satisfy them. Otherwise, the most popular song at Employee Karaoke Night might be the Rolling Stones' hit "(I Can't Get No) Satisfaction."

When applying the two factors motivation theory, a manager first might have to provide sufficient hygiene factors so that workers do not feel dissatisfied. Then, a manager can increase motivators to increase job satisfaction. This step may require redesigning jobs so that workers have opportunities for more achievement, recognition, growth, and responsibility. (Think about how this redesign connects to the discussion of organizing work and staffing in earlier chapters.) For example, repetitive data-entry keyboard jobs could be redesigned to include more task variety using telephones and other equipment. Career ladders could be developed for nurses (as discussed in Chapter 8) to motivate them with potential job-growth opportunities. A maintenance worker could be given more responsibility for scheduling preventive maintenance or selecting supplies. However, managers must ensure that workers have the ability to perform the increased job duties—training might be necessary. Further, extrinsic dissatisfiers must be minimized or else they will interfere with job design motivators.

VROOM'S EXPECTANCY THEORY

The motivation theories discussed thus far have been *content theories,* which suggest people are motivated to fulfill their unmet human needs. These unmet needs can be fulfilled by the *content of work*. Our focus now turns to the *process theories,* which focus on the *context in which work is done* and how people think and feel about work. These feelings motivate (or demotivate) people to work.

The first process theory is expectancy theory, which was developed by Victor Vroom (1964) and others. This approach is based on work effort, performance, and outcomes. In its simplest form, it can be understood as "I exert work effort to achieve performance that leads to valued work-related outcomes" (Hellriegel and Slocum 2011, 177). Let's consider an example.

1. Latasha figures out whether her *work efforts are tightly connected to her performance*. Does she expect that her efforts would be enough to create the necessary job performance? Or will other factors (e.g., lazy coworkers, broken equipment) interfere with her hard work and achieving excellent performance?

2. Latasha considers to what extent her *work performance would obtain a certain outcome*. Is the outcome tightly connected to her job performance? If she produces excellent job performance, will she really get that reward? Or does the outcome depend on something more than her performance—such as a supervisor's personal preference or the HCO's profits?

3. Latasha considers how strongly she *wants a certain outcome* (e.g., bonus pay, promotion). She bases her desire on how much she values each outcome.

Taken together, this approach argues that a worker will wonder if her *effort* will produce the *performance* needed to obtain a *valued outcome*. The more she feels that the answer is yes, the more she will be motivated to work.

As you may have already realized, the value or attractiveness of rewards varies according to people's unique needs. Suppose two workers—Ricardo and Quinn—work in a hospital's information systems department in Northridge, California. Ricardo wants personal growth and new experiences, whereas Quinn prefers other types of rewards. As an incentive, the hospital offers to send one worker to the Health Information and Management Systems Society conference. Ricardo would value that as a reward more than Quinn would.

Research generally supports this theory, although it has some weaknesses (Fottler et al. 2006). The expectancy theory assumes that workers (e.g., Latasha) rationally and logically do such mental calculations—but they might not. Also, even if workers try to rationally calculate the value of rewards, they might easily misjudge the connection between effort and performance or between performance and outcome. Finally, some people feel things are not within their control and instead are mostly influenced by other forces and events . . . so why bother? If workers perceive favoritism or a biased boss, applying expectancy theory will be less effective. This theory, like others, is culturally biased and thus works better in some countries (e.g., the United States, Canada) than others (e.g., Brazil, China) based on how much workers feel they can control their work and behavior (Hellriegel and Slocum 2011). As a manager, you can use this approach to motivate workers as long as you realize its limitations. Workers may put forth the effort you want if they feel (expect) their work will lead to the performance level that will earn them desired rewards.

ADAMS'S EQUITY THEORY

John Stacey Adams (1963) developed the equity theory based on people's desire to be treated fairly (equitably). This theory has two main elements: inputs and outcomes. A worker's inputs are the education, experience, skills, knowledge, efforts, and so forth brought to the job. Outcomes are the pay, benefits, recognition, and other rewards received for performing the job. A worker considers her outcomes received compared to her inputs given to the job and then judges whether the ratio seems fair. She also compares that ratio to the inputs and outcomes of other workers and judges whether it all seems fair. Have you ever gone through this process? Here is an example:

1. Sean, a health insurance sales representative, considers his education, years of experience, sales ability, and knowledge of the healthcare market that he brings to his job. He considers his pay, benefit package, and other rewards.

2. Sean knows the background of some of the other sales reps at his company. From conversations and other sources, he has a pretty good idea what Megan, Brandon, and Danielle are earning. He mentally sizes up the outcomes-to-inputs ratio of each sales rep.

$$\frac{\text{Sean's outcome}}{\text{Sean's inputs}} \quad \frac{\text{Megan's outcome}}{\text{Megan's inputs}} \quad \frac{\text{Brandon's outcome}}{\text{Brandon's inputs}} \quad \frac{\text{Danielle's outcomes}}{\text{Danielle's inputs}}$$

3. Sean figures he compares fairly (equitably) with Megan and Brandon. Sure, Brandon makes more money, but he has much more experience than the others, so it seems fair. But Sean is annoyed to think that Danielle's ratio is much higher than his and everyone else's. In his opinion, she is getting about the same pay despite having a lot less education, experience, and sales ability. He feels it is unfair, and he becomes dissatisfied. Of course, this feeling is based on Sean's *perceptions* and judgments. The secondhand information might be incorrect. He might not really know the full story about his coworkers. Nonetheless, he makes his judgments. This manner of judging fairness is not ideal, but workers often use it.

Inequity causes a worker to feel tension and become motivated to resolve the inequity. If Sean feels underpaid, he becomes motivated to seek increased rewards (e.g., pay, time off, work schedule) or else reduce his work effort to match (in his mind) his rewards. He might slack off and take long breaks. Some workers will leave the organization if they cannot achieve equity with their current employer. Some employees deviously increase their rewards by stealing supplies or using company equipment for personal purposes. Inequity can work in the other direction, too (Borkowski 2011). If Danielle becomes aware of all this information, she may feel overpaid. Perhaps she will feel tension (guilt) about the inequity and work extra hard to feel she really does deserve her pay.

Inequitable situations arise in healthcare, especially when workers compare themselves to similar workers in other organizations. Labor markets for some jobs are unstable, and pay scales are moving targets. (Recall the earlier chapters on staffing, recruitment, and compensation.) A nurse or pharmacist might find a peer getting a better deal somewhere else because that employer was frantic and paid a high starting salary for an essential position. Paying a higher salary upsets the outcomes-to-inputs ratio for the position. Workers might compare not only material outcomes, such as vacation days, but also subjective outcomes, such as praise from the boss.

Earlier chapters explained that HCOs sometimes use contract workers or agency staff, and this arrangement also can create feelings of inequity. Consider a hospital that has many vacant nurse positions and thus contracts with a nursing agency to provide nurses. Desperate to get enough nurses, the hospital pays the agency a lot of money, and the agency uses it to offer above-average wages to hire nurses. Although the agency nurse is paid more per hour than the full-time hospital nurse, the agency nurse might not initially do as much work because she is not as familiar with the hospital and has to learn. Equity theory predicts the demotivation of a full-time hospital nurse who learns that the agency nurse gets paid more while (initially) doing less.

Managers should pay attention to equity theory and realize how much workers compare themselves with others. **A challenge for managers is to get workers to consider all of their rewards rather than just pay.** Sometimes, a worker feels her lower pay is unfair when compared to someone else's pay without realizing that she also gets more weeks of vacation and better health insurance than the other person. Managers should remind employees about their total compensation. Managers must also realize that workers compare their work effort to other workers' efforts. Good workers quickly become frustrated and feel tension from inequity if they have to work with lousy coworkers. If the HCO leaders do not motivate (or replace) the low performers, the high performers are likely to leave the organization to relieve their tension. Then, the HCO loses good workers and is left with lousy ones. Hmmm, what's wrong with this picture?

LOCKE'S GOAL-SETTING THEORY

Edwin Locke (1968) theorized that goals would motivate people. Research has confirmed his theory—under certain conditions. Motivation from a goal increases when these factors occur (Fottler et al. 2006; Hellriegel and Slocum 2011):

◆ People know what the goal is.

◆ People accept the goal and are committed to work for it.

◆ People have the knowledge, ability, and resources to attain the goal.

◆ The goal is challenging yet attainable.

◆ The goal is specific, not vague and general.

◆ The goal is of manageable size and complexity; if not, it is broken into smaller subgoals.

◆ People receive enough feedback on progress toward the goal.

Managers may assign goals to a worker, let the worker set the goals, or cooperatively set goals with the worker. All these approaches can be effective for motivating workers. This theory might seem relatively simple, yet it requires thought and planning. A leader must carefully take three steps to set this theory into action (Borkowski 2011).

1. *Set the goal.* This step is not as simple as it might seem. If the goal is too easy to achieve, it will not motivate the worker. If it is too hard to achieve, it will create frustration, demotivation, and negative feelings toward the manager. Each employee is unique. Highly confident workers respond better to a harder goal than do workers with low self-confidence. A manager must know her employees well. Internal and external factors, such as laws, accreditation standards, consumers' demands, and community standards, may have to be considered in setting a goal. Thus, deciding the proper goal takes careful judgment.

2. *Obtain the employee's acceptance of the goal and commitment to accomplish it.* If the employee helped set the goal or provided input for it, acceptance and commitment are more likely. Prior success in achieving goals also contributes to acceptance of new goals.

3. *Provide necessary support and resources to enable goal achievement.* This could include training for a new skill; breaking a goal into smaller, doable steps and activities; and providing supplies, equipment, time, information, and so forth. The manager must support an employee by giving regular feedback regarding goal progress.

This approach to motivation can work well in HCOs. Let us consider a government-funded behavioral health clinic. As a result of the economic recession, the state government has less money and must cut funding for the clinic by 10 percent. Meanwhile, recession-related financial struggles have caused people to experience more stress, depression, and behavioral health problems. Because of these factors, the clinic supervisor meets with her four counselors to set goals for the number of clients each counselor will see per week. The staff, after some discussion, sets a goal of increasing client visits per counselor by five visits per week for the next six months (after which the goal will be reevaluated). All counselors commit to this goal, although the supervisor senses hesitation by two of them. They all brainstorm ideas that could help achieve this goal. The supervisor arranges for the clinic's scheduling coordinator to provide a weekly report to each counselor so that they can monitor progress. Later in the week, and then at least monthly, the supervisor meets individually with each counselor to give feedback (and seek counselors' feedback) on progress toward the goal.

SKINNER'S REINFORCEMENT THEORY

The final approach to motivation comes from B. F. Skinner's (1969) work and research on behavior modification. Skinner assumed that people learn from and become motivated by the consequences of their behavior. **In a work setting, managers can increase or decrease the frequency of a specific work behavior by using consequences. When applied properly, consequences reinforce desired behaviors at work.** When employees learn a favorable consequence of a specific behavior, they become motivated to repeat that behavior.

Let's consider a basic explanation of reinforcement theory (Hellriegel and Slocum 2011) and how a leader can use it. Application of the theory becomes more complicated when managers try to decide on the timing, frequency, and type of consequence.

1. The theory begins with a *stimulus*—a leader's rule, policy, instruction, or goal that informs a person what should be done. A leader stimulates a person to behave a certain way. The leader can also inform the person of which consequences will occur if the person does (or does not) behave the desired way.

2. The stimulus is followed by a *response*, which is the person's behavior or action.

3. That response is followed by a *consequence*—a leader rewarding or punishing the person. Depending on what the consequence is, it might increase or decrease the frequency of that response in the future. The consequence motivates the person to respond a certain way.

Sports coaches use this method with players and teams. Duke University men's basketball coach Mike Krzyzewski has won four National Collegiate Athletic Association championships and is a master motivator. Coach K (as he is known) uses reinforcement theory. He sometimes reminds players before a game to go after every loose ball—beat your opponent to the ball! Then during the game, even a star player who often appears in highlight films might get Coach K's harsh, penetrating scowl if that player does not make enough effort chasing a loose ball. Alternatively, the coach will verbally praise a player who hustles to chase a loose ball even when the team has a big lead with only a minute left to play. As a leader, Coach K uses both positive and negative consequences to motivate players.

1. A leader *gives something positive* (e.g., verbal praise) as a consequence of behavior. This action reinforces the behavior and makes it *more likely* to reoccur. Leaders use this method to reinforce desired behavior.

2. A leader *removes something negative* (e.g., running the usual exhausting sprints during practice) as a consequence of behavior. This action reinforces the behavior and makes it *more likely* to reoccur. Leaders use this method to reinforce desired behavior.

3. A leader *gives something negative* (e.g., a harsh scowl) as a consequence of behavior. This action makes the behavior *less likely* to reoccur. Leaders use this method to decrease unwanted behavior.

4. A leader *removes something positive* (e.g., being in the game's starting lineup) as a consequence of behavior. This action makes the behavior *less likely* to reoccur. Leaders use this method to decrease unwanted behavior.

Who else uses reinforcement theory? Parents do, when raising children. Can you think of examples from your own childhood? Of course, managers also use reinforcement theory. Perhaps you have seen examples in a job or internship.

Leaders must think carefully about which behaviors are being reinforced or not reinforced—intentionally or unintentionally. Sometimes a leader accidently gives something positive and accidentally reinforces unwanted behavior (Hellriegel and Slocum 2011). For example, in a meeting the leader gives time and attention to a disruptive person, which reinforces disruptive behavior. The leader must remove the positive reinforcement—time and attention—so that the undesired behavior decreases and stops. Further, in the meeting the leader might forget to commend a helpful person who contributes good ideas. Because he does not positively reinforce that desired behavior, people may stop contributing ideas. During the meeting, the leader should thank someone who contributes good ideas—then that behavior will continue.

Reinforcement theory works best when there is a clear relationship between someone's response (to a stimulus) and the consequence. Big consequences are more noticeable than small consequences. Prompt consequences to behavior are more effective than delayed consequences. However, the consequence does not have to occur for every response. The relationship may vary, such as an initial reward for every response and then, after some improvement, a change to every fifth response. Connecting consequences to a specific number of responses seems to work better than connecting them to specific time intervals (Fottler et al. 2006), although consequences following short time periods can be effective. What really matters is that employees know how consequences are related to their behaviors.

Managers should be cautious about removing a positive consequence that employees have come to expect, because after a while employees assume it is automatic. Managers should also be cautious about punishments as consequences and clearly explain the reason for them. If employees perceive those consequences as unfair or undeserved, they will feel resentment, anger, and hostility that can jeopardize future working relationships or make the worker try to secretly "get back at" the boss. Managers should strive to reinforce good behavior, ensure they do not reinforce bad behavior, and avoid too often punishing bad behavior. Finally, as with other aspects of managing and leading, managers must realize that employees are not all alike. Again, managers need to know their employees as individuals to be able to apply the motivational theory when necessary.

Reinforcement theory is common in HCOs. For example, suppose a medical imaging supervisor in Lincoln, Nebraska, instructs all technologists to "get it right the first time" and avoid repeat scans. The technologists must ensure the patient is properly positioned so that the scans and images fully capture the area of interest and do not have to be repeated. This procedure will save the facility money and save the patient time, discomfort, and inconvenience. The supervisor's instruction is a *stimulus*. It stimulates a *response* from imaging tech Lucinda, who has had her mind on other things and behaved carelessly at times. After receiving the stimulus, she now pays more attention and works more accurately when performing imaging scans. For the next week, Lucinda has fewer repeats than usual and only has to redo three procedures. Her supervisor rewards her with verbal praise for this specific improvement. The praise is a *consequence* of fewer repeat scans, and it feels good to Lucinda. It motivates her to keep improving to continue getting the praise. For the following week, Lucinda has zero retakes and receives even more praise. Meanwhile, Jason (another imaging tech) has had to repeat many scans and has not done much to improve. The supervisor talks privately with Jason, emphasizes how patient care has been harmed by Jason's behavior, and advises Jason that if his work does not improve, he could be suspended without pay. To avoid this negative consequence, Jason begins improving his work. The next week, he "gets it right the first time" for 98 percent of his patients—a big improvement! The supervisor praises Jason, and that positive consequence further motivates him to behave as desired.

→ TRY IT, APPLY IT

Suppose you are a summer intern in the human resources department of a health insurance company. More than 500 employees work there in more than a dozen different departments. The president wants the company to reduce its energy use by 15 percent during the next two years to be more eco-friendly and to save money. Employees submit plenty of suggestions for how they could reduce energy by changing their behaviors and actions. But who wants to change behavior? Using the ideas in this chapter, explain how to apply three different theories of motivation to influence groups of workers to reduce their energy use. Discuss your ideas with several classmates. What are the pros and cons of your motivation approaches?

POWER AND POLITICS

The use of power is important for leading, influencing, directing, and motivating. For example, although not stated explicitly, reinforcement theory involves the use of power to give and remove consequences, rewards, and punishments.

In management, we can think of **power** as "the ability of one person or department in an organization to influence other people to bring about desired outcomes" (Daft 2013, 531) and "the ability to exert influence or control over others" (Hoff and Rockmann 2012, 191). To be more concise, power is the ability to influence others to achieve outcomes. Some people think authority is the same as power. The two words are related, but they do not mean the same thing. Recall from Chapter 2 that authority is the power formally given to a job position (not a person) to make decisions, take actions, and direct subordinates and expect obedience from them. Authority is established in the formal organization hierarchy. It is one type of power, but it is not the only type, as we learn in this section.

SOURCES AND TYPES OF POWER

Besides authority, what are some other types of power? There are several—some tied to individual *people* and some tied to individual *positions* in an organization. A *person* in an HCO—Maria or Kyle—can have more than one type of power. Additionally, *positions* in an HCO—director of information systems or head nurse of pediatrics—can have several types of power that may be used by the person in the position. The early work of John French and Bertam Raven (1959) identified legitimate, reward, coercive, expert, and referent powers. Power in organizations is based on resource control, decisional control, network centrality, and coping with uncertainty and problems (Daft 2013). These ideas are summarized in Exhibit 10.4. Note that types of power may overlap and are not independent of each other. Returning to the Here's What Happened at the beginning of this chapter, which of these types of power do you think Partners HealthCare managers would use?

ORGANIZATIONAL POLITICS

People who have power may use it with politics and political activity in organizations. We can think of **politics** as "the use of power to influence decisions" (Daft 2013, 543). **In organizations, managers may strive to gain favors and favorable decisions through politics.** Someone might say, "she is playing politics" or "he is very political" when describing a person who does these things. Managers may use political tactics such as persuasion, inspirational appeal, ingratiation, favors and gifts, emphasizing loyalty, and making threats (Hellriegel and Slocum 2011; Hoff and Rockmann 2012).

Suppose top managers of a large multispecialty medical group start talking about cutting staff to save money. Lindsey, manager of the neurology service, engages in

EXHIBIT 10.4
Types of Power

Personal Power

Type	Definition	Examples
Reward	Give something that is valued	Give praise, money, friendship, a ride to work
Coercive	Punish, penalize, reprimand	Insult, scold, reduce wages
Expertise	Provide needed knowledge, skills, ability	Calculate return on investment, set up a new tech device
Referent	Entice someone to reverently follow (often by using charisma and emotion)	Behave and communicate in a compelling emotional way that inspires others to follow

Positional Power

Type	Definition	Examples
Legitimate	Authorize decisions, take actions, direct subordinates, and expect obedience from them	Assign work to subordinates
Reward	Give something that is valued	Give praise, promotion, pay raise, bigger office, reserved parking place
Coercive	Punish, penalize, reprimand	Reduce pay, take away reserved parking
Resource control	Give, remove, use, assign valued resources that others depend on	Control equipment, funds, information, staff, space, time
Decision control	Control when, how, by whom, and within which limits decisions will be made	Tell subordinates they can only recommend rather than make the final decision, allow staff to decide the work schedule but not the prices for services
Network centrality	Be in the flow of information ("in the loop") and connected to key people	Serve on key committees to know and affect what is going on
Coping with uncertainty and problems	Resolve uncertainty and solve big, unexpected, threatening problems	Quickly arrange extra hospital staff when a bus accident occurs on the nearby highway

SOURCES: Information from French and Raven (1959) and Daft (2013).

organizational politics to influence top managers not to cut her staff. She reports to the managers how much revenue and profit her neurology service brings in. She suggests that if her staff is cut, then patients' procedures will be delayed, patients will go elsewhere, and revenue will decrease. Then she asks physicians who order lots of neurology tests to "have a word" with the top managers about no layoffs for the neurology staff.

Although some may consider organizational politics and political games to be inappropriate and unethical, these activities can be positive or negative—for good or bad purposes (Daft 2013; Hellriegel and Slocum 2011). When managers use power in ways that are contrary to the organization's goals, policies, and rules (as happens when power is used for self-serving purposes), politics is negative. In that case, employees (including managers) think playing politics is bad—or nasty, dishonest, sleazy, manipulative, deceptive, or self-serving. Yet politics may be used positively, such as to influence stakeholders to resolve a tense, long-standing conflict that has paralyzed an HCO. Politics is a normal part of organizational life, and HCO managers should expect it. Managers have power, and they use it to influence decisions, overcome disagreements, and resolve conflicts so that the HCO can achieve its goals and mission.

New managers tend to focus on getting experience with projects yet often are not aware of the politics that surround their projects (Dye 2010). Being unaware of organizational politics can cause problems for the managers—and their HCOs. The examples that follow can help new managers recognize when people are playing politics (Mintzberg 1983a; Bewley 2008):

◆ *Insurgency:* Employees work together to resist legitimate authority, such as by only loosely following work schedules and policies.

◆ *Counterinsurgency:* Managers thwart an insurgency, such as by assigning the insurgents miserable work schedules and tasks.

◆ *Empire building:* A manager expands his domain and control by getting the chief executive officer to give him responsibility for inspecting and approving the safety of everyone's work areas.

◆ *Whistleblowing:* Employees send information about the organization to the local newspaper and post it on websites to reveal that the organization has enough money to avoid the announced layoff of 20 employees.

There are other ways of playing politics to gain power, including verbally attacking people, blaming people for problems, claiming credit for successes, manipulating information, building a base of support and loyal followers, carefully managing self-image, ingratiating ("apple polishing"), and doing favors so that later someone "owes you" (Borkowski 2011). As a manager, be aware of politics, watch for people using these methods, and learn how to use politics appropriately.

WHEN WILL POWER BE USED?

Power is more likely to be used in certain situations (Daft 2013; Fottler et al. 2006), such as those in the following list. Examples from HCOs are included.

♦ Important decisions (what new clinical equipment should be bought?)

♦ Difficulty in assessing performance (which mental health counselor is best?)

♦ Uncertainty and disagreement (who will be laid off and lose their jobs?)

♦ Incompatible conflicting goals (reduce costs but add service on weekends)

♦ Decentralized, diffuse power (each department head decides who in the department gets bonus pay at the end of the year)

♦ Interdependence, coordination (coordination among clinical care staff and across departments to improve patient engagement)

♦ Structural change (adding a new director of social media to help promote the organization)

♦ Management succession (what to do when the outpatient care manager retires next year)

♦ Limited resources and budgets (funds are available to cover only half of the requests for new iPads)

♦ Different attitudes, values, and subcultures (managers and physicians think differently about time urgency)

WHEN WILL POWER BE ABUSED?

Employees and groups sometimes use power and engage in political behavior to achieve what is good for themselves—even if it is contrary to the organization's goals, values, and ethics or harms the organization. For example, a manager might use his official organizational position to hire his friend as an overpriced marketing consultant even though that decision hurts the organization.

In some situations, power is more likely to be abused (Daft 2013; Fottler et al. 2006). Examples of such situations, including some from HCOs, are listed below. Managers should try to prevent the abuse of power by eliminating or minimizing these situations in their HCOs.

♦ Information ambiguity (rumors and secondhand gossip, rather than data)

♦ Fuzzy means to ends (uncertainty about which methods produce the best client satisfaction)

◆   Overly centralized decision-making structure (executive director makes all the decisions)

◆   Scarcity of rival coalitions (no group challenges the medical staff)

◆   One-sided interdependencies (the marketing supervisor depends on the webmaster more than the webmaster depends on the marketing supervisor)

◆   Complacent organizational culture (employees come to work, put in their time, collect their pay, and do not care about much else)

ONE MORE TIME

Management involves leading, and leading involves motivating. Motivation must happen at all levels of an HCO, beginning at the top and flowing through the organization. People are different and do not respond equally to the same motivators. Thus, a manager should first assess the situation and people. Second, a manager should choose appropriate motivation methods to fit the situation and people.

Leaders can apply content theories of motivation, which focus on the human needs that people have. These approaches include (1) Maslow's needs hierarchy theory, (2) Alderfer's ERG theory, (3) McClelland's learned needs theory, and (4) Herzberg's two factors theory. Leaders can also apply process theories of motivation, which focus on the context in which work is done and how people think and feel about work. These approaches include (1) Vroom's expectancy theory, (2) Adams's equity theory, (3) Locke's goal-setting theory, and (4) Skinner's reinforcement theory.

Who has power? Individual people have power, and individual positions (jobs) in organizations have power. Power is not constant, and there are different sources of power in organizations. The power sources may change as circumstances change. Leaders can become better managers by paying attention to which workers have which types of power and how they use those powers. Managers should use power to enable the organization to achieve its goals. However, some managers abuse power for their own purposes.

People in organizations engage in politics to increase power and influence for their preferred goals, which may or may not match organizational goals. The use of politics is evident with informal groups, whose members often engage in political behavior to achieve what is good for their own group even if it is contrary to the organization's goals.

ⓣ FOR YOUR TOOLBOX

- Maslow's needs hierarchy theory
- Alderfer's ERG theory
- McClelland's learned needs theory
- Herzberg's two factors theory
- Vroom's expectancy theory
- Adams's equity theory
- Locke's goal-setting theory
- Skinner's reinforcement theory
- Power (personal and positional)

FOR DISCUSSION

1. Discuss the differences between content theories and process theories of motivation.

2. Describe one content theory and one process theory that you would like to use as a leader. Do you think either of these theories would work for everyone in your work unit?

3. Which motivation theory do you think would be the most difficult to implement in an HCO? How could a manager overcome those difficulties?

4. Compare and contrast the different sources of power discussed in this chapter.

5. Think of different jobs in a HCO. Which sources of power do you think each of those jobs would have?

6. Which type of power appeals to you? Which would you feel least comfortable using?

7. What can managers do to minimize abuse of power in an HCO?

CASE STUDY QUESTIONS

These questions refer to the Integrative Case Studies at the back of this book.

1. I Can't Do It All case: Using at least two of the motivation theories discussed in this chapter, explain how Mr. Brice could motivate his vice presidents to make more decisions.

2. Ergonomics in Practice case: Using at least two of the motivation theories in this chapter, explain how Mr. Montana could try to motivate his staff to use the new lift system.

3. Taking Care of Business at Graceland Memorial Hospital case: Using at least two of the motivation theories described in this chapter, explain how Mr. Prestwood could try to motivate Mrs. Thompson to support the proposed policy change.

4. I Can't Do It All case: Referring to the types of power in Exhibit 10.4, describe which types of power you think Mr. Brice could use to achieve his desired outcomes.

5. Taking Care of Business at Graceland Memorial Hospital case: Referring to the types of power in Exhibit 10.4, describe which types of power you think Mr. Prestwood could use to achieve his desired outcomes.

 TRY IT, APPLY IT

You and a friend are driving home for the weekend. During the trip, you talk about things you want to do someday. Your friend says he wants to get students to join him in building a Habitat for Humanity house. He knows you are taking a course that involves management, so he asks you how to motivate students to join him. Use the information from this chapter to offer him specific advice.

CHAPTER 11

LEADING: CULTURE AND ETHICS

Clarifying the value system and breathing life into it are the greatest contributions a leader can make.

Thomas Peters and Robert Waterman,
management consultants

Studying this chapter will help you to

➤ define culture in an organization;

➤ explain why culture is important for managing HCOs;

➤ learn how to interpret culture in an organization;

➤ identify factors that create and shape culture in HCOs;

➤ explain why subcultures exist within a culture in an HCO;

➤ define ethics;

➤ describe four different types of ethics in HCOs; and

➤ explain how to lead, create, and maintain desired cultures and ethics in HCOs.

HERE'S WHAT HAPPENED

Changes outside of Partners HealthCare (in its external environment) forced changes inside the healthcare organization (HCO). Thus, managers had to lead thousands of employees to change. In the process, managers were helped by their organizational culture—the values, norms, and guiding beliefs that were considered correct at Partners. The HCO had developed a culture that valued technology, innovation, openness, preparedness, and adaptiveness. This culture had evolved over the years because of leaders who emphasized and rewarded this culture. Also, past success with technological innovations and adaption had reinforced innovation and adaptation as "the way we do things around here." When employees tried to figure out what really mattered at work and how to succeed in their jobs, they were influenced by the organization's cultural emphasis on technology, innovation, and adaptation. This shared set of values, norms, and beliefs was appropriate for an HCO that had to adapt to frequent changes in its external environment. It helped managers lead employees through change. If Partners's culture had not valued innovation and adaptation, managers would have struggled to lead employees to change.

Learning what happened at Partners HealthCare helps us realize that leading HCOs requires careful management of organizational culture and ethics. It is among the most important work leaders do *at all levels* of an HCO, as we learn in this chapter. This might surprise people who view culture and ethics as the "soft side" of management or perhaps even optional. Yet experienced managers know that the culture and ethics of an organization determine how the organization performs, whether it accomplishes its goals, how satisfied stakeholders are, and whether the organization thrives and survives. This is especially true for HCOs.

This chapter explains what culture and subcultures are and how to interpret them. The chapter discusses factors that create and influence culture in HCOs. Using that knowledge, we then learn how to change and re-create culture to achieve new plans and goals. Next, the chapter focuses on ethics (which is part of culture) and several types of ethics that guide behavior and decisions in HCOs. The chapter explains how leaders can create and maintain the ethics they feel are needed. Leaders at the top of the HCO create and maintain ethics for the overall HCO. Then, leaders in departments, teams, and other organizational units also create and maintain the right culture and ethics in their specific areas. When you are a manager, you will have this responsibility in your department and HCO.

WHAT IS CULTURE?

You have probably heard of culture, such as the Chinese culture or the culture of professional sports. We talk about the culture of a group of people, such as the Chinese or professional athletes. The same can be said about the people in an HCO. They are a group of people and they have a culture.

The **culture** in an organization is "the set of values, norms, guiding beliefs, and understandings that is shared by members of an organization and taught to new members as the correct way to think, feel, and behave" (Daft 2013, 392). As we saw earlier in the Here's What Happened, culture helps people understand what matters and how things are done in an organization. Culture helps answer questions such as: What does it take to get ahead in this HCO? Is it OK to call people by first names? What is the dress code? Does creativity matter here? What does matter here? Several points can explain culture:

◆ Culture is shared and learned.

◆ Culture evolves gradually and does not change quickly.

◆ Culture is mostly invisible, so it is interpreted by observing and listening to what can be sensed.

◆ Culture guides behavior and is powerful in doing that.

Managers should never forget this last point. In fact, some managers feel that "culture trumps strategy" because culture is so powerful. For example, the executive director of an HCO tried to implement a new strategy of innovation that conflicted with the long-term culture of "we do not like mistakes." Innovation requires trying new ideas, some of which might not succeed. So what happened? The culture prevailed. The strategy of innovation failed. Culture trumped (beat) strategy. People were afraid to try new ideas that might not work and would be viewed as mistakes. Managers then realized they first had to change the organization's culture so that employees would feel it was acceptable (and safe) to try new ideas that might not succeed. When Baylor Health Care System and Scott & White (a multispecialty academic medical center) considered a merger in Texas, did they first examine the balance sheets, income statements, and financial status of each HCO? Nope. They first examined the culture of each HCO to decide if the two cultures could fit together and work as one (Jacob 2013). That lesson is important when we recall from Chapter 1 that in the future many hospitals, medical groups, insurers, ambulatory clinics, long-term care facilities, and other HCOs will form mergers, alliances, networks, integrated delivery systems, accountable care organizations, and other collaborative structures. If their cultures clash, their strategy will not succeed. **Culture trumps strategy.**

Culture
The values, norms, guiding beliefs, and understandings shared by members of an organization and taught to new members as the correct way to think, feel, and behave.

WHAT CAUSES AND CREATES CULTURE?

How do organizations—such as your college, your favorite store, and HCOs—end up with the cultures they have? What causes and creates culture? Why does culture differ among HCOs? For example, why do some HCOs have a cautious, risk-averse culture while others have an innovative, risk-taking culture? Culture is partly a result of leaders deciding which norms, behaviors, and values they want in the HCO. But there is more to it than leaders deciding which culture they *want.* Strong forces and factors determine what the culture actually *will be,* and it might be different from what managers want it to be. Some factors shape culture regardless of what managers want or do not want. Many external and internal forces and factors influence the cultural values, norms, and beliefs of an HCO (Borkowski 2011; Daft 2013; Evans 2009; Hellriegel and Slocum 2011). The forces and factors appear in the following list with examples that are relevant for HCOs. A model of these forces and factors is shown in Exhibit 11.1.

1. External laws, standards, demands (e.g., nondiscrimination laws, accreditation standards, public demands for eco-friendly green behavior)

2. Organization mission (e.g., mission to improve the health status of all people in the local community)

3. Organization structure (e.g., highly centralized structure in which most decisions are made by the president)

4. Rewards and punishments (e.g., recognition at an employee banquet for excellent patient care, suspension from work for one day without pay after continual tardiness)

5. Training and education (e.g., online tutorials on how to save energy and recycle waste on the job)

6. Physical work setting (e.g., bland, cold, sterile building that does not inspire interpersonal warmth)

7. Beliefs, values, and norms of formal leaders (e.g., the senior vice president believes that too much competitive drive might cause employees to behave unethically)

8. Beliefs, values, and norms of informal leaders (e.g., a longtime employee telling new employees during lunch what she believes really matters in the HCO)

9. Beliefs, values, and norms of employees (e.g., a dental worker values cleanliness)

10. Ceremonies, symbols, rituals, and activities (e.g., diplomas and continuing education certificates displayed in the clinic)

11. Stories and legends (e.g., the story about how Alice made it to work despite three feet of snow—or was it four?—back in the winter of 1993 because her patients were counting on her)

12. Language (e.g., the blunt, no-nonsense way Alex, the new data analyst, talks)

Exhibit 11.1
Model of the
Forces and Factors
That Influence
HCO Culture

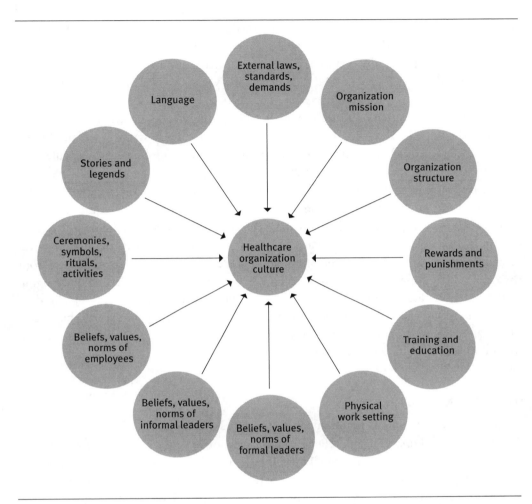

SOURCES: Information from Borkowski (2009); Daft (2013); Evans (2009); and Hellriegel and Slocum (2011).

PURPOSE AND BENEFITS OF CULTURE

When managers develop the right culture for their HCO, it can help achieve the organization's mission and goals by helping employees know what to do (Daft 2013). A culture helps workers understand the HCO and adjust to it. It helps employees figure out what to do in situations that are not covered by specific rules, standards, and policies. **Culture can strongly influence employees to work, act, think, feel, and behave a certain way to help the organization.** In the Here's What Happened at the beginning of this chapter, we saw that managers must develop a culture that supports the organization's mission, vision, values, and goals. In that way, the culture will benefit the organization.

The healthcare field has been learning from other fields just how important culture is to achieve safety. Consider this frequently cited example: In a tragic, stunning accident, the space shuttle *Columbia* exploded as it returned to Earth and disintegrated, killing all seven crew members. The "shuttle accident report concludes that no specific individual was at fault, but many individuals were influenced by the culture of the organization as a whole" (Haraden and Frankel 2004, 21). In its early years, the National Aeronautics and Space Administration (NASA) had a safety-first culture, but then NASA moved to a low-cost and high-productivity culture in which safety was given less attention. As another example, the organizational culture of the New York City subway system was found to be a big factor in the deaths of subway workers. In this culture, not following safety rules had become acceptable behavior (Neuman 2007).

Think about these examples. Then think about safety in HCOs, where there have been too many medical errors, wrong amputations, burns from unsafe equipment, and other accidents and problems. Some of these problems happened because organizational culture did not place enough emphasis on safety excellence and performance. Instead, some HCOs emphasized more production and lower costs. Now, because of pressure from the external environment, the culture of HCOs in general has been gradually changing so that safety is valued more. When Sentara Healthcare in Norfolk, Virginia, realized its patient safety had to improve, it knew the HCO had to value safety more in all that it did. Thus, safety is now more than a priority or goal at Sentara—it is a core value of the culture that permeates the HCO (Birk 2009).

INTERPRETING CULTURE

An organization's members figure out the culture based on what can be seen and heard. The actual underlying cultural beliefs, values, and norms (e.g., "Honesty matters" and "You have to be creative to get ahead") cannot be seen. However, based on what employees see and hear, they might infer that honesty matters and feel that you have to be creative to get ahead. Because people interpret an organization's culture based on what they can see and hear, conflicting signs or mixed signals can confuse them.

For example, managers want a culture of competence. The written dress code explains how employees should dress to convey competence. But a new employee sees that workers often do not follow the written code. So employees look, listen, wonder, ask, infer, think, and learn by trial and error to determine what the culture *really* is and "what really matters around here." Some factors that influence culture (see Exhibit 11.1) can be seen and heard and thus offer useful sources of information for interpreting the culture. The following list includes some of these factors, along with examples (see also the model in Exhibit 11.2):

1. Organization structure (e.g., management's official standards, rules, policy manuals, organization charts, and protocols for how things should be done)

2. Rewards and punishments (e.g., an award for zero workplace injuries in the past year)

3. Physical work setting (e.g., closed office doors, which suggest that managers are not open to hearing from employees)

4. Actions, words, and behaviors of informal leaders (e.g., Jenna, an informal leader on the third shift, tells a new employee, "We don't work too hard on this shift")

5. Actions, words, and behaviors of formal leaders (e.g., a vice president visits each of the HCO's nine community clinics every month)

6. Actions, words, and behaviors of employees (e.g., a bereavement counselor comforts family members)

7. Ceremonies, symbols, rituals, and activities (e.g., the Medical School dean presents diplomas at commencement)

8. Stories and legends (e.g., a favorite story in the maintenance department about Rick who "told it like it is" to the executive director)

9. Language (e.g., the sincere language used in the "Annual Report to Our Community")

SUBCULTURES

When everyone in the organization interprets the culture the same way and describes the culture in similar terms, the culture is strong and consistent. This type of culture has the advantages of employee harmony, working in the same direction, and presenting a

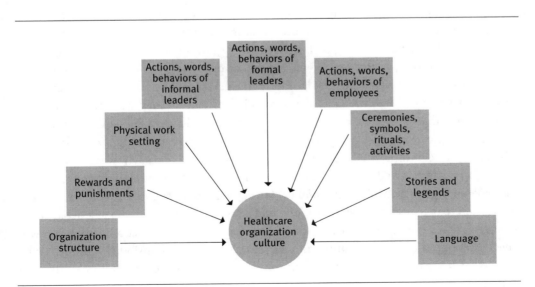

EXHIBIT 11.2
Model for Interpreting an HCO's Culture

consistent image to customers. However, a strong and consistent culture may have some disadvantages, too. Think about larger organizations with many departments that have different purposes and functions. In Chapter 4, we learned that because of the kind of work they do, some departments should be mechanistic whereas other departments should be organic. Thus, within the same organization, different departments may have different cultures. **Leaders should strive for the HCO to have a strong overall culture yet also allow for variation within departments that need their own subcultures.** For example, an accounting department has a bureaucratic, rule-driven culture, while the marketing department has a loose, creative culture. Yet both of these **subcultures** should support the overall organizational culture as much as possible.

Subculture

Culture of a distinct part of an organization (e.g., a department or team) that exists within the organization's culture.

HERE'S WHAT HAPPENED

James L. Zazzali and colleagues (2007) studied the satisfaction level of 1,593 physicians in 52 medical group practices across the United States. Organizational culture accounted for variances in their satisfaction levels. Group participatory culture was favorably linked to how satisfied physicians were with the human resources, technology, and price competition of their medical group. Hierarchical bureaucratic culture was unfavorably linked with how satisfied they were with management decision making, price competition, and practice competitiveness. Rational, task-oriented culture was unfavorably associated with physicians' satisfaction with human resources and price competition. Developmental risk-taking culture was not associated with physicians' satisfaction. The medical group practices displayed several different kinds of organizational culture. Those cultures were related to differences in how satisfied physicians felt about their group practice.

As we see in the preceding Here's What Happened, organizational culture affects physician satisfaction. This point is important for managers whose HCO is affiliating with physicians by buying or merging with their medical groups (a trend noted in Chapter 1). Hospitals and health systems usually have different organizational cultures than medical groups do—especially small medical groups with just a few physicians. In merger situations, managers must intentionally plan what kind of culture they want for the merged organization. Then they must decide to what extent they will allow subcultures to form— such as in acquired medical group practices. They must strive to develop (or, if it already exists, allow to continue) a culture that strengthens physician satisfaction.

Top managers and leaders must balance between (1) developing a strong, consistent, overall organizational culture and (2) letting individual facilities, subunits, departments, and teams develop their own individual subcultures. When you are a department manager, team captain, group leader, shift supervisor, or work unit coordinator, you will have to develop the right subculture for your unique area of responsibility (without drifting too far from the HCO's overall culture). The next section explains how to develop culture.

MANAGING AND SHAPING CULTURE

To successfully lead an organization, managers must deliberately shape and influence the culture so that it helps achieve the mission and goals. We can connect this task with strategic planning, which we studied in Chapter 3. Recall that in the "Where are we now?" (first) stage of planning, managers assess the organization's current mission, vision, and values. Let's consider a primary care group that is a traditional physician-centered practice in which physicians decide what to do for patients. The group analyzes its environment and realizes that stakeholders and the healthcare reform law are rewarding patient-centered medical homes. They realize that becoming a patient-centered practice is a great opportunity and say, "Let's do it!"

In the "Where should we be going?" (second) stage of planning, the managers set a goal to develop the patient-centered medical home approach. Pop quiz: What must happen in the third stage of strategic planning? Did you say "implementation"? If so, good for you! To implement the patient-centered medical home approach, the managers will have to change the culture from physician-centered to patient-centered. Physicians and other healthcare workers will have to think, feel, and behave differently than they do in their current, traditional approach. They will have to allow patients to join physicians as partners in deciding how to treat patients' medical problems. They will have to communicate more openly and completely with patients. These changes will require a different culture—a different "correct way to think, feel, and behave." Changing the culture will take time and effort for physicians and others who traditionally have been paternalistic (deciding *for* the patient) rather than patient-centered (deciding *with* the patient). If a medical group practice in Albany, Georgia, wants to become a patient-centered medical home, it will need a patient-centered culture to guide physicians and others to behave that way. Without the proper culture, managers will not be able to implement their planned goal. Culture will trump the strategy.

What tools and methods could managers use to implement a culture change so that the new patient-centered culture takes root in the medical group practice? How can managers and leaders shape their culture? (Hint: Look at Exhibit 11.1.) By managing the forces and factors that create the culture, managers can shift the culture to a different set of beliefs, norms, and values. For example, the medical group's managers can reward employees who involve patients as partners in patient-centered care. They could withhold rewards from those who cling to the old paternalistic approach. (Does this sound like motivation theory from Chapter 10?) Managers can train staff how to communicate more openly with patients by sharing clinical information that previously was kept from them. Managers can model the new culture by demonstrating patient-centered behavior in their daily work. They can state the new patient-centered values in the medical group's mission, vision, and values statements.

Top managers, such as those at Partners HealthCare in the opening Here's What Happened, implement culture changes for the HCO as a whole. Leaders of departments, groups, teams, committees, and smaller work units do the same for their parts of the organization. In implementing such changes, they must support the overall culture. Yet they must also consider the unique characteristics of their unit and perhaps create a sub-culture. As noted earlier, different departments might need different behaviors and norms to support their unique goals, stakeholders, and work methods. Lower-level managers and leaders must recognize this need.

Managers and leaders can shape and influence culture, though it takes persistent work. Premier Health Alliance is a national network of about 2,300 hospitals and 63,000 other healthcare facilities in the United States. It surveyed members about their experiences with implementing electronic health records in their HCOs. Changing from paper to electronic health records requires changes in norms, behaviors, values, and beliefs—a culture change. A prominent finding was that "cultural changes have proved to be far more challenging than technology issues or budgetary concerns" (DeVore and Figlioli 2010, 665).

"Clarifying the value system and breathing life into it are the greatest contributions a leader can make. Moreover, that's what the top people in the excellent companies seem to worry about most" (Peters and Waterman 1982, 291). Those words—still true today—come from the classic book *In Search of Excellence.* The book offered lessons for how to improve American industry after it lost its competitive edge to companies in other countries.

 TRY IT, APPLY IT

Suppose you work for Acme Medical Supply, Inc., which sells medical and health supplies to HCOs in a large metropolitan area. The company's 140 employees range in age from 18 to 67 and come from several generations. They don't work well together. For example, some workers disrespect older or younger workers. Some don't share information or cooperate. After declining service and sales, a new owner buys the company. The new owner thinks if employees work *with* others rather than *against* others, then sales and service will improve. List seven to ten suggestions for how Acme could change its culture to achieve the new owner's plans. Then, discuss your ideas with classmates.

Ethics
Values and moral principles about what is right and wrong.

Autonomy
An ethical principle that includes individual privacy, freedom of choice, and self-control.

WHAT IS ETHICS?

We now turn to ethics, which is part of values. We learned that values are part of culture, so ethics is also part of culture. **Ethics** is the set of values and moral principles someone holds about what is right and wrong (Daft 2013). These values and principles are essential. "Effective leaders are almost always values driven" (Dye 2010, xii.). Although there are many ethical principles for HCOs, Rosenau and Roemer (2008) identify three fundamental ones that have long guided healthcare services. The principle of **autonomy** includes

Exhibit 11.3
Types of Ethics in HCOs

Types of Ethics	Examples
Medical ethics guides right/wrong in the practice of medicine and clinical care	• Remove life support equipment from a terminally ill ICU patient • Conduct experimental medical research on humans in an academic medical center
Professional ethics guides right/wrong for a profession	• Maintain confidentiality of private information obtained in professional work • Act in the best interests of clients served by a counseling clinic (rather than act in one's personal best interests)
Managerial ethics guides right/wrong in the practice of management	• Make management decisions for the good of the wellness center (rather than just make the easiest decision) • Avoid false advertising of a nursing home's services
Social responsibility ethics guides right/wrong for the good of society	• Reduce the amount of toxic waste produced by the hospital • Provide unprofitable health services that the community needs

individual privacy, freedom of choice, and self-control. **Beneficence** includes doing good, not doing harm, and promoting the welfare of others. (Doing no harm is sometimes identified as a separate principle called *nonmaleficence*.) **Justice** includes fairness and equality.

In HCOs, ethical questions and situations arise often. Some are obvious (e.g., informed consent for a medical procedure) and some are subtle (e.g., what to tell the boss about a problem). Leaders and managers of HCOs must be concerned with **medical ethics**, **professional ethics**, **managerial ethics**, and **social responsibility**. Examples of these types of ethics are listed in Exhibit 11.3. Although each type is distinct, some types may overlap at times.

Ethics Problems

Every day, organizations, businesses, and HCOs deal with a wide range of situations involving ethical behavior and judgment. Managers do not always handle these situations well, as reflected in news headlines. HCOs deal with more ethical situations than many other organizations because of the ethics of medicine and health. Here are examples of ethical situations that arise in HCOs:

Beneficence
An ethical principle that includes doing good, not doing harm, and promoting the welfare of others.

Justice
An ethical principle that includes fairness and equality.

Medical ethics
Ethics that guide right and wrong in the practice of medicine.

Professional ethics
Ethics that guide right and wrong for a profession, such as the nursing profession.

Managerial ethics
Ethics that guide right and wrong in the practice of management.

Social responsibility
Ethics that guide right and wrong for the good of society.

◆ A medical director at a health insurance company must decide whether to cover experimental treatment for a cancer patient.

◆ A president, vice president of finance, and vice president of human resources at a medical supply company discuss which employees will be laid off.

◆ A physician worries that if she becomes employed by a healthcare system, she might be pressured to place profits above patient care.

◆ A hospital president realizes that more emphasis on population health would reduce needed revenue from a profitable hospital service.

◆ A long-term hospital patient tries to "friend" several physicians and nurses on Facebook.

◆ A surgeon must decide what to tell a man whose spouse was seriously harmed by a medical error.

◆ A clinic's marketing director considers exaggerating the benefits of a new pain therapy treatment.

◆ A professor of community health reviews assessment data and sees wide disparities in access to care and in health status.

◆ A new employee wonders if the HCO will keep the promises it made to him during the job interview.

◆ A manager of an indigent care clinic must decide how to use limited funds, staff, and facilities to care for its huge patient population.

◆ A board member wonders if the proposed costly merger would really achieve all the benefits and savings that consultants promised.

◆ A 16-year-old drug abuser is brought to the emergency department by his friends, who plead with the staff not to call his parents.

◆ A company, eager for a prominent physician to use its new product, invites the physician to speak at an all-expenses-paid conference in Hawaii.

Conflict of interest
A situation in which a person's self-interest interferes with that person's trusted obligation to another person, organization, profession, or purpose.

Ethical dilemma
A situation in which any decision or course of action will have an undesirable ethical outcome.

Moral distress
A situation in which an organization's constraints prevent a person from doing what she thinks is ethically right.

As the list shows, clinicians, managers, executives, and other HCO workers can face troubling ethical problems, questions, and uncertainty. Some involve a **conflict of interest**. An **ethical dilemma** is especially troubling because no matter what the worker does, someone will suffer. For example, some HCOs consider requiring all workers to get a flu shot to help protect patients. But some employees believe that mandatory flu shots violate their autonomy and self-determination (Nelson and Lahey 2013). Some employees struggle with **moral distress**, in which an organization's constraints prevent them from doing what they think is ethically right. (Hamric, Epstein, and White 2014). For example, a nurse is told to care for so many patients that she feels she cannot give them all the care they need. When these ethical problems are not handled well, they can harm workers and their HCOs. If Vince feels doubt about how to handle a difficult situation with ethical implications—such as mandatory flu shots or being assigned to care for too many patients—it creates stress and negative harmful emotions. The negatives can, in turn, cause job performance problems and perhaps cause a person to quit the job.

Managers and leaders in HCOs must strive to ensure that employees, physicians, volunteers, and others understand (and follow) appropriate ethics. In addition, managers should ensure that their HCOs have resources, structures, and processes to help people handle difficult ethical situations. These resources are needed to enable the HCO to achieve its mission, vision, values, and goals. The next section discusses how managers perform these tasks.

SOURCES OF ETHICS

In broad terms, the ethics of an HCO comes from three general sources:

1. The people in the organization

2. The organization's external environment

3. The organization itself

Ethics starts to develop early in people's lives. Take a few minutes to think of where your own ethics and morality came from. Perhaps they came from people who influenced you as you grew up—parents, relatives, peers, teachers, leaders of youth organizations, and religious and faith leaders. Even characters in novels, movies, and TV shows can influence what we view as right and wrong. How about laws and legal requirements? Yes, those shape our ethics as well. Maybe you thought of social norms and cultural values in the community where you grew up. Perhaps you sensed what was considered right and wrong based on who got in trouble at school. Some current events and news headlines also make us think about right and wrong.

Personal ethics and morals formed while growing up become part of a person's ethics at work. Thus, to create an ethical HCO, managers must try to hire people who already have the desired ethics. As discussed in Chapters 7 and 8, careful interviewing can help detect who is likely or unlikely to respect a patient's confidential information and how someone would respond to a salesman's offer of free tickets to a Boston Red Sox game.

Besides personal ethics that people bring into an HCO, sources outside of the HCO also affect what is deemed right and wrong in the organization. These sources include laws, regulations, court decisions, and Joint Commission accreditation standards, to name a few. We know that people bring their personal ethics to work and may also form work ethics based on ideas from external sources. Managers should realize that professional codes of ethics are external sources of ethics that guide members of many professions, such as nursing, engineering, pharmacy, accounting, occupational therapy, law, teaching, healthcare management, and other fields. Professional codes of ethical conduct may override an HCO's policies and guidelines when members of a profession feel more allegiance to their profession and its guidelines than to the HCO and its guidelines.

The American College of Healthcare Executives (ACHE) is the largest professional association for healthcare managers. Like some other professional organizations, the ACHE has carefully prepared a code of ethics that it distributes to its members. This code (see Exhibit 11.4) details the manager's ethical responsibilities to the profession, patients, organization, employees, and society. Take a few minutes to read the code to better understand managers' ethics in healthcare. Managers can use this code to guide appropriate managerial conduct for a wide range of ethical situations. Other professional associations, such as the Medical Group Management Association, the Healthcare Financial Management Association, and the Association of University Programs in Health Administration, also provide ethical guidance related to healthcare management. Some employers have created a social media code of conduct to help employees avoid violating ethical principles when using social media.

Exhibit 11.4 Code of Ethics of the American College of Healthcare Executives

American College of Healthcare Executives *Code of Ethics**

PREAMBLE

The purpose of the *Code of Ethics* of the American College of Healthcare Executives is to serve as a standard of conduct for members. It contains standards of ethical behavior for healthcare executives in their professional relationships. These relationships include colleagues, patients or others served; members of the healthcare executive's organization and other organizations; the community; and society as a whole.

The *Code of Ethics* also incorporates standards of ethical behavior governing individual behavior, particularly when that conduct directly relates to the role and identity of the healthcare executive.

The fundamental objectives of the healthcare management profession are to maintain or enhance the overall quality of life, dignity and well-being of every individual needing healthcare service and to create a more equitable, accessible, effective and efficient healthcare system.

Healthcare executives have an obligation to act in ways that will merit the trust, confidence, and respect of healthcare professionals and the general public. Therefore, healthcare executives should lead lives that embody an exemplary system of values and ethics.

In fulfilling their commitments and obligations to patients or others served, healthcare executives function as moral advocates and models. Since every management decision affects the health and well-being of both individuals and communities, healthcare executives must carefully evaluate the

* As amended by the Board of Governors on November 14, 2011.

(continued)

Exhibit 11.4
Code of Ethics
of the American
College of
Healthcare
Executives
(continued)

possible outcomes of their decisions. In organizations that deliver healthcare services, they must work to safeguard and foster the rights, interests and prerogatives of patients or others served.

The role of moral advocate requires that healthcare executives take actions necessary to promote such rights, interests and prerogatives.

Being a model means that decisions and actions will reflect personal integrity and ethical leadership that others will seek to emulate.

I. THE HEALTHCARE EXECUTIVE'S RESPONSIBILITIES TO THE PROFESSION OF HEALTHCARE MANAGEMENT

The healthcare executive shall:

A. Uphold the *Code of Ethics* and mission of the American College of Healthcare Executives;

B. Conduct professional activities with honesty, integrity, respect, fairness and good faith in a manner that will reflect well upon the profession;

C. Comply with all laws and regulations pertaining to healthcare management in the jurisdictions in which the healthcare executive is located or conducts professional activities;

D. Maintain competence and proficiency in healthcare management by implementing a personal program of assessment and continuing professional education;

E. Avoid the improper exploitation of professional relationships for personal gain;

F. Disclose financial and other conflicts of interest;

G. Use this *Code* to further the interests of the profession and not for selfish reasons;

H. Respect professional confidences;

I. Enhance the dignity and image of the healthcare management profession through positive public information programs; and

J. Refrain from participating in any activity that demeans the credibility and dignity of the healthcare management profession.

II. THE HEALTHCARE EXECUTIVE'S RESPONSIBILITIES TO PATIENTS OR OTHERS SERVED

The healthcare executive shall, within the scope of his or her authority:

A. Work to ensure the existence of a process to evaluate the quality of care or service rendered;

B. Avoid practicing or facilitating discrimination and institute safeguards to prevent discriminatory organizational practices;

C. Work to ensure the existence of a process that will advise patients or others served of the rights, opportunities, responsibilities and risks regarding available healthcare services;

(continued)

EXHIBIT 11.4
Code of Ethics
of the American
College of
Healthcare
Executives
(continued)

D. Work to ensure that there is a process in place to facilitate the resolution of conflicts that may arise when values of patients and their families differ from those of employees and physicians;

E. Demonstrate zero tolerance for any abuse of power that compromises patients or others served;

F. Work to provide a process that ensures the autonomy and self-determination of patients or others served;

G. Work to ensure the existence of procedures that will safeguard the confidentiality and privacy of patients or others served; and

H. Work to ensure the existence of an ongoing process and procedures to review, develop and consistently implement evidence-based clinical practices throughout the organization.

III. THE HEALTHCARE EXECUTIVE'S RESPONSIBILITIES TO THE ORGANIZATION

The healthcare executive shall, within the scope of his or her authority:

A. Provide healthcare services consistent with available resources, and when there are limited resources, work to ensure the existence of a resource allocation process that considers ethical ramifications;

B. Conduct both competitive and cooperative activities in ways that improve community healthcare services;

C. Lead the organization in the use and improvement of standards of management and sound business practices;

D. Respect the customs and practices of patients or others served, consistent with the organization's philosophy;

E. Be truthful in all forms of professional and organizational communication, and avoid disseminating information that is false, misleading or deceptive;

F. Report negative financial and other information promptly and accurately, and initiate appropriate action;

G. Prevent fraud and abuse and aggressive accounting practices that may result in disputable financial reports;

H. Create an organizational environment in which both clinical and management mistakes are minimized and, when they do occur, are disclosed and addressed effectively;

I. Implement an organizational code of ethics and monitor compliance; and

J. Provide ethics resources and mechanisms for staff to address ethical organizational and clinical issues.

(continued)

EXHIBIT 11.4
Code of Ethics
of the American
College of
Healthcare
Executives
(continued)

IV. THE HEALTHCARE EXECUTIVE'S RESPONSIBILITIES TO EMPLOYEES

Healthcare executives have ethical and professional obligations to the employees they manage that encompass but are not limited to:

A. Creating a work environment that promotes ethical conduct;

B. Providing a work environment that encourages a free expression of ethical concerns and provides mechanisms for discussing and addressing such concerns;

C. Promoting a healthy work environment, which includes freedom from harassment, sexual and other, and coercion of any kind, especially to perform illegal or unethical acts;

D. Promoting a culture of inclusivity that seeks to prevent discrimination on the basis of race, ethnicity, religion, gender, sexual orientation, age or disability;

E. Providing a work environment that promotes the proper use of employees' knowledge and skills; and

F. Providing a safe and healthy work environment.

V. THE HEALTHCARE EXECUTIVE'S RESPONSIBILITIES TO COMMUNITY AND SOCIETY

The healthcare executive shall:

A. Work to identify and meet the healthcare needs of the community;

B. Work to support access to healthcare services for all people;

C. Encourage and participate in public dialogue on healthcare policy issues, and advocate solutions that will improve health status and promote quality healthcare;

D. Apply short- and long-term assessments to management decisions affecting both community and society; and

E. Provide prospective patients and others with adequate and accurate information, enabling them to make enlightened decisions regarding services.

VI. THE HEALTHCARE EXECUTIVE'S RESPONSIBILITY TO REPORT VIOLATIONS OF THE *CODE*

A member of ACHE who has reasonable grounds to believe that another member has violated this *Code* has a duty to communicate such facts to the Ethics Committee.

SOURCE: Reprinted by permission of the American College of Healthcare Executives (2011).

What is the third source of ethics in an HCO? The HCO itself. Think back to the earlier part of this chapter. We learned that an organization's culture includes values, and values include ethics. The ethical climate is the "shared perceptions of how ethical issues should be addressed and what is ethically correct behavior for the organization" (Rorty

2014, 12). This part of the culture—the ethical climate—can strongly influence HCO employees and shapes their sense of right and wrong in the HCO. An HCO will decide on certain ethical principles and emphasize them. The principles become part of the ethical climate and organizational culture that evolve over time. These principles may be decided at a strategic planning retreat, approved in a staff meeting, declared by the chief executive officer following a crisis, identified while developing organizational culture, advocated by an employee, developed after ethics problems, or determined in other ways.

However, an HCO faces barriers when developing, maintaining, and actually behaving according to an appropriate ethical climate (Mills 2014):

- Many employees feel allegiance to the ethics of their professions and subcultures.

- Employees are culturally diverse, and what seems right to some employees may seem wrong to others.

- Many stakeholders exert pressures and demands on HCOs and push and pull it in different directions.

CREATING AND MAINTAINING ETHICS IN AN HCO

The top leaders and managers of an HCO are responsible for creating and maintaining the ethics of the organization. However, they do not, and should not, make all the decisions about ethical issues that arise in the HCO. **Senior managers should create organizational structures, processes, and cultures that enable managers, supervisors, employees, physicians, staff, and others at all levels of the organization to make ethics decisions in their areas of responsibility.** Senior managers take the lead in creating and maintaining ethics for the entire HCO; managers at lower levels take the lead in their own departments and work units. For example, the president of Apple Health Insurance is responsible for the ethical performance of the entire company. Shannon, the company's small business sales supervisor, is responsible for ethical performance of her sales team.

How can leaders create structures, processes, and cultures to strengthen ethical performance throughout their HCOs? Think back to earlier parts of this chapter and to prior chapters to fully appreciate the approaches listed in Exhibit 11.5.

Looking ahead to Chapter 13 on decision making, managers can use decision-making principles, tools, and methods for ethical decisions. Leaders must create a fair process in which decision makers carefully consider the views and values of all stakeholders who might be affected by a decision. When there is an ethical dilemma, decision makers must understand and reflect on conflicting views and values. Before making a decision, the decision makers must also consider the consequences of possible decisions and how they would affect all stakeholders. These procedures ensure that the conflicting values of

Approach	Principles, Tools, and Methods
Organizing the HCO	• Organize work, tasks, positions, groups, systems, and resources to support the HCO's ethics, and support people dealing with ethical questions. • Organize an ethics advisory committee or create an ethicist position to advise employees, physicians, supervisors, and others who want help with ethical dilemmas or distress. The committee or position should be available for all HCO-related ethics situations (not just medical ones). • Write and promote ethics rules, policies, processes, procedures, and a code of ethics—all to guide employees in ethical situations. Ensure that the documents are based on input from appropriate stakeholders rather than from just managers or certain interests. Include processes for how to avoid ethical problems, how to reach out for help (e.g., to an advisory committee) when ethical questions arise, and how to make ethical decisions. • Appoint a compliance officer or position. Monitor compliance and the HCO's ethical performance. Hold employees and others accountable for compliance with ethical standards, principles, policies, and codes. • Organize hotlines and whistle-blower mechanisms and processes for employees to report possible violations of the HCO's ethics. When violations are reported or found through monitoring, investigate and take appropriate action to prevent reoccurrence. Follow up with involved stakeholders. • Allocate sufficient resources to implement the structures, processes, positions, policies, and ethical climate for the intended ethical performance. To the extent possible, strive to allocate available resources in such a way that ethical problems, dilemmas, and distress are lessened.
Staffing the HCO	• Write job descriptions to reflect or even explicitly state ethical principles. • Award merit pay, incentives, and other compensation to influence positive ethics. • In annual performance reviews, evaluate workers for how well they follow ethical standards. Evaluate managers for how well they and their staffs follow ethical principles. • During orientation of new staff, emphasize ethical principles and explain how to get help when facing ethical questions.

EXHIBIT 11.5
Approaches to Creating and Maintaining Ethics

(continued)

Approach	Principles, Tools, and Methods
Staffing the HCO *(continued)*	• Train and educate staff about the HCO's ethical climate and principles. Ensure employees know the structures, processes, and resources available for how to handle ethical situations. • Require managers to do an ethics self-assessment annually to monitor their own ethics and identify possible improvements. • Ensure that employees feel safe when asking ethics questions or reporting ethics violations. • Provide counseling to employees, such as for moral distress, post-traumatic stress, or grief related to ethics situations.
Leading the HCO	• State clearly and often the HCO's ethics and ethical climate. • Be a role model of the HCO's ethics. Live the HCO's ethics. Personally support the desired ethics—even if that is politically difficult because of stakeholder disagreement. • Lead the development of an appropriate ethical culture and climate. Create a culture in which asking ethical questions and discussing ethics problems becomes "the way we do things here." Avoid a culture that emphasizes teamwork so much that an employee who has ethical concerns remains silent in order to be a team player. • When leading meetings, allow time for participants to ask questions and express concerns about the ethics of an issue or decision. • Motivate employees by using reinforcement, goal setting, Maslow's needs, and other approaches to drive ethical behavior. • Use a leader's power: Highly ethical leaders may have referent charismatic power (in addition to other powers) when influencing others about ethics. • Regularly monitor the ethical performance of the HCO.

Procedural justice
A process to resolve
ethical conflicts based
on fair procedures that
consider competing
values of all affected
groups.

the people who will be affected are considered *before* the decision is made. That approach supports fair ethical decisions and is known as **procedural justice**. "At the foundation of organizational ethical decision making is the application of procedural justice—organizations should rely on a deliberative process to foster fairness through a clear understanding of all competing values in response to a particular ethical conflict" (Nelson 2005, 9). This approach would be useful for responding to the types of future challenges, issues, and developments identified in Chapter 1—such as health disparities, mergers, population trends, use of social media, patients' engagement in their health, physician employment, reducing costs, and genetics in healthcare. A final step that leaders can take to strengthen ethics in their HCOs is to establish procedural justice to guide managers, committees, and others in making ethical decisions. Chapter 13 explains more about how to make such decisions.

Managers can use many tools and methods to lead with—and enhance the ethics of—their HCOs. Clarifying the value system and breathing life into it is especially important (Peters and Waterman 1982), as are incentives and celebrating the right behavior (Gilbert 2013). Managers must lead with their values and ethics—even when it seems difficult and requires "going against" the crowd.

 CHECK IT OUT

The American College of Healthcare Executives (ACHE) provides many resources to its members, some of which are available at its website. An Ethics Self-Assessment survey is available at www.ache.org/newclub/career/ethself.cfm. This survey poses statements to rate yourself on, such as, "I fulfill the promises I make" and "I respect the practices and customs of a diverse patient population while maintaining the organization's mission." Healthcare managers can use the Ethics Self-Assessment to consider their own ethics related to healthcare leadership. Students can use it to learn more about ethics in HCOs.

ONE MORE TIME

Culture in an organization is the shared and learned values, norms, guiding beliefs, and understanding among the organization's members. It evolves from forces inside and outside the organization. Because an HCO's culture is mostly invisible, employees interpret it by observing and listening to what goes on in the HCO. Culture strongly affects staff behavior, goal achievement, stakeholders' satisfaction, and the HCO's performance and survival. To successfully lead an organization, managers must deliberately shape and influence the organization's culture so that it becomes what they think is best for the organization, given its environment, mission, goals, plans, and so forth. Culture change is not easy, but it can be done by managing the forces and factors that affect the culture. Managers and leaders should try to develop a strong, consistent culture throughout the entire HCO. Yet, they must also let departments, work units, and teams develop their own subcultures (within the main culture) that are best for these individual parts of the organization.

An organization's culture includes its ethics, which are moral principles of right and wrong. Managerial ethics, medical ethics, professional ethics, and social responsibility ethics are all important for HCOs. In HCOs, ethics come from personal ethics of staff (especially leaders), external sources such as accreditation standards and laws, and the organization itself. Leaders can use management tools and methods to shape ethics and culture.

FOR YOUR TOOLBOX

- Model of forces and factors that influence HCO culture
- Model for interpreting an HCO's culture
- Code of ethics
- Procedural justice
- Approaches to creating and maintaining ethics

FOR DISCUSSION

1. Discuss the factors that shape culture in HCOs. Why do individual HCOs have different cultures?

2. How can you interpret the culture of an organization? Interpret the culture of your college or university.

3. Describe examples of subcultures within an HCO culture. What are the pros and cons of having subcultures?

4. Discuss examples of medical ethics, professional ethics, and managerial ethics in HCOs.

5. Discuss ethical problems you have heard of in the news. Why do you think these problems occurred?

6. Which approaches for creating and maintaining ethics in HCOs do you think are most important? Why?

7. What captured your interest in the ACHE Code of Ethics? How do you feel about the ethical responsibilities of the healthcare management profession?

CASE STUDY QUESTIONS

These questions refer to the Integrative Case Studies at the back of this book.

1. I Can't Do It All case: How would you describe the organizational culture of Healthdyne? Using Exhibit 11.1, identify specific forces and factors that Mr. Brice could manage to change the culture.

2. Taking Care of Business at Graceland Memorial Hospital case: Analyze this case by considering possible problems of medical ethics, professional ethics, managerial ethics, and social responsibility. What are some possible ethical questions or problems?

3. Disparities in Care at Southern Regional Health System case: Suppose the health system sets a goal of reducing disparities by 15 percent during the next three years. Identify ethical questions and concerns pertaining to autonomy, beneficence, and justice.

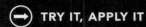 TRY IT, APPLY IT

Return to the Ethics Problems section of this chapter and review the examples of ethical situations that arise in HCOs. Then return to Exhibit 11.5 and review approaches managers can use to create and maintain ethical behavior in their HCOs. Which approaches, principles, tools, and methods would you use for specific ethical situations? Discuss your ideas with classmates and justify your answers.

CHAPTER 12

CONTROLLING AND IMPROVING PERFORMANCE

You can't manage what you don't measure.

Common management expression

Studying this chapter will help you to

➤ define and describe control;

➤ identify types of performance that managers must control in healthcare organizations;

➤ explain how managers control organizational performance;

➤ describe a three-step approach for control; and

➤ explain control tools and techniques.

HERE'S WHAT HAPPENED

Managers measured the performance of Partners HealthCare and realized not all expectations were met. Some aspects of performance did not compare well to standards and expected performance levels. At Faulkner Hospital (part of the Partners health system), 27 percent of discharged heart failure patients had to be readmitted within 30 days. That outcome was too high and worse than the national rate. Managers saw a need to improve quality of patient care for heart failure. They redesigned the patient care process for treating heart problems and then continued to measure outcomes. The redesign used telehealth to enable Partners' staff to monitor heart patients at home after discharge from the hospital. In this new approach, staff also taught patients self-care for their heart problems so they could stay healthy. After making the improvements, managers continued to measure readmission rates. They also measured other aspects of performance, such as how much patients learned about their heart failure, were able to control their heart health problem, and were confident they could independently manage their heart failure. Results showed a 51 percent decrease in heart failure readmissions, high patient satisfaction, and $8,155 net savings per patient because of reduced readmissions.

As evident in the preceding Here's What Happened, managers must control their organization's performance. Partners' managers realized some performance was "out of control" when they compared actual results to planned results. So they made changes to improve performance, remeasured the results, and brought performance "in control."

How do managers control and improve performance? This chapter explains how. The chapter begins by defining and describing the management control function. Controlling and improving performance is the fifth and final management function (as we learned in Chapter 2), and it interacts with the other four functions. It is part of four of the ten managerial roles identified by Henry Mintzberg (described in Chapter 2): the roles of monitor, entrepreneur, disturbance handler, and resource allocator. Next, the chapter discusses types of performance that managers must control in healthcare organizations (HCOs) and explains how managers control organizational performance using a three-step approach plus some interesting control tools. The chapter concludes with information about controlling quality, which is an especially important kind of performance that stakeholders demand be better controlled in HCOs.

WHAT IS CONTROL?

"Controlling is an essential function for all managers in the organization by which they monitor performance and take corrective action when needed" (Dunn 2010, 585). When is corrective action needed? **When performance does not meet expectations and standards, managers must make corrections.** Thus, managers do three things to **control** performance:

Control
To monitor performance and take corrective action if performance does not meet expected standards.

1. Set standards and expectations.

2. Monitor and judge performance compared to the standards and expectations.

3. Make improvements if standards and expectations are not met well enough.

What are some examples of control? A thermostat is a mechanical device that controls the performance of a heating/cooling system to achieve a preset expected temperature. In this example, there is one dimension of performance: temperature. Often, we are interested in several dimensions of performance, such as when we drive a car and control it. The car itself measures its speed, fuel consumption, engine temperature, and other dimensions of performance. We measure other dimensions, such as the direction of travel, the comfort level, and our progress toward the expected destination. We compare the speed measurements to speed standards posted on signs, and we adjust the car's performance if necessary. We steer the car so that it performs according to the expectations we have based on Google Maps. All these actions enable us to control *multiple dimensions of performance* to accomplish our goal of getting to work/class/home safely, on time, and without a speeding ticket. The driving example involves both mechanical and human control systems.

Organizations are not machines. They are composed of people rather than machine parts, which makes control more challenging. Fortunately, effective methods are available that managers can use to control their organizations. The methods are not as simple and as responsive as turning a steering wheel or stepping on a brake pedal. However, they do work. We next examine dimensions of control in HCOs and then study control methods for HCOs. Although managers do not use a steering wheel, they do use management tools to steer their HCOs. What have you already learned from this book that you could use to steer performance in an HCO? Try to list at least five tools.

CONTROL IN HCOS

HCOs constantly control many dimensions of their performance. Name an HCO, and then list a few dimensions of performance you think it should control. (Hints: Think of the six aims of *Crossing the Quality Chasm* that were reported in a Chapter 5 Check It Out box, and reread the Here's What Happened at the beginning of this chapter.) Here are some types of performance that HCOs control:

◆   Costs, productivity, efficiency, and value

◆   Customer satisfaction, convenience, quality, safety, and waiting time

◆   Employee satisfaction, morale, retention, and growth

The Institute of Medicine (2001) set six goals for the US healthcare system to "cross the quality chasm" and become more efficient, effective, equitable, safe, timely, and patient centered. The healthcare system and many HCOs are trying to control and improve these six aspects of performance (McKinney 2011). The HCOs also control financial performance, such as measuring actual spending, comparing it to a budgeted amount, and then adjusting spending if it is too far from budget. (Perhaps you use this approach for your own spending.)

Another view of control in HCOs involves three dimensions of performance that all managers should know: structure, process, and outcome. These dimensions were developed by Avedis Donabedian (1966) primarily for medical care but then were extended to other kinds of work.

◆ **Structure measures**: These measures include available resources, staff, equipment, competencies, inputs, facilities, and characteristics of the HCO. They reflect how the organization is (or was) set up (but before someone presses the "on" button). The rehabilitation facility is accredited, the medical group has electronic health records, and the public health department has two health inspectors.

◆ **Process measures**: These measures include what work is (was) done and how, as well as what activities are (were) involved. They reflect the HCO in action (after someone presses the "on" button). The outpatient surgery center verified insurance information for 87 percent of its patients, the hospital made 17 medication errors, and the telehealth program remotely monitors the pulse and blood pressure readings of 349 rural patients.

◆ **Outcome measures**: These measures include what happens (happened) as a result of the structures and processes. They reflect the results and effects. The physician group achieved 5 percent growth in pediatric market share, 90 percent of cardiac rehabilitation patients were able to return to work, and 12 percent of hospital patients were readmitted within 30 days.

Structure measures
Measures of resources, staff, equipment, competencies, inputs, facilities, and characteristics of the organization; how the organization is set up.

Process measures
Measures of the work that is done, how it is done, and the activities performed.

Outcome measures
Measures of results and effects.

Managers traditionally focused on structure measures because they could be more easily controlled (Flood, Zinn, and Scott 2006). Patient care workers focused on process measures because they could control their work activities. Patients paid the most attention to their outcomes. Today, stakeholders are focusing more on outcomes. As we learned in Chapter 1, stakeholders have begun actively holding HCOs accountable for better value (an outcome). This practice will become more common in the future. HCOs' performance will become more transparent (open and visible) as more assessment data are made available online for everyone to see. This trend will drive HCOs to further analyze, redesign, and improve healthcare structures and processes for better outcomes: value, quality, and cost.

To control the performance of an entire HCO, managers must control the structure, process, and outcome performance of individual parts of the HCO. These parts include departments (e.g., laboratory), work units (e.g., microbiology), shifts (e.g., second shift), and workers (e.g., lab tech). Managers must also control how the many parts work together (the coordination we studied in Chapter 5) because organizations are systems of interrelated parts (as we learned in Chapter 4). **Managers should realize that quality problems are often caused by the system rather than by a person.** Quality expert W. Edwards Deming believed that only about 15 percent of quality problems were caused by faulty workers, whereas the other 85 percent were caused by faulty systems, processes, and management (Warren 2014). In HCOs, managers are realizing this situation and adjusting how they manage their organization and how they try to improve quality. For example, at Moses Cone Health System in Greensboro, North Carolina, leaders have created a "just culture" of justice and fairness for quality problems. This approach holds employees responsible for their own gross misconduct and negligence but not for system problems and errors beyond their control, such as those resulting from faulty work processes. When a serious patient safety problem occurred at Moses Cone, managers recognized that it was because of how the work processes were designed. They took responsibility for redesigning the work processes rather than blaming an individual therapist. In the long run, this approach allows everyone to be more open in identifying and fixing system problems without fear of blame and punishment (Birk 2010).

A Three-Step Control Method

Managers can use three steps for control. These steps should be viewed as a continual cycle because the steps never stop.

Step 1: Set Standards and Expectations

Managers often set standards and expectations when they perform other management functions. In Chapter 3 we learned that managers plan goals and decide what they want to accomplish during the next year, month, week, shift, and so forth. During implementation planning and project planning, they set targets such as

- 50 clients per day;
- at least 4 percent return on investment this fiscal year; and
- new building space leased by June 1.

Suppose Greg manages a community health education center in Omaha, Nebraska. He sets expectations for which classes will be offered, when each new class will begin, and how many people will enroll in each class. Greg creates standards when he organizes jobs and work, such as a standard of 24 hours to respond to a customer's inquiry. He sets staffing targets, such as less than 10 percent annual employee turnover. Managers like Greg should make their targets SMART: specific, measurable, achievable, realistic, and time related.

Managers set targets, expectations, and standards based on external and internal factors. External factors include accreditation standards, licensure requirements, government regulations, and industry standards. For example, The Joint Commission, the International Organization for Standardization, and the Malcolm Baldrige National Quality Award all have criteria for quality in HCOs. **Benchmarks** are best practices among a group of HCOs, such as best cancer survival rates and best employee satisfaction scores. Websites now publicly report data about HCOs' prices, quality, outcomes, and other measures. Managers might ask, "What are our competitors doing, and what do our customers expect?" to understand the expectations for performance targets. All these external sources of data and information influence managers as they set their performance targets.

Benchmark
The best level of performance for a group.

Internal factors are also considered when setting expectations and targets. Managers must consider costs and how much money they have to spend, which leads to setting spending targets and budgets. They consider internal leadership capabilities and organization culture that influence goals and targets. Recall from Chapter 3 that the strategic planning process requires an HCO to identify its strengths and weaknesses. Managers must consider these factors when setting a realistic target (rather than a wild dream).

Stakeholders—both internal and external—influence managers as they set targets and expectations. Internally, if employees express frequent complaints about parking and demand improvement, managers may set targets of adding 50 parking spaces by December 1 and increasing employees' satisfaction with parking to 90 percent. Externally, when lenders set target dates for repayment of loans, a physician recruiting company must accept those targets. **Managers should consider expectations of stakeholders when setting targets for performance.**

After considering external and internal factors, managers set targets and expectations for the future. The targets are reflected in organization documents, such as budgets, staffing plans, job descriptions, policies, rules, inventory stock levels, and Gantt charts. Some documents are formal, such as the strategic plan and official budget. Others are casual, such as a handwritten note saying, "Answer the phone before the third ring."

STEP 2: MONITOR AND JUDGE PERFORMANCE

The second step in control is to judge performance by comparing "actual" to "expected."

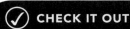

CHECK IT OUT

As part of control, managers compare performance of their HCO with that of similar HCOs. One way they compare is by using publicly available online data. These data are provided so that people can be better informed when they buy and consume healthcare. Managers of HCOs can use other HCOs' data to see how well the organization is doing, find the "best" performance in the area, and determine what might be a reasonable target to strive for next year. One national website, Hospital Compare (www.hospitalcompare.hhs.gov), offers performance data that one can use to compare hospitals in an area for specific types of clinical care. Many states provide comparative benchmarks and performance data for hospitals, nursing homes, surgery centers, home care agencies, or physician practices. Two examples are Florida Health Finder (www.floridahealthfinder.gov) and Illinois Hospital Report Card (www.healthcarereportcard.illinois.gov).

Suppose Nina manages a clinic in Tallahassee, Florida. While preparing a budget, she remembers that she had previously set a target of serving 25 patients per day at her clinic. Now she wonders how her clinic is doing. She must measure the actual number of clinic patients served per day and compare that number to 25 to determine if performance was better than, worse than, or equal to the target.

As a manager, you will be responsible for measuring performance in your area of responsibility. If you do not measure how your department is doing, you cannot successfully manage it (as the quote that begins this chapter tells us). Which measures are best? It all depends, of course! As a manager you will help decide which dimensions of performance should be measured and controlled.

There are many ways of measuring and presenting data to monitor performance and comparing it to expectations, standards, and targets. Measures should provide useful information and be accurate, easily understood, calculated the same way over time, and easily available (Spath 2013). Managers often use quantitative measures, such as counts, frequencies, percentages, ratios, averages, and other numerical data. These data can be presented in charts, graphs, tables, and other visual displays that help managers see the main points. Examples are shown in Exhibits 12.1 through 12.5.

Some people say that every picture tells a story. One textbook author says that every chart, graph, and exhibit tells a story. What story do you think is told by each of these exhibits? Managers use a line graph (sometimes called a run chart) to show performance data trends, such as trends for communicating X-ray reports (Exhibit 12.1). Managers use a bar graph (sometimes called a bar chart) to show and compare performance data, such as performance data for multiple hospital units (Exhibit 12.2). Managers use a pie chart to show how all performance data are divided into data categories—for example, how all patient complaints are divided into five categories of complaints (Exhibit 12.3). Managers use a control chart to show actual performance data and trends—such as actual rejected

Exhibit 12.1
Line Graph or
Run Chart

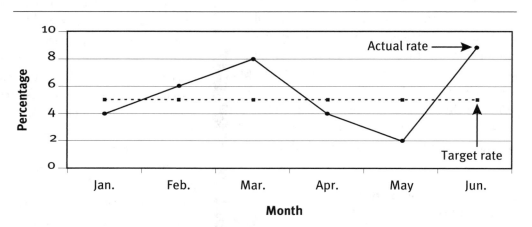

SOURCE: Spath (2013).

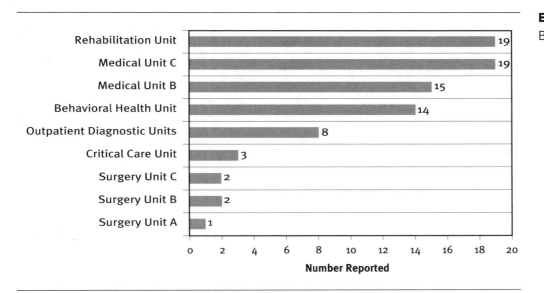

EXHIBIT 12.2
Bar Chart

SOURCE: Spath (2013).

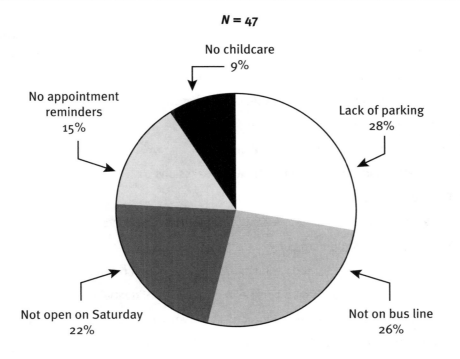

EXHIBIT 12.3
Pie Chart

SOURCE: Spath (2013).

EXHIBIT 12.4
Control Chart

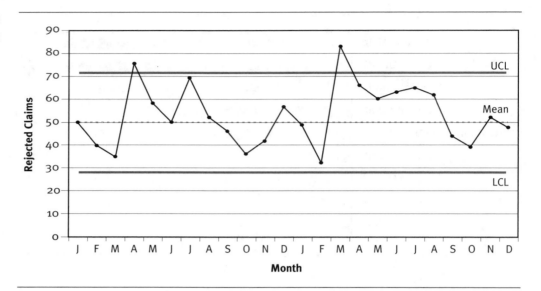

SOURCE: Spath (2013).

EXHIBIT 12.5
Table of Data

Survey Questions	Mean Score N = 47
Overall, how would you evaluate:	
1. The quality of the mental health services you received	3.5
2. The helpfulness of the staff members	3.0
3. The courtesy shown you by the staff members	3.8
4. Staff's attention to privacy during treatment sessions	4.0
5. The professionalism of the staff members	3.9
6. The extent to which your mental health needs were addressed	3.6
7. The availability of appointments	3.5
8. The effectiveness of the medication and/or treatment you received	3.8
9. The degree to which staff members respected your confidentiality	4.1
10. Opportunities to participate in decisions about your treatment	3.9
Scale: 1 = Poor 2 = Fair 3 = Good 4 = Very Good 5 = Excellent	

SOURCE: Spath (2013).

insurance claims—compared to performance standards. An upper control limit (UCL) and lower control limit (LCL) (shown in Exhibit 12.4 as thick gray lines) define the range within which performance is considered normal. Within this range, performance can vary and still be considered normal (Spath 2013). A center mean line (shown in Exhibit 12.4 as a dashed gray center line) is another standard for comparison. Managers use a tabular report (sometimes called a table of data) to show performance data, such as patient satisfaction results, in a readable format (Exhibit 12.5). Another example of a tabular report is shown in Exhibit 5 of the Partners HealthCare case, which appears in an appendix at the back of this book.

Many HCOs use scorecards and dashboards to report performance measures in a single report. These graphics generally report performance for a specific period, such as a day, a month, or a year. They may show any number of measures (e.g., the ones found throughout this chapter), depending on which measures managers decide to include. The graphics can be produced by computer software and easily revised to show different measures selected by the managers at any level of an HCO. **Balanced scorecards** were first developed in the 1990s to present a balanced view of an organization, rather than only a financial view. The scorecards typically include measures in four categories (Kaplan and Norton 1996):

1. Financial (e.g., revenue and return on investment)

2. Customer service (e.g., new customers and client satisfaction)

3. Internal business processes (e.g., inventory levels and production errors)

4. Potential for growth and learning (e.g., new services and employee retention)

Balanced scorecards
Reports with performance measures for finances, customer service, internal business processes, and growth/learning; other kinds of measures may be used.

Some HCOs use more categories to focus on additional dimensions of performance. Managers can add measures that are important and remove measures that have become less urgent. For example, at a home health care business that is near bankruptcy, managers could include "cash on hand" and "billed revenue" in the dashboard or scorecard. After the business becomes more financially stable, they could remove those measures and replace them with newer measures, such as "patient engagement."

Where do all the data for these graphics come from? Managers can gather data from inside their HCO as well as from outside sources. Internally, medical records, financial accounts, and registration files have lots of data about customers and services. Departmental records have data about the work that is produced (e.g., lab tests, webpages, surgical procedures, medical supplies, meals). Many data are automatically entered into digital databases that managers can search. More data are available through surveys, such as patient satisfaction surveys and employee attitude surveys. These surveys might be quantitative, with check boxes or numerical ratings (e.g., scale of 1 to 5). Or, they might be qualitative, allowing for comments and explanations beyond a single number. Qualitative data also come from organized focus groups, customer interviews, conversations, tweets, phone calls, e-mail, and other feedback from stakeholders. Managers obtain external data from licensure agencies, accreditation surveys, government databases, customers, supply chain partners, and other stakeholders and sources.

HCOs are using digital "big data" tools to quickly gather, sort, combine, and analyze enormous amounts of data from internal and external sources. Managers use what they learn from big data analytics to then improve performance. The examples that follow describe how managers use data analytics to manage HCOs (May 2014):

◆ At Memorial Healthcare System in Broward County, Florida, managers combine multiple data sources and then use predictive modeling algorithms to forecast utilization of health services during the next five years. This practice enables managers to better plan strategy and resources.

◆ At Memorial Healthcare System in Broward County, Florida, managers check the many suppliers of each of its HCOs against hundreds of external databases to identify potential fraud, conflicts of interest, and other problems.

◆ At Beth Israel Deaconess Medical Center in Boston, managers improve population health in a community by identifying members of an accountable care organization who did not have colorectal cancer screenings and then using targeted letters and calls to reach them.

If you take a job in an existing department or program, there will probably be some measurement systems in place (although you might want to update them). If you are helping to start a new program or HCO, you will have to create systems to gather performance data. Some data capture could be centralized for the whole HCO, such as for patient billing. Other data capture might be decentralized to individual departments, such as recording numbers of departmental procedures done per day. You may have to set up data records for customer complaints, waiting times, and procedure completion times.

Nowadays, many data are automatically captured by computers, barcode scanners, and other devices. Automatic data capture can help, but it can also create problems if too many unnecessary data are captured and reported for managers to sort through. Data for some measures might not be easily available because they are confidential, scattered across many departments, or not routinely collected. Will you have to set up new data collection processes? If so, will employees feel these processes waste their time by interfering with their "real" work? Good, valid, reliable data are usually not free, so managers must ensure the value of the data exceeds the cost of accurately collecting and processing it.

STEP 3: MAKE IMPROVEMENTS WITH CORRECTIVE ACTION

When the second control step (monitoring) shows performance does not meet expectations, then managers must take the third control step—corrective action. Managers must correct the performance problems and steer the HCO toward the expected performance standards. **Corrections can be made by applying the management tools, methods, principles, theories, and techniques discussed in earlier chapters.**

Managers can reconsider the goals and expectations set in the planning stage and decide if they are still realistic. Maybe a law changed or a new competitor emerged. Perhaps managers were far too optimistic in setting goals (as often happens). For many reasons, managers might realize that a target or expectation should be changed. (Of course, managers should not simply change the target every time performance misses the target!)

When managers feel their targets are reasonable and should be maintained, then they must change the organization's structure, processes, culture, staff, or other components that will lead to satisfactory performance. What are some possibilities? Think back to previous chapters. Managers might have to adjust the job design, work design, organization design, decentralization, standardization, coordination, culture, motivation, training, staffing ratios, schedules, rules, processes, performance appraisals, and motivations. Review the For Your Toolbox at the end of each chapter and the defined terms throughout the chapters to think of other possibilities. Remember that HCOs are systems of interrelated, interdependent parts. If one part is changed, other parts will be affected and might also have to change for the system to perform well.

Researchers have studied the "unfulfilled promises" of healthcare information technology systems (Kellermann and Jones 2013). Why did actual performance not match the expected performance of these systems? Because human work processes were not changed to fit the new technology. For HCOs and their new technological systems to reach performance targets, work processes had to be redesigned, workers had to be trained in the new processes, and incentives had to be provided to motivate the workers.

Managers have plenty of possible adjustments that they *could* make. Which ones *should* they make? That depends on the situation. It is a problem to be solved, and the tools in this book can help. Chapter 13, which discusses problem-solving methods, will help.

Managers can use a **cause-and-effect diagram** (also called a **fishbone diagram**) to analyze causes of performance. Exhibit 12.6 is an example of a cause-and-effect diagram. This tool can be used to drill down to factors that contribute to good performance or bad performance. The performance is stated in the "fish head" on the right side of the diagram. The fish skeleton is on the left of the fish head and flows into the head. In Exhibit 12.6, the horizontal spine of the fish connects to four diagonal fishbones that represent four types of factors that might contribute to the problem in the fish head.

The four main fishbones (or categories of factors) are the

Cause-and-effect (fishbone) diagram
A tool that visually identifies which factors might affect performance.

1.   environment in which the work is performed,

2.   equipment used to perform the work,

3.   procedures done to perform the work, and

4.   people who perform the work.

EXHIBIT 12.6
Cause-and-
Effect (Fishbone)
Diagram

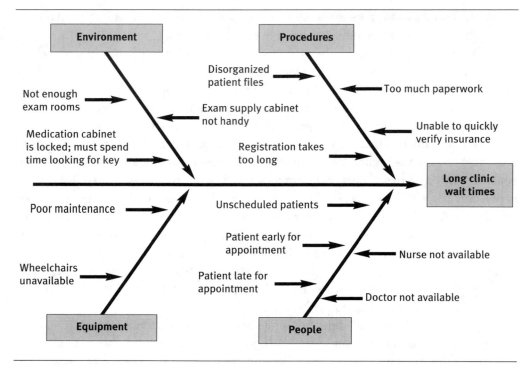

SOURCE: Spath (2013).

These four types of factors can be used to diagnose causes of performance problems. Managers can add other fishbones if necessary for additional categories of factors.

Managers and staff brainstorm *possible* factors in each of these four categories that *might* cause the performance problem. In Exhibit 12.6, "disorganized patient files" is a factor in the Procedures category that might cause the problem of long clinic wait times. Managers could drill down to identify subfactors that might cause the disorganized files factor. Although not shown in the exhibit, "lack of staff training" could be a subfactor that causes the "disorganized patient files" factor, which in turn causes the problem of long clinic wait times. After the group has suggested possible factors and subfactors, they use data to figure out which ones are most likely causing the problem. Data and information gathered in the second step of the control method can help them uncover the problem.

Managers may use a **flowchart** (or process map) to visually see the work processes and then improve them by taking corrective action. A flowchart is shown in Exhibit 12.7. This tool enables managers to identify, arrange, and analyze the flow of steps required to complete a process, such as registering a new clinic patient. Managers can use a flowchart to initially plan a work process or to revise an existing process. Causes of process problems may be apparent. Perhaps steps should be added, deleted, combined, rearranged, or simplified to make the process easier, faster, less complicated, more accurate, less error prone, more convenient, less costly, or better in some other way.

Flowchart
A tool that identifies and shows in sequence the flow of steps required to complete a process; also called a process map.

EXHIBIT 12.7
Flowchart

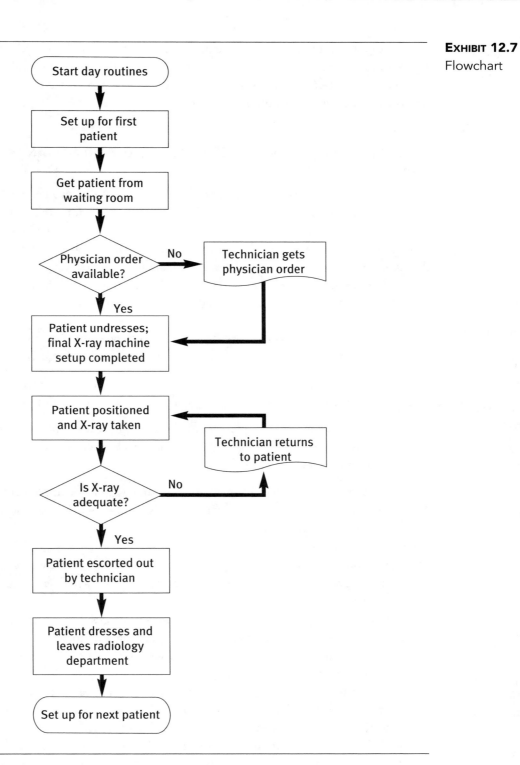

An interesting way to diagnose problems is to prepare a flowchart of how the work process was originally *designed* and then compare it to a flowchart of how the work is actually being *performed*. Managers may discover differences that should be corrected. These charts force managers to think through work processes and how to improve them.

RELATED APPROACHES TO CONTROL AND PERFORMANCE IMPROVEMENT

To summarize what we have learned in this chapter so far, managers control by setting standards and expectations, monitoring and judging actual performance compared to standards, and improving performance if necessary. This three-step approach is an excellent general control model. Managers sometimes use variations of it, and several are briefly discussed in this section. Managers have successfully used these variations in HCOs.

The **Plan-Do-Check-Act (PDCA) cycle**, sometimes called the Plan-Do-Study-Act (PDSA) cycle, involves four main steps (Spath 2013; Warren 2014).

1. *Plan:* Managers plan goals and objectives they want to achieve, including how to implement the plan (who will do what, where, and when).

2. *Do:* Managers implement the plan on a small scale and see what happens, noting problems and gathering data about the implementation.

3. *Check:* Managers analyze data to check (study) what happened, assess how well results match plans, summarize lessons learned, and decide if plans and implementation should be changed.

4. *Act:* Managers make changes and continue with more implementation and more PDCA, gradually fine-tuning until the goals and objectives are accomplished.

Managers should keep cycling through these steps until the goals have been implemented. Each step and cycle enables managers to try, learn, adjust, try again, learn again, and adjust again, as needed.

Reengineering is done to improve business processes that involve tasks and activities from multiple departments that must work well together to accomplish an end result for customers (Daft 2013). It often starts from scratch with a clean-slate approach to prevent getting trapped in preexisting ideas about how to do work. Reengineering has been applied to performing a surgical procedure that requires a team of workers from several departments. Processing health insurance claims is another application of reengineering. Reengineering is supposed to improve performance by adjusting organization structure, coordination among workers and departments, training, motivation, and culture to enable workers to serve customers more effectively.

Plan-Do-Check-Act (PDCA) cycle
A control model in which managers plan goals, do things to implement plans, check implementation, and act to improve implementation to achieve goals.

Reengineering
Redesigning and improving work processes that involve multiple departments that must work together to accomplish a result.

Lean production is an approach used to reduce waste and increase efficiency and speed. It may also improve quality. The Lean approach focuses on what is valuable to customers and then designs work processes to produce value for customers. While this method makes sense, it is not always done. For example, some work processes are designed to produce value for other stakeholders, such as when work is designed to make things more convenient for employees. Lean methods also strive for perfection and zero repeat work caused by errors. Work is analyzed using flowcharts, fishbones, and other methods to detect and reduce waste from delays, unnecessary movement, unnecessary repeat work, and extra work that does not add value (Spath 2013).

Six Sigma takes basic methods discussed earlier and applies them with greater rigor to reduce variation and defects in business processes. The five steps used in Six Sigma are sometimes referred to by the acronym DMAIC (Warren 2014):

1. **D**efine customers and their problems and desired outputs.

2. **M**easure what is happening.

3. **A**nalyze causes of defects and problems.

4. **I**mprove work processes and measure changes until satisfactory.

5. **C**ontrol the process with continued monitoring.

Lean production
Design of work processes to reduce waste, increase efficiency and speed, and thereby produce more value for customers.

Six Sigma
Performance improvement that aims to reduce variation and defects in work processes.

CONTROLLING PEOPLE

Controlling and improving performance involves people, so we also should think about controlling people. This book has already presented many approaches for controlling human behavior. What are some ideas (tools) you can think of from previous chapters? Leadership, supervision, motivation, performance appraisals, power, authority, rewards, punishments, data, job descriptions, training, culture, values, structure, and rules. Excellent—you thought of many useful tools! And remember the point from earlier in this chapter: Performance problems are often caused by the system rather than by the person. When trying to control employee behavior, consider the bigger picture and system the employee is in. It might lack essential resources or not enable easy coordination among departments. When controlling staff, some managers ask employees: Are there any obstacles in your workplace that prevent you from doing a terrific job?

Managers can use these tools to control people *appropriately* to help control organizational performance. We know people are not all alike, so what works for Miraya might not work for Tony. What works for baby boomers may not work as well for Generation Y workers. Professional workers may expect more self-control and peer control than authoritarian control of performance. In general, organizations have been changing to rely more on organization culture and values and less on bureaucratic rules and supervision to guide employees' performance (Daft 2013). When employees strongly embrace organization values, their performance is controlled more by those values and less by managerial authority and supervision.

Another important trend is the increased use of evidence, valid data, analytics, benchmarks, and monitoring systems to help workers know their current performance—often in great detail and frequency. Even physicians who have historically relied on their own professional judgment are now using these tools to improve their performance (Calayag 2014).

Finally, for managers to successfully control their HCOs, they must control themselves and their own performance. This book has briefly offered some ideas for improving one's performance and will return to this topic more fully in Chapter 15 on professionalism. As a manager, you should continually strive to improve your own performance to contribute more to the HCO, serve as a role model, and manage others effectively.

 TRY IT, APPLY IT

Think of examples of controlling performance in your daily life. Do you control your use of time? Use of money? Academic performance? Performance in a sport or hobby? If so, describe how you control. Are there pros and cons to your control methods? Discuss this topic with your classmates.

HERE'S WHAT HAPPENED

Geisinger Health System in Pennsylvania applied performance control methods that led to remarkable improvements in quality. One approach was to reduce variation in clinical processes by creating a standard approach for all physicians and employees to follow. Heart surgery is now done by following a checklist of 40 specific steps based on best practices from the American Heart Association and the American College of Cardiology. Although surgeons first rejected this approach as "cookbook medicine," they realized it improves their results and their patients' health. It also reduces costs by getting the process right the first time. Before the standard approach was adopted, different surgeons had different surgical processes. This variability led to confusion and errors by employees who assisted different surgeons. Further, these different processes were not all based on best practices. Now, with standard processes based on best practices, Geisinger has elevated its heart surgery process and reduced the variability that confused employees. These actions have improved heart surgery results and costs (Connolly 2009).

Managers at all levels of an HCO must control performance of their work units, departments, and the entire organization. They control performance by following a three-step process: (1) set standards and expectations, (2) monitor and judge performance compared to standards, and (3) improve performance if necessary. This approach is used to control many dimensions of performance, such as costs, value, productivity, quality, satisfaction, health status, and dozens of others. Managers should pay attention to structure measures, process measures, and outcome measures of performance. Although outcome measures have become more important recently, all measures are important. Managers can use internal and external data and information to set standards that are SMART: specific, measurable, achievable, realistic, and time related.

Managers must collect, analyze, and display data to compare planned to actual performance. Data collection systems must be created, and data can be organized in charts and graphs for interpretation. If performance is unsatisfactory, then control tools, such as cause-and-effect diagrams and flowcharts, should be used to analyze causes and develop possible solutions. These solutions are likely to require organizational adjustments to job design, work design, organization design, decentralization, standardization, coordination, culture, motivation, training, staffing ratios, schedules, rules, procedures, policies, decision making, and other components. The Plan-Do-Check-Act cycle, reengineering, Lean production, and Six Sigma methods can help control and improve quality and other dimensions of performance in HCOs.

(T) FOR YOUR TOOLBOX

- Three control steps
- Structure, process, and outcome measures
- Benchmarks
- Line graph (run chart)
- Bar graph (bar chart)
- Pie chart
- Control chart

- Tabular report (table of data)
- Cause-and-effect (fishbone) diagram
- Flowchart
- Plan-Do-Check-Act (PDCA) cycle
- Reengineering
- Lean production
- Six Sigma

FOR DISCUSSION

1. Define and explain "management control" in your own words.

2. What are some types of performance that a manager would have to control for a home health care agency? A health insurance company? A primary care clinic? An outpatient surgery facility? A mental health counseling center? A medical supply store?

3. Explain how control is related to planning, organizing, staffing, and leading.

4. Describe the three-step approach to management control. Which step do you think would be the most difficult? What could you do to make that step easier?

5. Compare and contrast what a manager can show in a line graph, bar chart, pie chart, and control chart.

6. Discuss how a manager can control employees to make necessary changes in an HCO.

CASE STUDY QUESTIONS

These questions refer to the Integrative Case Studies at the back of this book.

1. Decisions, Decisions case: Suppose University Memorial Hospitals decides to build and operate its own day-care center. First, list five possible stakeholder expectations of the new center. Second, describe how you would gather data to monitor performance toward fulfilling those expectations.

2. Decisions, Decisions case: Six months after its opening, parents complain that the day-care center smells bad and looks dirty. Prepare a cause-and-effect diagram to diagnose possible causes of the problem. Which data would you collect to further analyze the performance problem?

3. Ergonomics in Practice case: Referring to the specific control methods in this chapter, explain how Tim Montana is trying to control performance at Riverlea Rehab. Which methods do you think are being used in this case?

4. Disparities in Care at Southern Regional Health System case: Using the specific control methods outlined in this chapter, explain how you would *set standards and expectations* for reducing disparities. Using the methods outlined in this chapter, explain how you would *measure and judge how well the standards and expectations are met.*

TRY IT, APPLY IT

1. Pick a healthcare organization (e.g., Acme Home Care).

2. Identify the organization's many stakeholders (e.g., family of a patient receiving home care).

3. List the stakes/expectations of each stakeholder (e.g., patient's family expects no cancelled home care visits by Acme Home Care).

4. Name at least two measures to assess how well the organization met each stakeholder's expectations (e.g., number of appointments cancelled by Acme Home Care).

5. Would you want to weight any stakeholders or their expectations so that some would count more than others in judging organizational effectiveness? Why or why not?

6. Discuss your performance measurements with classmates.

CHAPTER 13

MAKING DECISIONS AND SOLVING PROBLEMS

A problem well-stated is a problem half-solved.

John Dewey, philosopher and
pioneer of educational reform

LEARNING OBJECTIVES

Studying this chapter will help you to

➤ define and describe decision making;

➤ discuss who makes decisions;

➤ explain the rational decision-making approach and its limits;

➤ explain satisficing, intuition, incremental, evidence-based, political, and garbage can approaches to decision making;

➤ identify barriers to decision making; and

➤ explain how to resolve conflict.

HERE'S WHAT HAPPENED

Partners HealthCare faced serious problems in the areas of quality of care and financial risk. At all levels of the organization, managers had to make decisions to solve
these problems and resolve conflicts. They had to diagnose problems, consider alternative ways to solve them, and decide which solutions to try. Yet even before they
performed these steps, managers first had to decide who should make the decisions
and which decision-making approaches to use. Should they use a rational approach,
a political approach, an evidence-based approach, an intuitive approach, or some
other approach? Making one decision often led managers to have to make other
decisions. For example, managers decided to use telehealth to solve the readmission problem—and that led managers to have to decide who, when, where, and how
to actually implement telehealth technology. They had to decide on new positions,
responsibility and authority for positions, whom to hire, work schedules, patient
care policies, and other matters. Conflict was inevitable, and when some nurses
and primary care physicians resisted, the Connected Cardiac Care Program managers resolved those conflicts. To address these issues, they first had to decide which
approach to use to resolve conflict—accommodating, compromising, collaborating,
or something else.

Managers at Partners HealthCare continually made decisions, solved problems,
and resolved conflicts to achieve the organization's goals and mission. These
activities are a big part of what managers do at every level of a healthcare organization (HCO). **Although decisions at higher levels have bigger consequences than
decisions at lower levels, managers at all levels make decisions to solve problems and
resolve conflicts.** Thinking back to earlier chapters, you can imagine the decisions, problems, and conflicts that HCO managers have to handle.

Managers make decisions to perform all five main management functions—planning, organizing, staffing, leading, and controlling. Several of Henry Mintzberg's management roles (discussed in Chapter 2) involve making decisions and solving problems:
monitor, disturbance handler, resource allocator, and negotiator. Decision making affects
management activities described in other chapters. Conversely, management activities in
other chapters affect how decisions are made. For instance, recall that organizing work
includes centralization and decentralization of authority—that affects how decisions are
made throughout an organization. Think how different leadership styles and organizational cultures affect decision making, problem solving, and resolving conflict.

How do managers make decisions? Well, how do *you* make decisions? Flip a coin?
Throw a dart? Compare the pros and cons of several options? Just do what worked before? Follow instincts? Go with the first idea that comes to mind? All of the above? None of the above?

This chapter teaches how managers at all levels of an HCO can make decisions to solve problems and resolve conflicts. First, it describes decision making and identifies the types of decisions. Then it explains several approaches that managers use to make decisions. The main approach, which is based on rational thinking and analysis, is not always feasible. Thus, managers often use other methods, which are explained in the chapter. Barriers to effective decisions and trends in decision making are also discussed. The final section of the chapter discusses how to resolve conflict, which involves making decisions.

DECISION MAKING AND DECISIONS

Decision making is "choosing from among alternatives to determine a course of action" (Liebler and McConnell 2004, 141). This definition focuses on choosing from alternatives—making up your mind. Organizational decision making is "the process of identifying and solving problems" (Daft 2013, 478). This definition includes two activities: (1) *identifying problems*, which involves judging an organization's performance and noting deficiencies, and (2) *solving problems*, which considers alternative courses of action and then chooses and implements one of them. Daft's definition of decision making goes beyond choosing an alternative. It also embraces implementation of the chosen action, which forces managers to make decisions that are realistic and can be implemented! Some writers (e.g., Liebler and McConnell 2004) do not directly include implementation in their definitions. However, their decision-making processes do include steps for evaluating implemented decisions. Based on the preceding discussion, in this book **decision making** is a process of choosing from among alternatives to determine and implement a course of action.

Note that decision making is a process. Decision makers usually go through a series of steps over a period of time. This process can help managers make good decisions. However, multiple steps also mean more ways for decision making to go wrong and leave people wondering, "What were they thinking?" Also, note that decision making is tied to problem solving. **We solve problems by making decisions, and we make decisions to solve problems.** Finally, note that decision making overlaps with control, which includes monitoring performance and making decisions about how to improve performance problems. Thus, control and decision making are studied in consecutive chapters—Chapters 12 and 13.

Managers have to make two types of decisions and solve two types of problems (Daft 2013). **Programmed decisions** are well defined, routine, recurring, easily diagnosed, and easily solved with standard rules, formulas, and procedures. These decisions can be made with high confidence that the chosen alternative will succeed and solve the problem. For example, when should I see a dentist? How many custodians should we hire for the new retirement home? On the other hand, **nonprogrammed decisions** are new, unusual, hard to define and understand, and hard to diagnose. They present fuzzy alternatives with uncertain cause and effect. For example, when the United States enacted the Patient

Decision making
Choosing from among alternatives to determine and implement a course of action.

Programmed decisions
Decisions that are well defined, routine, recurring, easily diagnosed, and easily solved with standard rules, formulas, and procedures.

Nonprogrammed decisions
Decisions that are new, unusual, hard to define, and hard to diagnose; they present fuzzy alternatives with uncertain cause and effect.

Protection and Affordable Care Act in 2010, staff in HCOs throughout the country wondered, "How will this health reform affect us and what should we do?" They struggled to define the decisions to be made, to describe alternative courses of action, and to anticipate how alternatives might play out and with which consequences. The new healthcare reform law had many fuzzy parts, and it was not clear how the reforms would affect HCOs and their stakeholders. Recall from Chapter 3 that nonprogrammed problems and decisions often arise during strategic planning.

Do you suppose managers use the same decision-making methods for programmed and nonprogrammed decisions? Think about this question as you study the decision methods in this chapter.

Who Makes Decisions?

Individuals at all levels of an organization make decisions, and so do groups, committees, teams, and HCOs. Experienced senior managers make decisions, and so do inexperienced managers in their first week on the job. Think of the previous chapters and the decisions managers have to make for planning, organizing, staffing, leading, and controlling. To refresh your memory, and to help you understand how those functions relate to decision making, look through some chapters and jot down a few decisions that managers would have to make. (Meet you back here in five minutes.)

We can categorize decisions as *individual* and *organizational*. Individual decisions are made by a single person—such as you, a webmaster, a physician, or a marketing coordinator. Organizational decisions are made by groups of people in an organization—such as a website design task force, the department of pediatrics, or an informal group of new managers who think the marketing coordinator pushes too much work onto them. Group decisions have become more common as a way to bring many kinds of expertise into the decision process. Another benefit of group decisions is that more stakeholders are involved in the decision, and it will thus have more support. However, as we saw in Chapter 6, more people means more time and cost.

Physicians are involved in many of an HCO's decisions, so a manager should remember that physicians tend to be independent. Dr. Loie Lenarz is the senior medical director for Fairview Clinics and is responsible for 22 primary care clinics in Minnesota. She explains, "Most of what we do in clinical practice reinforces our sense that when we're with the patient, we're on our own. On our own we need to gather data, assess what's important and what's not, and make a decision" (Silversin and Kornacki 2000, xxi). This approach carries over to other aspects of work such that organizational and group decision making does not come naturally to physicians. On the other hand, managers are used to getting input from others for decisions and are more comfortable with organizational decisions. Managers must recognize this difference and strive to help physicians when they are involved in organizational decisions.

A manager who is dealing with a problem must determine who will make a decision to solve it. It might be the manager, others, or the manager and others. A manager should clearly tell others which one of the following five approaches should be used for a particular decision (Connelly and O'Brien 2007, 56):

1. *Authoritative:* I will decide on my own without your input.

2. *Consultative:* Give me your advice; then I will decide.

3. *Participative:* Give me your input and help me think through this problem.

4. *Consensual:* We will decide this together and reach a consensus.

5. *Delegated:* You decide without me.

Think back to the leadership chapters (Chapters 9, 10, and 11). Which leadership style would you associate with these decision-making approaches?

(→) TRY IT, APPLY IT

As a manager, your involvement in making a specific decision can range from high to low. Think of examples from your life in which you used each of these five approaches— authoritative, consultative, participative, consensual, and delegated. Then, think of a future situation in which you would be likely to use each of these five approaches. Discuss your examples with classmates. This practice will help you recognize that your amount of involvement in decisions will vary.

METHODS FOR MAKING DECISIONS

Managers can make decisions using different approaches. Some of them are used by individual managers, some by groups, and some by individuals and groups. We begin with the rational approach, which will seem familiar to many people. It is common, yet idealistic, and it is sometimes hard to follow completely. After studying this method, we will learn why it is hard to follow fully and then consider other approaches.

RATIONAL DECISION MAKING

As the name suggests, the rational approach to decision making is based on logical reasons and deliberate analysis to arrive at the best decision. This approach makes sense, although it is idealistic. In the real world, in the midst of a busy workday, managers may find it hard to faithfully follow the rational approach. Thus, people tend to "kind of" follow this method yet take a few shortcuts along the way. You have probably "kind of" used this method to make a choice, such as which college to attend. Individuals, groups, committees, and teams use this method in organizations.

The rational approach consists of the following eight steps (Daft 2013):

1. *Monitor the decision environment:* review external and internal information, check results, and detect performance problems.

2. *Define the decision problem:* describe a detected performance problem by gathering more information about it, such as who, what, where, and when.

3. *Specify the decision objectives:* state what is to be accomplished by the decision, and identify the desired outcomes.

4. *Diagnose the problem:* analyze information to determine why the problem happened, and figure out causes of the problem.

5. *Develop alternative solutions:* state what could be done to solve the problem— what are the options?

6. *Evaluate the alternatives:* judge how well each alternative solution would achieve the decision objectives and outcomes, and consider pros and cons and likelihoods.

7. *Choose the best alternative:* select the best alternative to achieve the decision objectives.

8. *Implement the chosen alternative:* put the chosen alternative into effect—make it happen.

Other writers present similar approaches, and some combine steps. The first four steps *identify the problem* and the decision that must be made. Identifying the problem is important, as reflected in the quote at the beginning of this chapter. The last four steps *solve the problem* by making and implementing a decision. Each of these eight steps builds on what was done in the previous steps. Decision makers are supposed to do the steps in sequence, from 1 to 8. However, they sometimes back up to redo earlier steps. See Exhibit 13.1 for an application of the rational approach to a daily-life decision and to an HCO decision.

Chapter 11 discussed ethics problems and suggested that managers should have in their HCOs a process for deciding how to resolve ethical problems. Managers and ethics committees can and do follow a process similar to this rational model. They define the problem, diagnose it, develop alternative solutions, consider the pros and cons of those

Exhibit 13.1

Examples of the
Rational Decision-
Making Process

Rational Decision-Making Steps	Daily-Life Example: A Place to Rent	HCO Example: Lab Productivity
1. Monitor the decision environment	Apartment listings show rental rates are starting to go up	Internal reports show lab tests performed per tech declined 4 percent this year and are now 7 percent below industry standards
2. Define the decision problem	On September 1, rent for my 1-bedroom apartment will rise to $900/month	Tests/tech are 3 percent above standards on 1st shift and 8 percent below standards on 2nd shift; automated tests/tech equal standards; manual tests/tech are 11 percent below standards
3. Specify the decision objectives	Spend no more than $800/month on rent during next academic year	Lab tests/tech should equal industry standards for our kind of lab tests and equipment
4. Diagnose the problem	Landlords have to cover their rising costs; my apartment will be upgraded with new appliances	2nd-shift chief tech job vacant; 2nd-shift workload declined 9 percent since last May 1
5. Develop alternative solutions	Negotiate an $800 rate with landlord; move to a cheaper 1-bedroom apartment; join friend in a 2-bedroom apartment for $500/month/person	Promote a 2nd-shift tech into chief tech job to supervise staff; create a productivity incentive system on 2nd shift; advertise the lab to bring in more work on 2nd shift
6. Evaluate alternatives	Consider cost, location, safety, independence, and comfort	Consider costs, feasibility, effects on entire lab, and likelihood of increasing 2nd shift's tests/tech
7. Choose the best alternative	Move in with friend	Promote a 2nd-shift tech into chief tech job to supervise staff
8. Implement the chosen alternative	Let current lease expire, sign new lease, move my stuff, and notify family and friends	Promote tech, provide supervisory training and mentoring, and monitor results

solutions, pick the one they think is right, and implement it. Participants in this process give extra attention to ethics by considering (Nelson 2005)

◆ the values and preferences of all stakeholders who would be affected by the decision,

◆ the ethical consequences of alternatives,

◆ which ethical principles (e.g., beneficence) support each alternative solution, and

◆ whether an alternative solution violates an ethical principle (e.g., justice).

For the rational model, managers need data (often lots of data) with which they can analyze and evaluate problems and alternative solutions. Where do the data come from? How do managers evaluate alternative solutions? They use quantitative and qualitative methods and often combine them rather than rely on only one approach (Daft 2013; Hellriegel and Slocum 2011; Ledlow and Stephens 2009):

Quantitative Data and Methods

◆ Files, reports, databases, records, scorecards, and other sources inside an HCO have useful data, as do external reports, websites, and databases.

◆ Computer programs with probability models, linear programming models, decision trees, mathematical formulas, scheduling systems, statistical programs, and comparison matrices help in analyzing information and evaluating alternatives. Internal staff and external consultants can assist managers with these methods, and newer computer software has become more user-friendly for novices.

Qualitative Data and Methods

◆ Discussions, interviews, focus groups, and conversations with people inside and outside the HCO provide information. They are useful for evaluating ideas and alternative solutions.

◆ Delphi technique, nominal group technique, brainstorming, intuition, devil's advocate approach, expert opinion, and pro/con discussions can help in evaluating alternative solutions to a problem. External consultants and internal research staff in larger organizations can assist managers with these methods.

Note that internal staff positions might help the actual decision makers. Do you recall line and staff positions from the earlier chapters on organizing? Staff workers (at the direction of line managers) use specialized skills, abilities, and expertise to support the line managers and decision makers. For example, researchers and decision analysts gather information, analyze it, compare alternatives, run decision-making software to calculate consequences of alternatives, set up linear programming models, and so forth. With today's computer software, new managers can learn how to do some of this quantitative data analysis. Online software and apps also enable managers to do qualitative analysis online. Results are distributed without identifying individuals, so participants are anonymous. Compared to traditional methods, e-methods such as e-brainstorming produce more participation and more willingness to offer "wild ideas" because there is less concern about "sounding stupid" or saying something the boss would not like (Hellriegel and Slocum 2011).

An organization must strive to have its information available at the right time in the right place in the right form for the right people. Doing this requires effective **knowledge management**—a system for finding, organizing, and making available an organization's knowledge, including its experience, understanding, expertise, methods, judgment, lessons learned, and know-how (Daft 2013; Hellriegel and Slocum 2011). It includes both codified knowledge in written documents and tacit knowledge in people's heads. Tacit knowledge is insight, know-how, intuition, experience, judgment, and expertise. Compared to codified knowledge, it is harder to find, gather, organize, store, and make available to others in the organization—yet tacit knowledge comprises much of an organization's unique, valuable knowledge. Managers use information technology (IT) to manage codified knowledge relatively easily. Managing tacit knowledge is more challenging, and it depends on person-to-person interactions, professional networks, and face-to-face connections. Managers must facilitate these relationships so that employees can easily find and interact with people who have the right tacit knowledge. Face-to-face meetings, team huddles, and conversations are useful. Managers can also invest in telecommunication systems, Skype, FaceTime, and other IT to enable conversations for sharing tacit knowledge.

Knowledge management
A system for finding, organizing, and making available an organization's knowledge, including its experience, understanding, expertise, methods, judgment, lessons learned, and know-how.

LIMITS OF RATIONAL DECISION MAKING

Rational decision making makes sense, and managers often use it as they make decisions and solve problems. But sometimes managers do not rely on it. Why? **Human ability to be rational is limited. The human brain can only process a limited amount of information, consider a limited number of factors, and evaluate a limited set of alternatives.** Even the brains of world-champion chess grandmasters eventually become "full" and cannot consider one more alternative move. Further, human brains are not robotic; they are biased by personality, emotions, personal values, experiences, situations, and pressures. Also, some problems are just too complex to accurately describe and diagnose. Finally, in today's complex world and organizations, there may not be enough time to gather all the information, much less analyze it. The result is **bounded rationality.** There are limits (boundaries) to how far rational decision making can go. Then what happens?

As a result of bounded rationality, managers sometimes make decisions using other approaches. They may use satisficing, intuition, incremental, evidence-based, political, and garbage can decision making. These approaches are explained next.

SATISFICING

Herbert Simon (1957) is often credited with developing the satisficing approach, which argues that people are not capable of making the best decision among all possible alternatives. **Because of bounded rationality, people cannot (and do not) make the choice that will maximize outcomes and results.** Instead, they conduct a limited search for alternatives and choose an early solution that will achieve their minimum acceptable results. They **satisfice**—that is, they decide on a satisfactory alternative that will suffice. A manager "kind of" follows the rational model but hurries along, takes shortcuts, and settles on a solution that is good enough. For example, Rachel might just follow simple decision rules that have worked in the past. This approach is simpler and faster and requires fewer resources and disagreements than the ideal pursuit of the best solution. Managers realize better alternatives might exist, yet they also realize not all problems need the best solution—they just need an acceptable solution (Liebler and McConnell 2004). Individuals often satisfice when making individual decisions.

Some organizational decisions are made by groups and coalitions (rather than by just one person). These groups are also likely to satisfice. For organizational decisions, there are even more barriers to the rational approach than for an individual decision. With more people involved, there are more personal biases, hopes, fears, favors to repay, and so forth. It becomes challenging for all group members to analyze all possible solutions and agree on a best solution. Some groups cannot even agree on what "best" means! People want to finish the decision-making meeting to get back to other work that is piling up. So they look for a simple solution that everyone can live with, even though it might not be the best solution. To enable the process, a group member might informally confer with a few other members before a meeting and compromise toward a satisficing solution.

INTUITION

Instead of using rational analysis, individuals sometimes make a decision by using **intuition**. Dr. O'Neill examines numerical lab values and other diagnostic test results, and then considers hunches based on his years of experience. **Intuition is commonly used, especially when time is short, problems are complex, precedents do not exist, and facts are scarce** (Borkowski 2009). Some situations are just too fuzzy to make rational choices. Even when rational decision making can be used, managers may supplement it with intuition. A

Bounded rationality
Limits to human rational decision making.

Satisfice
To decide on a satisfactory alternative that will suffice, although it might not be the best.

Intuition
Knowing or deciding based on experience, hunches, or unconscious processes rather than on rational thinking and reasons.

---

manager in Fort Pierce, Florida, might use the rational approach and tentatively decide to hire Alan as a new community outreach specialist. However, before she tells the human resources director her decision, she wants to "sleep on it" and see if she still feels comfortable with the decision in the morning.

The origins of intuition are not fully understood, although experience seems to help it develop. People may not be able to fully explain their intuition or justify intuitive decisions. Yet, they may use it with good results. Intuition can be developed, and a manager can practice intuitive thinking by paying more attention to her inner mind and her feelings about choices. Managers should try to develop the intuitive approach to complement the rational approach for decisions.

INCREMENTAL

An HCO might begin a rational decision-making process but then proceed through the steps with pauses, restarts, a backup, interruptions, a redo, and gradual progress. For example, suppose decision makers at a dental clinic in Redwood City, California, face a parking problem. They move forward toward a decision but later feel their choice is unrealistic because they had not seriously considered neighborhood opposition. Eventually, they make a decision. But during implementation, the city zoning board changes its regulations, and now the clinic's decision might be illegal. Should the clinic proceed and seek an exemption, or should it back up and try again? The clinic's attorney says legal hurdles will take at least three months. The clinic decides to seek an exemption from the new zoning regulations and continue with its decision. It starts looking for ways to make up the lost time.

Sometimes decision making is incremental and does not follow an orderly sequence of steps. Managers might say, "If we try to figure out the whole solution, by the time we do, the situation will have changed, and we'll have to figure it out again." Managers take two steps forward and one back (and then maybe a step sideways and another step forward). Deciding what to do and implementing it becomes a trial-and-error process. They think, "Let's get started, and we'll keep figuring it out as we go." This approach works best in HCOs that value learning, experimentation, change, and innovation (which are discussed in Chapter 14). Some HCOs encourage this trial-and-error approach as a way to learn, especially for complex problems that are just too big to solve all at once. In 2010, many HCOs began incrementally deciding how to adapt to the new Affordable Care Act. They knew they would have to incrementally figure out what to do as more of the law was gradually implemented, courts ruled on legal challenges to the law, and the law was modified.

EVIDENCE-BASED DECISION MAKING

In an interesting trend adopted from the field of medicine, more managers have been using **evidence-based decision making**. This approach is similar to rational decision making but goes further. Managers use this approach to dig deeply and overcome their bounded rationality, blinders, biases, groupthink, flawed assumptions, and closed-mindedness (Hellriegel and Slocum 2011). The evidence-based approach begins with a careful statement (and restatements) of the problem to be solved. As new evidence is examined and logically applied to the problem, managers might further refine the problem. This intelligent approach searches for relevant information from multiple sources (Briner, Denyer, and Rousseau 2009):

Evidence-based decision making Making decisions based on systematically finding, evaluating, and applying the best relevant evidence to a clearly defined problem.

- ◆   External scientific research evidence

- ◆   Internal evidence from the local setting, context, or organization

- ◆   Experiences, expertise, and judgments of practicing managers

- ◆   Preferences, values, and views of relevant stakeholders who will be affected

In this informed approach, managers systematically acquire and use the best evidence available. They give careful attention to which evidence and information is relevant and how accurate, valid, and reliable it is. They give greater weight to some evidence than other evidence. This approach moves the rational process closer to the idealized version. Managers apply discipline and ask each other tough questions to avoid quick fixes, faddish answers, and educated guesses (Hellriegel and Slocum 2011; Kovner, Fine, and D'Aquila 2009). However, because of its systematic thoroughness, this approach takes more resources, time, and staff. Despite added costs and time, evidence-based decision making has become more common in HCOs during the past decade.

POLITICAL

The political approach to decision making is different from the evidence-based approach. A manager who uses a political approach relies on his flawed assumptions, biases, and closed-mindedness. Huh? Why would a manager do that? He would do it to reach a decision that is self-serving. He wants a decision that is good for him, and he is less concerned about what is good for others and the organization (Hellriegel and Slocum 2011). When managers have different interests, goals, ambitions, and values—without strong overarching commitment to the organization—they are likely to engage in political decision making to get their way. It is especially true in "win–lose situations," in which, for example, one person gets the big new office and everyone else does not.

Recall from earlier in the chapter the eight steps of the rational decision-making approach. At each step, a political decision maker might use bias, misinformation, and political tactics to gain advantage. She will define the problem so that it shifts blame to others but not to herself: "It's a finance problem, not a marketing problem." She will search for and use data that support her point of view or make her opponents look bad. When evaluating possible solutions to a problem, she will use methods that make her preferred solution look best. Each step of the rational decision-making process could be biased to tilt the decision in favor of her self-interests. Information is power, and unlike evidence-based decision makers, a political decision maker will only search for and use information that supports her goals. She will not share all information with others and will selectively use biased information that supports her opinion. She might even present rumors as facts.

This political activity was discussed in Chapter 10. It is common because people have different interests, goals, ambitions, and values—and they want to get their way. So, managers should expect this type of activity. Some HCOs use the evidence-based approach to thwart political decision making.

GARBAGE CAN

Garbage can decision making

Seemingly random organizational decision making resulting from evolving streams of problems, solutions, participants, and decision-making opportunities.

Garbage can decision making is even less sequential and step-by-step than the incremental approach. It does not even try to follow the rational model and could simultaneously consider multiple decisions to solve multiple problems. Garbage can decision making occurs in freewheeling, organic, chaotic, nonbureaucratic organizations with people, problems, and solutions all coming, going, and changing (Daft 2013; Ledlow and Stephens 2009). Imagine problems, solutions, people, and decision-making opportunities all mixed together (Daft 2013) during a meeting in an organization.

Lauren, a supervisor, is running a meeting that is supposed to be about weekend staffing levels, but some participants have brought other ideas ("garbage") to the meeting. Juan complains about the sick-pay plan. Bob mentions his pet peeve—parking. Gina suggests "free food Fridays" in the cafeteria, which is offered where her cousin works. All this leads someone else to wonder aloud, "How is employee morale around here?" Brittany says morale is fine in her department and asks if there is a morale problem in other departments. Gina now excitedly says her idea would improve the morale problem! Some people agree; no one asks for evidence. The food service supervisor is not at this meeting to comment on how Gina's free food idea would affect his department.

Meanwhile, guess what is happening in a different meeting downstairs? Some people who were at the April meeting are not at the May meeting, and vice versa. Some arrive late, leave early, take cell phone calls, and are not present for all discussions and decisions. Problems arise that have uncertain answers because of uncertain cause-and-effect relationships. Information is limited, obscure, and fuzzy. Thus, decision makers do not understand the causes of the problems or if proposed solutions will really solve the problems. If they do x, it might cause y, but then again it might cause z, or it might not cause anything. Managers will try a solution; if it does not work, they will try something else.

This garbage can decision making might seem surprising. Yet some organic, non-bureaucratic organizations use this method as an alternative to the rational process (Daft 2013). Managers should realize that it might occur in their HCO if meetings and the HCO are too loose, unstructured, and chaotic.

BARRIERS TO EFFECTIVE DECISION MAKING

Managers face barriers to decision making (Daft 2013; Dye and Garman 2015; Liebler and McConnell 2004). As a manager, strive to avoid these barriers:

◆ Not enough time, in a hurry

◆ Closed organizational culture, closed leadership style

◆ Risk averse, afraid to decide on a new idea, too much caution, stuck in a rut

◆ Avoidance, delay, procrastination

◆ Unwilling to confront problems, unwilling to confront the *real* problems

◆ Not seeking, getting, or using relevant information

◆ Wishful thinking, unrealistic optimism, hubris, overestimating ability to handle problems

◆ Unwillingness to admit a previous decision was wrong and is not working

◆ Not diagnosing a problem well enough to really solve it

◆ Accepting only favorable information, avoiding unfavorable information, rejecting useful information because of its source

◆ Biases, personal agendas, conflicts of interest

◆   Defining a problem in such a way as to be solved too easily and quickly

◆   Not involving the right people in the decision

◆   Using an inappropriate approach to decision making

◆   Groupthink, conformity, playing it safe, copycat thinking, copycat decisions

To avoid the last barrier, consider this classic advice from longtime management consultant, writer, and expert, Peter Drucker (1967, 148): "The first rule in decision-making is that one does not make a decision unless there is disagreement."

TRENDS IN DECISION MAKING

The external environment of most HCOs has become more complex and less certain. As a result, HCOs' decisions have also become more complex and less certain. HCOs face more nonprogrammed decisions that do not fit their playbooks. Compared to decisions made in the past, today's decisions usually involve more factors, more alternatives, more information, and more stakeholders' interests. Thus, some HCOs and decision makers use deliberate evidence-based decision making, involve more people, and make more group (rather than individual) decisions.

On the other hand, the environment has been changing rapidly, so HCOs feel they must make decisions rapidly. Pressure to make complex decisions quickly has led some managers to use more satisficing, intuition, and incremental decision making. HCOs are now more willing to allow trial and error followed by learning. They make an incremental decision, try it, learn from it, adjust, and try again. (Does this method remind you of the Plan-Do-Check-Act cycle in Chapter 12?) Some HCOs have begun actively encouraging a trial-and-error approach.

Finally, the workforce and decision makers in most HCOs have become more culturally diverse. **Decision makers should take the time to understand relevant views, concerns, and ideas of different cultures that are involved in a decision or that will be affected by the decision.** Doing so takes more time and patience amid pressure to make fast decisions.

These trends are general and do not apply to every situation and organization. However, managers should be aware of them.

RESOLVING CONFLICT

Conflict in an HCO can be managed with decisions. Conflicts and decisions have a reciprocal relationship—they affect each other. Decisions can help resolve conflict by diagnosing the conflict and then choosing and implementing an alternative course of action. And conflict can help improve decisions by generating new ideas, opening up closed thinking, and discouraging groupthink. Good decisions depend on first examining conflicting ideas, views, and alternatives. Conflict prevents harmful decisions based on groupthink (see Chapter 6), in which members quickly, politely, and superficially agree without considering different values and information. **Some conflict (but not too much) is good for HCOs and decision making. Conflict is normal and should be expected.** Next, we find out why it is normal and study how to manage it.

CAUSES OF CONFLICT

Conflict arises for reasons listed below (Daft 2013; Dreachslin and Kiddy 2006; Hoff and Rockmann 2012). Examples (including some in healthcare) are included.

- ◆ *Goal incompatibility:* decrease costs versus increase weekend staffing; innovation versus consistency

- ◆ *Differences in perceptions, values, beliefs, cognition, emotions, cultures, and views:* physicians and managers think differently; diversity exists among people in terms of gender, age, culture, education, status, and other characteristics

- ◆ *Task interdependence:* a nurse hands the surgeon a scalpel; the restaurant server impatiently waits for the cook to finish making a pizza

- ◆ *Resource scarcity:* there is not enough time, information, power, money, space, or equipment to meet everyone's needs; three employees requested an iPad, but only one is available

- ◆ *Unclear expectations:* people are not sure what to do or how or when to do it (often a result of incorrect or unclear communication); the policy says "perform equipment maintenance daily," but the first shift leaves the maintenance work for the second shift and vice versa

These causes of conflict occur naturally, so managers should expect them in their HCOs. Take a few minutes to think of examples in your life.

HERE'S WHAT HAPPENED

A man was interviewing for the chief operating officer position at a large regional medical center. During the job interview, a board member said there was conflict between physicians and managers. The board member then asked the candidate what he thought about that and if conflict happened in other hospitals. The applicant answered that conflict between physicians and managers is natural and common, and it sometimes can be useful. What is important, he added, is that the two groups are able to resolve conflict in a way that both groups accept and feel is fair.

INTERPERSONAL CONFLICT RESOLUTION STYLES

Kenneth W. Thomas and Ralph H. Kilman (1974) developed a model to resolve conflict that is seen in healthcare literature and practice (Borkowski 2011; Dreachslin and Kiddy 2006; Ledlow 2009). This model consists of five resolution styles—collaborating, competing, compromising, accommodating, and avoiding (see Exhibit 13.2). These five styles can be used in HCOs. Which approach should be used? That depends on *how assertive* and *how cooperative* someone chooses to be, which depends on the situation. In other words, the approach depends on *concern for oneself* and *concern for others*. Based on high, medium, or low assertiveness and cooperativeness, a person uses one of these five approaches to resolve conflict (Exhibit 13.3). Each of these approaches is sometimes appropriate and sometimes not appropriate. (The styles might remind you of the leadership styles in Chapter 9.)

A manager decides which style to use after evaluating the situation. In other words, the best approach is contingent (sound familiar?). When you are a manager or supervisor, you can use these guidelines to evaluate conflict and then choose the style that seems right for the situation. Studies have found that in general, though not always, managers who collaborate are more successful, are found more in high-performing organizations, and are viewed more positively by others than managers who do not collaborate (Hellriegel and Slocum 2011). In contrast, managers who compete or avoid are more likely to be viewed negatively. The studies showed that compromising was generally viewed positively by others. Results for accommodating were mixed, without clear conclusions.

SUGGESTIONS FOR MANAGING CONFLICT

When dealing with conflict, remember how emotional it can be! You have probably seen or been in a conflict when people were fervent about their points of view. This type of conflict

EXHIBIT 13.2
Five Styles for
Resolving Conflict

Collaborating	Competing	Compromising	Accommodating	Avoiding
Exchanging information and examining differences to reach a win–win situation (high assertive / high cooperative)	Forcing acceptance of your position while ignoring the needs of the other party (high assertive / low cooperative)	Both parties giving and taking something to reach a mutually acceptable solution (moderately assertive / moderately cooperative)	Playing down differences and emphasizing commonalties to satisfy the other party while neglecting your own concerns (low assertive / high cooperative)	Withdrawing or sidestepping the issue by not addressing the conflict (low assertive / low cooperative)

SOURCE: Information from Dreachslin and Kiddy (2006) and Hellriegel and Slocum (2011).

Collaborating is useful when	Competing is useful when	Compromising is useful when	Accommodating is useful when	Avoiding is useful when
• The outcome matters to everyone.	• The outcome is important to you.	• There is not time now for collaboration.	• The outcome does not matter to you but does to another person.	• The outcome does not matter to you.
• You want a win–win.	• Conflict involves essential rules or laws.	• Conflict involves incompatible goals.	• You know you are wrong.	• It is beyond your control or cannot be solved.
• There is time to carefully consider everyone's views.	• Conflict must be quickly settled, such as in an emergency.	• A quick though temporary resolution of a complex conflict is needed.	• You are unlikely to get your way; you pick your battles.	• It is not your responsibility.
• You want everyone committed to the solution.	• Conflict is with someone who takes advantage of cooperation.		• It's important to get along with others; peace matters.	• The conflict may resolve itself.
• Problem-solving expertise is available.	• Conflict involves an unpopular yet necessary matter.		• Yielding now can help you get something else later.	
			• You want others to try their ideas.	

EXHIBIT 13.3
Guidelines for Choosing a Conflict Resolution Style

SOURCES: Information from Hellriegel and Slocum (2011); Ledlow (2009); and Polzer, Neale, and Illes (2006).

happens when something important is at stake. So take a deep, calming breath if necessary, control yourself, and help others control themselves. Try to empathize and understand their needs, feelings, and anxieties. Managing conflict with people of diverse cultures can be especially challenging and may take more time, effort, and patience.

In conflict, people are likely to use power to get their way. Recall from our study of power, for instance, that someone may try to line up allies who will go to bat for a cause. Anticipate power games and organizational politics that were explained earlier in this chapter and in Chapter 10. Use your own power appropriately.

Apply the rational decision-making process to clearly state the conflict (problem), diagnose it, identify possible solutions, evaluate the solutions, and so forth. Keep it objective and problem focused (not person focused). Use data to support the process. Know what is negotiable and what is nonnegotiable; when possible, negotiate to reach an agreement.

A final suggestion is to seek expert help if necessary to resolve difficult conflicts that are harming you or the HCO. The expert could be someone in the HCO, such as the human resources director or a counselor who has experience in conflict resolution. Or, it could be an outside consultant, mediator, or arbitrator. An arbitrator allows disputants to present their views and input and then makes a decision (similar to a court judge) to resolve the conflict. A mediator leads conflicting parties through discussions, questions and answers, negotiations, and processes that guide them to decide for themselves how to work out the problem (Polzer, Neale, and Illes 2006).

ONE MORE TIME

Managers in an HCO make decisions to solve problems and resolve conflicts to achieve the HCO's goals and mission. Making decisions is a big part of what managers do at every level of an HCO to perform all five main management functions—planning, organizing, staffing, leading, and controlling. Decision making is a process of choosing from among alternatives to determine and implement a course of action. Some decisions are programmed (routine, common) whereas others are nonprogrammed (nonroutine, uncommon) and thus harder. The external environment has become more complex and less certain, so HCOs' decisions have also become more complex and less certain.

Managers sometimes make decisions alone but more often involve other people. They are likely to use the rational approach based on quantitative and qualitative data, deliberate analysis, explicit reasons, and striving for a best decision. This approach makes sense, yet managers may find it hard to follow completely because of bounded rationality. Thus, they might partly follow the rational method and then use satisficing, incremental, intuitive, evidence-based, or political approaches. A final approach, though not recommended, is garbage can decision making.

Conflict is natural in HCOs because of differences among people, differences among departments, scarce resources, work relationships, unclear expectations, and unclear communications. To resolve conflict, managers may collaborate with, compete with, compromise with, accommodate, or avoid the other person(s). The right approach depends on *how assertive* and *how cooperative* someone chooses to be, or how much *concern for oneself* and *concern for others* a person has. Although the collaborative style seems to work best in many situations, a manager should develop the ability to use each of the five conflict resolution styles when appropriate.

(T) FOR YOUR TOOLBOX

- Five approaches for who makes a decision
- Rational decision making
- Satisficing decision making
- Intuition decision making
- Incremental decision making

- Evidence-based decision making
- Political decision making
- Garbage can decision making
- Conflict resolution styles and guidelines for choosing a style

FOR DISCUSSION

1. How do you feel about using intuition rather than rational thinking to make decisions? Have you ever relied on intuition?

2. Is satisficing really appropriate for managers, or is it just being lazy?

3. Compare and contrast rational, incremental, and garbage can approaches to decision making. What is your opinion of these methods?

4. Which barriers to effective decision making have you observed or experienced in a club, team, or group? What could have been done to overcome those barriers?

5. Zach is a senior and has started thinking about jobs in HCOs. He wants to find an HCO that does not have conflict because it will be less stressful working there. What do you think of his idea?

6. Discuss the pros and cons of the five conflict resolution styles. Which style would you favor? How could you become better prepared to use all the styles?

CASE STUDY QUESTIONS

These questions refer to the Integrative Case Studies at the back of this book.

1. Decisions, Decisions Case: Explain which parts of the rational decision-making model are seen in this case.

2. Nowhere Job case: Explain how Jack could use the rational decision making process to decide if he should quit his "nowhere job." In your answer, refer to information from the case.

3. Disparities in Care at Southern Regional Health System case: This chapter presents seven approaches to decision making. Explain which (one or more) of these you think Mr. Hank should use to reduce the disparities.

4. Taking Care of Business at Graceland Memorial Hospital case: This chapter explains causes of conflict. Describe which of these are seen in this case.

5. Taking Care of Business at Graceland Memorial Hospital case: Referring to Exhibits 13.2 and 13.3, which of the five conflict resolution styles do you think should be used to resolve the conflict? Justify your answer.

 TRY IT, APPLY IT

At Partners HealthCare, managers tried to implement a telehealth program using electronic telecommunications and information systems to check vital signs and heart health of patients in their homes. Some nurses opposed the telehealth program and preferred the high-touch approach to patient care. Which of the conflict resolution styles presented in this chapter would you use to resolve the conflict? In class, form trios with classmates acting as telehealth manager, traditional high-touch nurse, and observer. Take turns role-playing the manager and nurse in a meeting to resolve the conflict. Afterward, the observer can give feedback and lead a discussion of what happened in the role-play.

CHAPTER 14

MANAGING CHANGE

Change is inevitable. . . . Change is constant.

Benjamin Disraeli, British prime minister and writer

LEARNING OBJECTIVES

Studying this chapter will help you to

➤ describe change in healthcare organizations;

➤ explain why so much change happens in healthcare organizations;

➤ contrast radical and incremental change;

➤ explain why people resist change and how managers can overcome resistance;

➤ describe the three-step approach to implementing small-scale change; and

➤ explain the eight-step approach to implementing large-scale change.

HERE'S WHAT HAPPENED

The Partners HealthCare system was engaged in extensive change to adapt to its changing external environment, satisfy its stakeholders, and fulfill its mission. Partners changed some of its strategic goals, patient care delivery, management systems, organization structure, clinical processes, communication policies, work technology, staff positions, and performance measurements. Some changes were radical, such as major redesign of patient care delivery, while others were incremental with only minor adjustments. To successfully make these changes, managers used change management methods. For instance, senior managers demonstrated support for the changes by committing funds and resources for them. Employee "champions" were identified who understood the changes and could rally others to accept and support them. Managers provided staff to implement new technology and processes. The managers gave the workers enough time to adapt to changes in their work. New patient care systems were pilot tested with 150 patients before expanding to more than a thousand. Managers evaluated many aspects of the changes and shared positive evidence to overcome resistance from some staff. Although the changes affected hundreds of employees, managers succeeded with changes so that Partners could improve health in its community.

As we learned in the opening Here's What Happened, healthcare organizations (HCOs) often change. In fact, they change continually. So much change occurs that some employees think that living with change is a survival skill for working in HCOs. While that might be true, merely surviving change is not enough for managers. **Because of their roles and responsibilities, managers must be able to lead and manage change for their HCO, not just survive it for themselves.** In this area, managers can make important contributions to their HCOs. Managers at all levels of an HCO must be able to successfully manage change. Because change is so common, this ability is important for managers' job success and career growth.

Think about changes mentioned in the opening Here's What Happened, changes described throughout this book, changes in the local news, and changes in your daily life. There always has been and always will be plenty of change! When changes in HCOs succeed, they can help people obtain healthcare and ultimately lead healthier lives. Managers who help plan and implement the changes feel positive emotions afterward—satisfaction, accomplishment, joy, and relief.

Unfortunately, some changes do not work out well. Less than half of the changes in HCOs succeed, and outright failure is more common than reported (Weiner, Amick, and Lee 2008). In these cases, managers feel negative emotions. As a manager, you will be more likely to succeed with change if you understand how to lead and manage change.

Managers deal with change when they perform the five management functions explored in this book. Planning, by nature, causes change as new goals and strategies are developed for the future. Organizing work, tasks, jobs, teams, and departments involves changing authority, responsibility, and supervisory relationships. Staffing involves change as new tasks are added to jobs, people retire and are replaced, and compensation changes. Leading and motivating also require change because people's motivational needs change. Controlling identifies performance that does not meet expectations and thus leads to change to meet performance targets. Two of Henry Mintzberg's ten managerial roles (discussed in Chapter 2) clearly involve change: entrepreneur and disturbance handler. Although change management is not a distinct management function, it is part of performing the five basic management functions studied in this book. Managers deal with change all the time.

This chapter discusses change in HCOs and why it is so common. We learn why people resist change and how managers can overcome resistance. Doing so prepares us to study how to implement change. First, we learn a three-step process to implement small changes. Second, we study an eight-step approach to implement large-scale organizational change. This chapter teaches how to adapt to change and to implement change in HCOs. You should learn to manage change well, because managers at all levels of an HCO need to do so to succeed in their jobs and careers.

CHANGE IN HCOs

Much of what goes on in HCOs involves change. Can you think of some examples of changes in HCOs? Why do you suppose those changes occurred?

Recall from Chapters 1 and 3 that changes in the external environment often drive changes in HCOs. Chapter 1 lists examples of external environmental changes that force HCO changes—such as patient-centered care, mergers, and social media. There have been (and always will be) many more changes in society, culture, technology, consumers, financing and reimbursement, populations, government policy, competitors' plans, scientific discoveries, industries that supply HCOs, schools that educate workers, economic conditions, and other parts of HCOs' environments. Those changes in the external environment force HCOs to change so that they can survive and thrive.

While much change is forced by external factors, sometimes change is driven by internal factors from within the organization. The network technician retires. The carpet in the lobby wears out. Cheryl discovers a daily pattern of narcotics missing from the pharmacy. Some of these factors are predictable, and some are surprises. Here, too, HCOs must make changes to survive and thrive.

Another reason for so much change is that one change leads to other changes. Most HCOs are complex with many interacting moving parts. When the storeroom changes its schedule for delivering supplies to the clinics, the clinics then change their procedures for using and ordering supplies. A medical supply business hears the demands from customers (in the external environment) for lower prices such as those offered by the competition (in the external environment). Kelly, the sales manager, decentralizes authority so that sales staff can more quickly adjust prices for customers. This sales department change causes Roberto in the accounting department to change corporate control mechanisms that monitor sales, prices, and revenues. These accounting department changes then cause changes in other departments. Each change results in another.

Managers and HCOs often have many projects underway. They might build a surgery facility, install a new computer system, prepare an inventory control system, or open a healthcare consulting office in Minneapolis. These projects are another source of change and require change management. Managers who have implemented health information technology (IT) and electronic health records made a good point in discussing their experience. They have emphasized that it is "important to see the effort as an exercise in change management, not an IT initiative" (DeVore and Figlioli 2010, 665). **Think of a project as managing change rather than as building a facility or installing computers.**

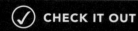

Radical change
Large, major revolutionary change.

Incremental change
Small, minor evolutionary change.

RADICAL AND INCREMENTAL CHANGE

Managers face two types of change: **radical change** that is revolutionary and **incremental change** that is evolutionary (Daft 2013). During the 1990s, change shifted (changed!) toward radical change as consultants told managers to get rid of their old business models and create entirely new ones. Consultants said the external environment had changed so much and so fast that minor adjustments would not be enough. Instead, major changes were required to survive in the future. But a few years later, leaders realized the downsides of radical, wholesale change (Abrahamson 2000; Wetlaufer 2001). What do you think happened? Rapid, extensive change left too little time for organizations and people to recover and restabilize. There was too much turmoil and instability for everyone to function normally. Employees were fearful and overstressed. Managers were so busy with change that they did not perform other necessary tasks and functions. Leaders realized that too much change implemented too quickly destroyed an organization's core competencies without successfully developing new competencies.

Since then, change in HCOs has become more incremental and less radical. Today, HCOs require some of each type of change. For example, both radical change and incremental change are needed to achieve the six aims for the US healthcare system presented in the *Crossing the Quality*

✓ CHECK IT OUT

How comfortable are you with change? When your club, job, college, family, or town announces a change, how do you usually feel? Tests can help people judge their readiness for change and how well they accept change. Managers may use these tests when leading change in HCOs because readiness for change is one factor needed for successful change. Some online tests take only a few minutes to complete—for example, The Seven Traits of Change-Readiness at http://www.ecfvp.org/files/uploads/2_-change_readiness_assessment_0426111.pdf (from a website for leadership class taught by Associate Professor T. J. Jenney at Purdue University: www.tech.purdue.edu/ols/courses/ols386/crispo/changereadinesstest.doc). Completing the test will help you learn about your readiness for change.

Chasm report (discussed in Chapter 12). Similarly, in the Here's What Happened at the beginning of this chapter, Partners HealthCare made incremental and radical changes. They had to manage the pace of these changes to avoid overwhelming everyone and harming the HCO's strengths.

RESISTANCE TO CHANGE

We learned that forces outside and inside an HCO push *for* change. Simultaneously, forces push back *against* change. The resistance comes from an essential part of every HCO: people who work there! Not everyone resists change, of course, but there will be some who push back and perhaps even try to stop the change. **Employees at all levels, including managers, may resist changes. Resistance might arise in the decision-making stage, the planning stage, the implementation stage, and probably in all other stages.** So when managers plan and lead change, they should expect resistance, noncompliance, and perhaps outright defiance. Some staff resisted change at Partners HealthCare in the Here's What Happened at the beginning of this chapter. Resistance is natural and part of the change management process. Be ready to address it.

WHY PEOPLE RESIST CHANGE

Pop quiz: Name the five human needs in Maslow's Hierarchy of Needs. This is an open-book quiz, so feel free to check Chapter 10 on motivation. After identifying these five needs, imagine a change that might interfere with your fulfillment of these five needs. You are not sure how the proposed change will play out, but you do worry that it might interfere with your fulfillment of these five human needs. Do you feel like resisting the change?

Thinking about Maslow's needs gives us a framework for understanding some reasons people resist change (see Exhibit 14.1). **People resist changes at work because they fear that these changes might reduce satisfaction of their human needs. They fear a possible loss of something they value.** Even though people do not know for certain that they will experience loss, they worry that they might lose something. The unknown and the uncertainty create fears and worry, which cause resistance. With these factors in mind, what should you do to help implement change when you are a manager?

Another reason people resist change is that they do not understand how it might benefit them. Exhibit 14.1 could be redone to show that a change might increase fulfillment of Maslow's needs. A change might lead to *more* job security, status, pay, and opportunity for self-fulfillment. Sometimes people do not perceive possible benefits, which leaves them worried about loss instead. Other times they resist change because they do not see the reason for it and do not understand why it is needed. They ask, "Why do we have to go through all this change?" or "What's the purpose?" When you are a manager, what should you to do to help implement change in these situations?

Exhibit **14.1**

Changes at Work
and Their Effects
on Basic Needs

Change at Work	Effect on Basic Needs
Job becomes routine and less fulfilling; job does not use your abilities; job provides less chance for professional growth	Less self-fulfillment; less self-actualization
Job becomes less important with lower status; job earns less respect from others; job has less power and prestige; job change reflects badly on you and your professional reputation	Less esteem; less respect from others
Job no longer involves working with favorite coworkers; loss of on-the-job friends and comfortable work groups; job now has a new unknown boss	Less affiliation, friendship, love, belonging
Job now involves unsafe, unhealthy work setting; job is less secure; work hours and pay might be cut; new unknown boss creates insecurity; less control of schedule and work setting; fear of failure in new job situation	Less security and safety
Job might be eliminated so paycheck (and survival) is less certain; job creates physical and mental stress	Less physiological survival; uncertainty about meeting basic needs such as food and shelter

Employees can understand the purpose of a change as well as likely gains and losses. Yet they still might resist. Why? Because they think the change is unrealistic or even impossible. They feel there are too many other things going on, not enough resources, or too many legal restraints to accomplish the change. These reasons *sometimes* are valid. For example, a medical office decided to change to open-access scheduling, which was expected to improve patient access to urgent appointments. The staff began implementing the change, but turmoil arose. The leader assessed the situation and then had to decide whether to push ahead or back off. He decided to back off the change rather than force it. He believed the open-access scheduling was still a good idea, but he acknowledged the staff did not understand it well enough to be able to implement it correctly. So he and the staff stepped back, revised the change plan, learned more, gained competence with it, and then tried again, which led to better results (Reinertsen 2014).

People resist change because of human habit and inertia. In physical science, **inertia** means that an object at rest tends to stay at rest and an object in motion tends to continue its motion. Energy is required to overcome inertia, either to change the motion of a moving object or to move a resting object. The same is true of people, jobs, work, and organizations. They develop motion—a usual work routine. Inertia sets in, and they keep

Inertia
An object at rest tends to stay at rest and an object in motion tends to continue its motion; this principle applies to work in organizations.

moving pretty much the same way. Some employees even say, "I'm on autopilot." If they are expected to change their daily routine, they will have to use new energy and effort to overcome the inertia of their usual way (Drafke 2009).

Finally, some people resist change to spite or get revenge on a boss or organization. A worker who feels mistreated and has a grudge can resist or even sabotage change out of revenge. Workers may feel their actions are justified and resist change openly or secretly (Drafke 2009).

As was noted earlier, employees do not all view change the same way. Some dread it whereas others can't wait for it to begin! Let's consider an outpatient diagnostic testing center. For a single proposed change, such as adding evening appointments for customers, employees may range from high resistance to high support. The manager communicates the same information to all employees. But each employee has a unique personality, past experiences, biases, current life stresses, and other factors that, for *some* people, can impede proposed change.

ORGANIZATION CHARACTERISTICS THAT MAY IMPEDE CHANGE

Like people, organizations also have unique personalities, past experiences, biases, current life stresses, and other factors that, for *some* organizations, can impede change. Recall from Chapter 4 that organizations have structures that range from mechanistic to organic. Do you recall which type has rigid specialized tasks and strict hierarchy, control, rules, and authority? Hopefully, you recall the mechanistic type. That structure impedes change. On the other hand, the organic structure has flexible shared tasks and loose hierarchy, control, rules, and authority. The organic structure enables change. Other structural barriers that impede change include unclear goals, roles, responsibility, and accountability. Recall from Chapter 11 what comprises organization culture: values, norms, guiding beliefs, and understandings shared by members as the correct way to think, feel, and behave. Some organizations have cultures in which employees believe they are not allowed to question their bosses, dare not make mistakes, and should respect tradition. That culture has some advantages, but it also has the disadvantage of impeding change. On the other hand, some cultures value innovation and learning, and employees respect creative new ideas. That culture surely supports change.

Other characteristics of organizations can also impede change (Hellriegel and Slocum 2011; Longenecker and Longenecker 2014). Organizations that have limited resources and tight budgets are less able to try new ideas and spend money on change that might fail. Some organizations lack the leadership, trust, teamwork, and cooperation needed for change. Organizations in frequently changing environments feel more pressure to change than do organizations in stable environments. Finally, some organizations have commitments such as contracts with labor unions, vendors, and physicians. Some have entered into group collaborations, joint ventures, partnerships, and affiliations. All these organizational commitments—some of which may last for many years—impede change.

HEALTHCARE CHARACTERISTICS THAT IMPEDE CHANGE

We next consider several characteristics of healthcare that can impede change in HCOs. In general, the pace of successful change in healthcare and HCOs has been slow. Quality improvement in healthcare has lagged behind quality improvement in other industries (Nembhard et al. 2009). Adoption of health IT has been sluggish and performance has been disappointing (Kellermann and Jones 2013). The healthcare characteristics in Exhibit 14.2 help to explain why. These statements are general and do not apply to every worker or every HCO. However, managers should pay attention to these characteristics when they attempt change in HCOs.

HOW PEOPLE RESIST CHANGE

People may resist change aggressively or passively, directly or indirectly, and openly or secretly. At one extreme, workers may be open and even aggressive about resisting change. An example is when unionized workers refuse to work because of a change, go on strike, and take to the streets in protest. An individual worker may refuse to comply with a change, such as when an employee feels a change is unsafe. Refusal, of course, can lead to punishment, so it is not common. Yet it occurs sometimes and may lead managers to reconsider a change. Direct aggressive resistance is easier to detect, which also makes it less common. **Workers are more likely to resist indirectly.** They usually want to be seen as team players who support upper management and do not make waves. So workers resist a change without directly refusing to comply. Instead, they take more sick time and arrive

EXHIBIT 14.2
Healthcare
Characteristics
That Deter Change

Characteristic of Healthcare	How the Characteristic Deters Change
Involves risk to patients amid high uncertainty	Staff is averse to experimentation needed for successful change
Staff interactions are based on hierarchy, rules, professional identities, and status	Staff does not naturally collaborate, which is needed for organizational changes
Identity and self-image are strongly linked to one's profession and only weakly to one's organization	Staff interest in organizational change may be weak
Relationships between healthcare staff and managers are based on transactions, self-interests, and conflicting goals	Hard for healthcare staff and managers to pursue shared organizational change

SOURCE: Information from Nembhard et al. (2009).

late when they do go to work. Resistance may also be seen in minor violations of rules, sloppy work, less work, and barely acceptable work. This approach is less confrontational and harder for managers to connect to a specific change.

Some workers resist a change in their current job by changing to a new job. For example, Donna, a secretary, takes a different job in the same HCO to get away from a change that is happening only in her department. Her marketing department moved out of the health insurance company's building to leased office space downtown near the media. Since then, Donna has felt isolated from her friends who work in other departments. So she transfers to a different secretary job in the company's main building and now can have lunch with her friends again. Some workers resist or escape changes in their HCOs by taking jobs at different organizations.

People exhibit different degrees of sincerity in their resistance. Some people may speak up to stop a change that they sincerely believe (rightly or wrongly) will harm people or the HCO. Recall from Chapter 8 that employees have a right to protection from harm, and they have some rights (within boundaries) to express their views about work. On the other hand, as mentioned, some people resist change as a form of revenge. Their opposition to change is not sincere.

In the long run, people are usually better off accepting an organization change than fighting it. Continued resistance can make a worker obsolete and unable to function in the new work world. Knowledge, skills, and attitudes become outdated. Workers, especially managers who lead other workers, should accept that change is inevitable and will soon be coming to a workplace near them. Lower-level managers and supervisors who adjust to change, and help their staff adjust to change, are respected by high-level executives.

How to Overcome Resistance to Change

Managers must work to minimize resistance to change and then overcome what resistance occurs. This action is especially important when undertaking large-scale change that will affect many people throughout an HCO. Dealing with possible or actual resistance might be frustrating to eager managers who want to get on with implementing the change. Yet, if managers do not do enough in the front end to minimize resistance, it will haunt them later.

So what should managers do? Following are some suggestions, which draw from earlier chapters and other writers (Borkowski 2011; Drafke 2009; Hellriegel and Slocum 2011; Longenecker and Longenecker 2014). These ideas are grouped under four broad, interrelated categories:

1. Involve people in planning and implementing change at the appropriate time.

2. Explain the change to employees and other stakeholders.

3.   Apply leadership principles and methods.

4.   Realize that people change at different times and speeds.

These ideas work best when managers have trusting relationships with others and have the organizational structure, culture, resources, and flexibility to enable change. If these factors are missing, managers will struggle to overcome resistance because people will not believe them nor feel safe trying new ideas. The organization and employees first should be ready for change.

Involve people in planning and implementing the change at the appropriate time. This activity begins in the planning stage of management when problems are solved and decisions made. Managers should involve the right people in making plans and decisions so that they "buy in" to the decision and will support it. When planning an implementation schedule (see the Gantt chart in Chapter 3), think about who will be affected by the change and who is needed to help it succeed. If the medical lab must move to a new location, involve the lab staff in planning the move. That will strengthen their commitment to the change and help create a realistic plan and schedule. The timing for involving people will vary depending on the change, the people, the relocation timing, and other factors. A manager needs good judgment (which can be developed through experience) to determine when to involve which people. If in doubt, involving people sooner is usually better than doing so later.

Explain the change to employees and other stakeholders who will be affected by the change and whose support is needed. This recommendation is related to the first one. As implementation proceeds, a manager must explain the change to a wider group of people who need to know about it. The timing for this explanation will vary depending on how particular people will be involved, how crucial their support will be, and the extent to which they were involved in the actual decision to change or the plans for implementation.

As patiently as possible, explain the who, what, why, where, when, and how of the change. Emphasize the purpose of the change and make a compelling case for it. Suggest how it might affect specific groups of people, such as second-shift workers, clerical staff, workers with fewer than ten years of seniority, and patient care staff. Try to reduce uncertainty by addressing pros and cons. Be ready to answer "What's in it for me?" Include lead time for people to get information, think about it, and follow up later with questions. People who resist are unlikely to change overnight, so allow them time to come to terms with the change. Be prepared for questions and answer them sincerely. Empathy will help, and so will honesty. Superficial buzzwords and vague promises will not help. Multiple forms of communication may be required depending on the change, number of people involved, and other factors. Allowing people to express their feelings, acknowledging their feelings, and acting on their feelings can help overcome resistance. (Chapter 15 on professionalism and communication offers more advice for effective communication.)

Managers should be willing to "change the change." That is, they should change the planned change when it seems necessary to resolve people's valid concerns. In the earlier example, the medical office manager did "change the change" by revising the planned schedule for implementing the new open-access scheduling.

Apply leadership principles and methods. Think back to earlier chapters on leadership, conflict resolution, motivation, power, and culture. Use knowledge and tools from those chapters to implement change and overcome resistance. For example, identify clear, compelling goals. Identify and clarify tasks, roles, responsibilities, and accountabilities for the change. Apply conflict-resolution methods appropriately. Strive for win–win collaboration, but be flexible at times. Compromise and negotiation can help overcome resistance. If workers resist because they think two weeks is not enough time to make the change, consider negotiating more time. Being rigid and using authority to force implementation of change might sometimes be necessary (e.g., compliance with a legal court decision). But it can irritate employees and cause indirect resistance, such as rule infractions and absence from work. Use sources of power, including authority, reward, and punishment, when appropriate to influence resisters. Apply principles of motivation. For example, a change might create opportunity for job growth or job autonomy that would motivate some workers. Leaders must be role models for change and help create a culture that supports change. Create a culture that values experimenting, trying new ideas, learning from mistakes, and taking reasonable risks. In this culture, workers will feel more secure about trying a change, not succeeding at first, and practicing until they get it right. Offer training and preparation for the change, and help people learn about it.

Realize that people change at different times and speeds. A manager should judge people's readiness for a proposed change. (This can be done with a change readiness survey such as the one in this chapter's Check It Out.) Think about groups in general and key individuals in particular who must help the change succeed. When judging the readiness of workers on a scale of 1 to 10, some will be rated 1, some 10, and many will be in between. Some people thrive on change and become bored without it; they might be ready for change before the managers are. Others wait to follow the crowd; they will be ready after a majority has tried the change and has told coworkers it is not too bad. Some people delay and avoid change for reasons given earlier. Manage the pace of change, but do not try to move everyone at the same pace. Support people as they proceed through the change process.

When you are a manager, realize that overcoming resistance to change is not the same as creating commitment to change (Weiner, Amick, and Lee 2008). Just because Alyssa does not resist changing to a new method of registering patients does not mean she supports it. Alyssa might not exert herself much for the change and might not help sell it to others. If the change falters, she may cut corners and not fully perform the new method. **Remember that lack of resistance is not commitment.** "I don't have a problem with it" does not mean "I am committed to making it succeed."

TRY IT, APPLY IT

Think about a change you know of in an organization. It might be an organization where you did an internship, held a part-time job, or go to college. Use what you have learned in this chapter to analyze how the change was managed. Was it a radical or an incremental change? Who led and managed the change? How was the change handled? Did some people resist, and if so, why? Describe what was done to deal with resistance. Discuss your ideas with classmates.

MANAGING ORGANIZATIONAL CHANGE

Prior literature and research on how to manage organizational change offer useful lessons and models. Taken together, these models emphasize the importance of a big-picture shared vision yet also a carefully developed implementation plan with flexibility to adapt (Kash et al. 2014). We will examine two models for change that are often used in organizations—including HCOs.

SMALL-SCALE CHANGE

Unfreeze
Create dissatisfaction with the current situation and motivate people to change.

Kurt Lewin (1951) developed a classic three-step approach to change that is still popular and effective today. The three steps are (1) **unfreeze**, (2) move, and (3) **refreeze** (see Exhibit 14.3). They are explained in this section, based on the work of Drafke (2009) and Borkowski (2011). An HCO business office example has been created to illustrate the three steps.

Refreeze
Lock in change and make it the new correct way of doing things.

Step 1: Unfreeze the current situation

◆   Clear out old ideas to make way for new ideas.

◆   Explain why change is necessary.

◆   Motivate people to want to change.

◆   Make people feel dissatisfied with the current situation.

◆   Alter the way people think about the situation.

◆   Help people see how the future could be better.

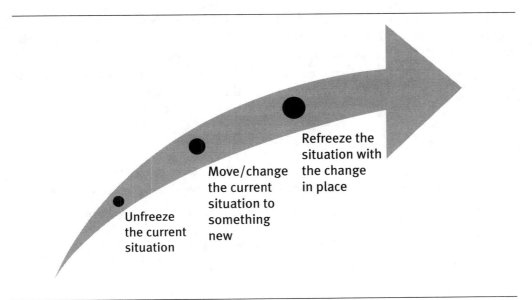

EXHIBIT 14.3
The Three-Step
Change Process

Refreeze the
situation with
the change
in place

Move/change
the current
situation to
something
new

Unfreeze
the current
situation

SOURCE: Information from Lewin (1951).

◆   Lead people to feel a change is possible and can succeed.

◆   Begin to overcome resistance.

If this step is done well, people will be committed to make the change succeed, and better yet, they will persist if difficulty arises.

Throughout the healthcare industry, many nonprofit health associations, charities, foundations, and interest groups raise funds to help people with a specific aspect of health. You have probably heard of some, such as the American Cancer Society, the American Lung Association, and the Children's Hunger Fund. Some are national, with state and local offices. Others are regional or local. They must work well with clients, donors, and other stakeholders who call their offices. Let's think about the business office at one of these HCOs in Cincinnati.

The business office manager, Mr. Remson, held a staff meeting. He reviewed surveys (used to monitor performance as part of the control process) that indicated people who called the business office were unhappy about staff performance. More specifically, survey responses revealed that the staff was not helpful or polite enough when taking phone calls from clients and families. He explained this situation to the 12 business office employees and also passed around a letter from a caller who wrote to complain about the staff. He explained that impolite, uncaring behavior (as perceived by the caller) harms the reputation of the business office and the entire HCO. Mr. Remson added that a bad image leads to fewer clients, fewer donations, and perhaps job losses and layoffs. He suggested that employees try "the mother test": Ask yourself, "Is this how I would want someone to talk to my mother?" Then he distributed telephone guidelines from a business etiquette book for the staff to follow. He asked for feedback, opinions, and input from each employee, and discussion followed. Mr. Remson expressed confidence in the employees and told them they could do better.

Step 2: Move (change the situation)

◆ Move into place the new methods, processes, techniques, structures, culture, policies, procedures, training, tools, work settings, and people for the change.

◆ Reorganize work, jobs, and tasks and the way they are performed.

◆ Exert energy and effort to overcome inertia and use what is new.

◆ Set control mechanisms to measure new performance.

This step applies management principles learned earlier in this book to move or change the situation. Work standardization is applied.

At the business office, each employee received a printed list of telephone etiquette standards to follow (e.g., answer a call by the third ring; before putting a caller on hold, ask if the caller would mind holding). Job descriptions were changed to specifically state that telephone etiquette was an important part of the job. Employees took turns calling each other pretending to be a client, and staff practiced the new standards. During practice calls, staff sometimes backed up for a redo as they learned the new procedures. There were funny moments. Mr. Remson continued to emphasize that customer service was a core value and that the new telephone guidelines taught the correct way to handle phone calls for excellent customer service.

Step 3: Refreeze the situation

◆ Link the new method to the rest of the organization.

◆ Reward and reinforce the change.

◆ Make the change the new normal and part of the daily routine.

◆ Stabilize the new way with repetition so that inertia sets in.

If this step is not done well, people will drift back to the old way if the new way becomes too hard.

At the business office, Mr. Remson continually emphasized the new telephone standards and commended staff when he heard them following the guidelines. He made a point of asking each employee (individually) about experiences with and feelings about the changes. Resistance faded, and employees seemed to get the hang of it. After the first week, the change was going well. They celebrated their progress with a cake, and an employee felt safe joking with Mr. Remson about one call she received.

All three steps must be done well for the change to take root and succeed. At the front end, inadequate unfreezing and lack of readiness to change are frequent causes of failure. If you are managing change, invest the time needed to prepare people and unfreeze the situation. This investment will be worth it. At the back end, sometimes too little effort is made to refreeze after change has begun. For example, a hospital executive attempted change with employees. After preparation, training, and other activities, the change began, but a few weeks later it was gone. "We provided two days of training, but it didn't stick," he said. The training wore off and seemed to never have happened. The executive asked, "What do we have to do to make change stick?" The answer: "Refreeze the situation."

EIGHT-STEP APPROACH TO LARGE-SCALE CHANGE

John P. Kotter (1996) developed a useful eight-step approach to create and sustain large-scale change in organizations. This approach builds on the three steps for small-scale change. Steps 1 through 4 unfreeze the old way, steps 5 through 7 move the processes along and install new ways, and step 8 refreezes the situation. The steps are described in this section (drawing from Borkowski 2011 and Weiner, Helfrich, and Hernandez 2006). Managers can use principles and methods from previous chapters when they perform these eight steps. For example, the chapters on leadership and organizing teams have useful ideas. Think about how the concepts you have learned would be useful in executing the eight steps.

Step 1: Establish urgency

◆   Show a real need that cannot wait any longer.

◆   Describe a real or potential crisis (e.g., bankruptcy).

◆   Create dissatisfaction with the way things are now.

◆   Describe a great opportunity or vision that must be pursued.

◆   Realize that merely identifying a problem does not create urgency.

Step 2: Create a guiding coalition

◆   Line up influential supporters at all levels of the organization.

◆   Enlist support of people whose input and commitment are needed to make change happen.

◆   Create a project team to implement the change.

Step 3: Develop vision

◆ Create a clear, simple, easily understood statement of what the future will be.

◆ Tell how the future can be better than the current situation.

◆ Provide a sense of direction that motivates people.

◆ Ensure the vision statement makes sense to people at all levels of the organization.

Step 4: Communicate the change vision

◆ Enable the guiding coalition to communicate the new idea and its benefits.

◆ Communicate in multiple ways, both formally and informally.

◆ Ask people what they know about the proposed change.

◆ Seek feedback and input from others about the change.

◆ Constantly repeat and reinforce the message.

Step 5: Empower broad-based action

◆ Give others permission to try the change.

◆ Revise policies, procedures, rules, and structures to enable the change.

◆ Let people take risks and learn from mistakes when trying the change. Provide training, practice, and support for the change.

◆ Support and reward the early adopters of the change.

◆ Continually work to overcome resistance.

Step 6: Create short-term wins

◆ Arrange some quick, easy successes with the change.

◆ Publicize and celebrate the early wins.

Step 7: Consolidate gains

◆ Reward success to keep the momentum going.

◆ Build on early successes to expand the change.

◆ Train more people to use the change.

◆ Show how success with the change is benefitting workers and other stakeholders.

◆ Redesign organization structure and processes to "lock in" early successes.

Step 8: Anchor new approaches in the culture

◆ Make the change part of what is valued and considered correct in the organization.

◆ Reward and reinforce the change to make it "the way we do things here."

◆ Hire and promote people who support the change.

◆ Ingrain the change in the culture to make it permanent.

Note that the second step—creating a guiding coalition—includes creating a project team to implement the change. Now is a good time to return to project management, which we studied in Chapter 3. Recall that project managers work to ensure assigned projects are completed within established constraints of time, budget, risks, scope, quality, and available resources (Project Management Institute 2013; Schwalbe and Furlong 2013). This work helps an HCO implement change. To ensure projects are completed, a project manager forms a project team based on the specific requirements of the project. It requires careful thought and choices (explained in Chapter 6 about teams). The project manager and team then use management tools and project management tools to implement the change (project).

The Here's What Happened in this chapter (and in other chapters) described Partners HealthCare managing change. The entire Partners HealthCare case study is in an appendix. By reading the case, you can see in more detail what Partners did to successfully implement large-scale change.

ONE MORE TIME

Managers at all levels of an HCO must successfully manage change. Change is constant, so this ability is important for managers' job success and career growth. Although change management is not a distinct management function, it is used when performing the five basic management functions: planning, organizing, staffing, leading, and controlling. Managers make changes in an HCO because of external factors, internal factors, and previous changes in the HCO. Some changes are radical and others are incremental; both types are needed.

People often resist change. Common reasons include fear of losing something, not understanding the purpose of change, not understanding benefits of change, and inertia. The resistance may be evident or hidden. To reduce resistance, managers should involve people in planning and implementing the change, explain the change to stakeholders, apply leadership principles and methods, and recognize that people change at different times and speeds.

Small-scale change can be implemented using Lewin's three steps: unfreeze, move, and refreeze. Large-scale change can be managed with Kotter's eight-step approach, which builds on the three steps for small-scale change. Managers should establish urgency, create a guiding coalition, develop vision, communicate the change vision, empower broad-based action, create short-term wins, consolidate gains, and anchor new approaches in organization culture. They can also apply project management techniques to keep change within budget and on schedule.

 FOR YOUR TOOLBOX

- Lewin's three-step approach to change
- Kotter's eight-step approach to large-scale change

FOR DISCUSSION

1. Why is there so much change in HCOs? How do you think change in HCOs is similar to or different from change in other kinds of organizations and businesses?

2. Compare and contrast radical change and incremental change. Which would you prefer?

3. Think about a change made by your college or workplace that you resisted. Why did you resist the change? Could the organization have done anything differently to reduce resistance?

4. Consider Lewin's three-step process. Which of the three steps do you think would be hardest to do? How might experience help develop a manager's ability to use this change process?

5. Describe with specific examples how at least five management principles, methods, theories, or tools studied in other chapters could be used in Kotter's eight-step approach for large-scale organizational change.

CASE STUDY QUESTIONS

These questions refer to the Integrative Case Studies at the back of this book.

1. Taking Care of Business at Graceland Memorial Hospital case: Why do you think Ms. Thompson resists compliance with the new Occupational Safety & Health Administration (OSHA) requirement? Explain how to use Lewin's three-step process at Graceland Memorial Hospital to implement change for compliance with OSHA.

2. Ergonomics in Practice case: Why do you think the staff at Riverlea does not like the lift system? Explain how Tim Montana could apply Lewin's three-step process at Riverlea to implement the new lift system.

3. Disparities in Care at Southern Regional Health System case: Explain how Mr. Hank could apply Kotter's eight-step process to implement change to reduce the healthcare disparities.

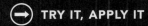 TRY IT, APPLY IT

Imagine that your college has not yet done anything to become green and eco-friendly. Describe how you could use Kotter's eight-step approach for large-scale change to help your college go green. Explain in detail how you would perform each of the eight steps.

CHAPTER 15

PROFESSIONALISM AND COMMUNICATION

It's a communication breakdown!

Common expression

LEARNING OBJECTIVES

Studying this chapter will help you to

➤ understand professionalism for managers;

➤ explain how emotional intelligence is needed for professionalism and management;

➤ explain how cultural competence is needed for professionalism and management;

➤ define and describe communication;

➤ identify types of communication in healthcare organizations; and

➤ apply a communication model to avoid communication problems.

HERE'S WHAT HAPPENED

Throughout all levels of Partners HealthCare, managers worked to achieve Partners's mission, vision, values, goals, and strategy. Their work required professionalism, emotional intelligence, cultural competence, and communication. Professionalism— living up to ethical and professional standards and being dependable, accountable, honest, fair, competent, and respectful—enables managers to work with others to serve their community and profession. Emotional intelligence enables managers to understand emotions in themselves and others and use that understanding to manage their behavior and personal relationships. Cultural competency helps managers understand and interact with people who are culturally different from themselves: patients, employees, volunteers, donors, community leaders, and other stakeholders.

Partners's managers communicated often. They communicated with people inside and outside the organization, and with individuals and groups. They spoke in quick hallway conversations and in carefully planned speeches. They wrote hurried texts and formal documents. They decided which information to share with which people by using which words in which media. Intentionally (and sometimes unintentionally), their behavior and appearance communicated messages about themselves. Communication enabled managers to accomplish goals, serve others, and help people live healthier lives.

As seen in the opening Here's What Happened, professionalism, emotional intelligence, cultural competence, and communication are important for a healthcare organization (HCO). They are also important for HCO managers at all levels— including new, entry-level managers. By now, you know that managers perform five functions: they plan, organize, staff, lead, and control. While performing these functions, they also perform ten management roles: figurehead, leader, liaison, monitor, disseminator, spokesperson, entrepreneur, disturbance handler, resource allocator, and negotiator. Managers at Partners HealthCare carried out these roles, and in your career you will too. By doing this work with professionalism, managers become more satisfied and successful in their jobs and careers. Professionalism involves emotional intelligence and cultural competency, which also improve managers' satisfaction and success. Of course, professionalism also requires communication—lots of it.

This chapter, the final one, focuses on professionalism and communication. It first teaches professionalism—what it means, why it is important, and how it is done. Both emotional intelligence and cultural competence are needed for and intertwined with the professional approach to management. Then the chapter shifts to a discussion of interpersonal communication. It defines communication and describes several important types of communication in HCOs. Next, it presents a model of the communication process to explain how to communicate effectively—and avoid a "communication breakdown." The process makes clear that managers can avoid problems by planning their communication process. The chapter ends with tips for improving communication.

PROFESSIONALISM

Professionalism is the "ability to align personal and organizational conduct with ethical and professional standards that include a responsibility to the patient and community, a service orientation, and a commitment to lifelong learning and improvement" (ACHE 2013, 2). It includes personal and professional accountability, professional development and lifelong learning, and contributions to the community and profession (ACHE 2013, 2). Character, conduct, and quality are basic components of professionalism (Benson and Hummer 2014).

To better understand this concept, let's return to the *Code of Ethics* of the American College of Healthcare Executives, which we saw in Chapter 11 (ACHE 2011). The preamble and the section directly pertaining to the healthcare management profession follow. Read the sections slowly, pause occasionally, and think about what they mean for you and your career.

PREAMBLE

The purpose of the *Code of Ethics* of the American College of Healthcare Executives is to serve as a standard of conduct for members. It contains standards of ethical behavior for healthcare executives in their professional relationships. These relationships include colleagues, patients or others served; members of the healthcare executive's organization and other organizations; the community; and society as a whole.

The *Code of Ethics* also incorporates standards of ethical behavior governing individual behavior, particularly when that conduct directly relates to the role and identity of the healthcare executive.

The fundamental objectives of the healthcare management profession are to maintain or enhance the overall quality of life, dignity and well-being of every individual needing healthcare service and to create a more equitable, accessible, effective and efficient healthcare system.

Healthcare executives have an obligation to act in ways that will merit the trust, confidence, and respect of healthcare professionals and the general public. Therefore, healthcare executives should lead lives that embody an exemplary system of values and ethics.

In fulfilling their commitments and obligations to patients or others served, healthcare executives function as moral advocates and models. Since every management decision affects the health and well-being of both individuals and communities, healthcare executives must carefully evaluate the possible outcomes of their decisions. In organizations that deliver healthcare services, they must work to safeguard and foster the rights, interests and prerogatives of patients or others served.

The role of moral advocate requires that healthcare executives take actions necessary to promote such rights, interests and prerogatives.

Being a model means that decisions and actions will reflect personal integrity and ethical leadership that others will seek to emulate.

I. THE HEALTHCARE EXECUTIVE'S RESPONSIBILITIES TO THE PROFESSION OF HEALTHCARE MANAGEMENT

The healthcare executive shall:

A. Uphold the *Code of Ethics* and mission of the American College of Healthcare Executives;

B. Conduct professional activities with honesty, integrity, respect, fairness and good faith in a manner that will reflect well upon the profession;

C. Comply with all laws and regulations pertaining to healthcare management in the jurisdictions in which the healthcare executive is located or conducts professional activities;

D. Maintain competence and proficiency in healthcare management by implementing a personal program of assessment and continuing professional education;

E. Avoid the improper exploitation of professional relationships for personal gain;

F. Disclose financial and other conflicts of interest;

G. Use this *Code* to further the interests of the profession and not for selfish reasons;

H. Respect professional confidences;

I. Enhance the dignity and image of the healthcare management profession through positive public information programs; and

J. Refrain from participating in any activity that demeans the credibility and dignity of the healthcare management profession.

What caught your attention when you read the *Code of Ethics* excerpt? Did you notice how it indicates proper *character* and *conduct* for HCO managers when they interact with other people? It also guides a manager's behavior when working alone. Professionalism means HCO managers behave in ways that earn trust, confidence, and respect. They are honest, fair, competent, and respectful of others. They serve others and their community. In their work, they follow professional standards and governmental laws, act in good faith, and are accountable for what they do. Professional managers continually develop by evaluating themselves, making improvements, and learning throughout their careers. Professional managers of HCOs realize how their actions, behaviors, and decisions affect the health, well-being, and lives of patients, employees, and many other people. This professionalism helps them and their HCOs contribute to the two fundamental objectives of the healthcare management profession (ACHE 2011):

1. Maintain or enhance the life, dignity, and well-being of everyone who needs healthcare.

2. Create a more equitable, accessible, effective, and efficient healthcare system.

Further, this professionalism helps managers achieve excellence in their life objectives.

You might think that this seems like a lot to do. You're right—it is a lot. Yet, on a day-to-day basis, as the objectives become habit, they become doable. Think of professionalism as doing a lot of the "little things" that maybe you already do. For example, common courtesy, dependability, and helping people are part of professional relationships. Maybe you often do these things; if so, you are on your way to becoming a professional manager. If you do these things only occasionally, well, that's a start to build on as you prepare for your career.

Which of the following words and phrases (ACHE 2011; Benson and Hummer 2014; Dolan 2013; Green 2013) describe you at work, in a volunteer activity, or on a group project?

◆ Trustworthy   ◆ Accepts criticism

◆ Engaged   ◆ Learns from mistakes

◆ Polite   ◆ Apologizes

◆ Dependable   ◆ Meets deadlines

◆ Pleasant   ◆ Avoids workplace gossip

◆ Listens well   ◆ Respects confidentiality

◆ Gives praise   ◆ Neat and clean

◆ Shares credit   ◆ Pursues excellence

◆ Accountable

These words and phrases reflect character and conduct often associated with professionalism. The more you exhibit these characteristics in your job, the more you will be perceived as a professional. Realize that employees pay attention to what managers do—and don't do. Consciously and unconsciously, workers watch and judge managers. They might not call it "professionalism," but workers judge the way managers conduct their work. Of course, nobody is perfect, including someone chosen as "manager of the year"! Even senior managers with twenty or more years of experience are still improving their professionalism.

Professionalism also means doing the "little things" to learn new skills and abilities for professional development. By reading this book, you are developing new skills. This chapter and others (e.g., Chapter 6 on behavior in groups and meetings and Chapter 11 on ethical behavior) help you develop your professionalism. Be sure to keep reading throughout your adult life. Also talk with knowledgeable people (in person, online, or on the phone), attend presentations, watch videos, observe other managers, tour HCOs, gather ideas using social media, participate in workshops, and be a lifelong learner in other ways. Realize that data, information, and knowledge may suddenly emerge and be relevant—and just as suddenly become irrelevant when it is replaced by something even newer. Thus, virtual networks, social media, blogs, tweets, and online discussions are essential (May 2013). All these actions are part of professionalism.

 CHECK IT OUT

The American College of Healthcare Executives (ACHE) is the premier professional association for healthcare managers. ACHE offers many resources to help managers (and future managers) develop themselves as professional healthcare managers. One good resource is the Professional Pointers section in ACHE's bimonthly magazine *Healthcare Executive*. The short, engaging Pointers pertain to topics such as trust in the workplace, career development, holding people accountable, effective meetings, overcoming undesirable behavior, introducing a speaker, adhering to deadlines, responding to ideas, and forgiving workplace grudges. It is a great resource for practical tips on professionalism.

EMOTIONAL INTELLIGENCE

We learned that professionalism includes a manager's personal character and behavior as well as her relationships with other people. This concept leads us to emotional intelligence (EI), which is a big part of character, behavior, and relationships with others.

Emotional intelligence is the "ability to recognize and understand emotions in yourself and others, and your ability to use this awareness to manage your behavior and relationships" (Kivland 2014, 72). Understanding the feelings and emotions of oneself and others—and then using that to guide action and behavior—is EI (Dye 2010).

Emotional intelligence
Ability to recognize and understand emotions in yourself and others, and then use this awareness to manage your behavior and relationships.

A manager must have good EI to have good professionalism and good management. Recall from Chapter 2 our definition of management: the process of getting things done through and with people. Because people (including managers) are strongly affected by emotions, a manager must understand both her emotions and other people's emotions to get things done through and with people. Recall from Chapter 1 the many different types of healthcare management jobs and HCOs. You will be better able to perform those jobs and work in those HCOs if you develop your EI. Plus, you will feel more satisfaction and fulfillment.

As originally developed (Goleman 1998) and applied to healthcare (Freshman and Rubino 2002), EI involves self-awareness, self-regulation, self-motivation, social awareness, and social skills. Self-regulation and self-motivation may be combined (into self-management) so that EI consists of four core skills (Kivland 2014):

1.   Self-awareness is the ability to perceive emotions accurately and be aware of them as they happen.

2.   Self-management is the ability to use emotional awareness to positively direct your behavior.

3.   Social awareness is the ability to understand people's emotions and needs along with organizational "mood" to deepen relationships and increase business outcomes.

4.   Relationship management is the ability to use awareness of your own and others' emotions to inspire and engage greatness.

EI has long been studied as traits, skills, and behaviors for leadership. Combining them into EI and applying the concept to workplace success gained prominence in the 1990s. Research at that time on hundreds of companies found that leadership success was linked more to people skills such as EI than to technical skills such as finance (Goleman 1998). That has become even truer today because organizations use more teams, groups, and collaboration—which requires good EI (Noe et al. 2015). This concept pertains to healthcare too. **Sensitivity to emotions (of oneself and others) and relationship skills are essential competencies for healthcare settings** (Kivland 2014). For example, think about how Partners HealthCare managers would rely on EI to interact with stakeholders while planning and implementing telehealth services in the Boston area.

Of course, managers are not the only people in an HCO who have EI. Everyone has it. Managers should realize that employees use EI to judge managers' emotions, behaviors, and relationships. Subordinates observe their supervisor and then share their EI perceptions with each other. Workers consciously study and unconsciously sense their manager's emotions and behaviors. They might ask peers, "What kind of mood is he in today?" Then they figure out the best way to relate to the boss—or in some cases avoid the boss! Managers with good EI create a positive vibe that attracts employees and strengthens them. Managers with poor EI create a negative vibe that drives away workers and weakens them. This vibe or mood tends to flow downward through the HCO. So a manager must use her EI to be aware of her emotions, to understand how her emotions affect her interactions with other people, and to understand how other people perceive her emotions and interactions. Then, if necessary, she can make adjustments so a positive vibe flows through the organization to strengthen the workforce. For example, some managers adjust their daily work schedule to allow more time for unexpected, urgent matters. Doing so reduces stress so the managers are more pleasant, calm, and attentive to others.

The preceding example illustrates that there are managers and leaders who have room for improvement when it comes to EI. Maybe you have seen or heard this type of manager in a group activity, a team project, a job, a social situation, or a business setting. A manager who improves his EI will improve professionalism, management, and job performance. As is true with other behaviors, skills, and competencies, managers can improve their EI with deliberate effort (Dye 2010). A good first step is to pay attention to emotions throughout the day—to become more aware. Managers should identify emotional triggers and keep track of what causes negative feelings. Causes can include stress, conflict, personal criticism, difficult people, or bad news. Note if behavior and mood change when a trigger occurs. Some people become aggressive, hostile, impatient, or withdrawn. Managers should take notes or keep a journal for a week. Honest feedback from others about emotions and interpersonal relationships is needed too. So managers must be open to feedback from staff and stakeholders. Managers who want to develop good EI actively seek feedback (rather than passively waiting for it to appear). Despite busy schedules, they are available, approachable, welcoming, and good listeners. They are open to good news and bad news. They accept praise and criticism. These characteristics help a manager understand how others perceive him. From there, he can adjust his behavior and interpersonal relationships. You may have heard this advice for dealing with emotions before: pause, take a deep breath, slowly count to ten, and get control of yourself. Many books and videos on this topic are available for EI professional development.

CULTURAL COMPETENCE

For a high degree of professionalism, a manager must also have **cultural competence**—the knowledge, skills, and attitudes needed to understand and interact well with people who are culturally different from oneself. People are diverse in many aspects of culture and identity, such as race, ethnicity, faith and religion, gender, sexual orientation, disability, personality, social status, age, geographic origin, and other characteristics (Molinari and Shanderson 2014). Diversity leads to differences in values, languages, behaviors, beliefs, appearances, and other aspects of life and work. Cultures may differ regarding status, verbal communication, authority, body language, sense of time, etiquette, professional behaviors, and seemingly minor things such as what to do when given a business card.

Cultural competence
The knowledge, skills, and attitudes needed to understand and interact well with people who are culturally different from oneself.

As you may have realized, cultural competence overlaps and is intertwined with professionalism and EI. Although they are different, they support each other. For example, the EI that you learned about in the prior section will help you be more culturally competent. Recall that EI includes social awareness, which is the ability to understand people's emotions and needs. EI skills and attitudes will help you understand and interact well with people who are culturally different.

Chapter 1 discussed how the future will bring more diversity to the American population

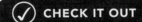

✓ CHECK IT OUT

The American College of Healthcare Executives, the American Hospital Association, the Institute for Diversity in Health Management, and the National Center for Healthcare Leadership together developed an excellent diversity and cultural proficiency assessment tool that managers can use to assess how well their healthcare organizations are prepared for diverse and culturally different people. The tool is available at www.aha.org/content/00-10/diversitytool.pdf.

and thus to HCOs' mix of patients, employees, and stakeholders. So in addition to being culturally competent herself, a manager must create a culturally competent organization. An HCO's buildings, equipment, staff, policies, structures, processes, and services should be sensitive to people of different cultures. Patients should be allowed to identify their cultural preferences, such as language requirements. Managers can use many tools, methods, techniques, and principles from this book to make their HCO more culturally competent, such as the following:

◆   During the strategic planning process, add cultural competency to the organization's mission, vision, values, and goals.

◆   Use project planning to plan projects to achieve this part of the mission.

◆   Assign cultural competency responsibilities and tasks to jobs and departments.

◆   Use staffing methods to ensure the HCO has the right staff, training, incentives, and appraisals to support cultural diversity and competence. Leadership and motivation theories will help.

◆   Use control methods to set standards, monitor performance, and adjust the HCO's structures and processes so that it becomes more culturally competent.

These principles will require decisions and change, so those tools and methods should also be used.

It might seem surprising, but the Golden Rule of treating others as you wish to be treated might not always be the best approach! For cultural competence, instead consider using the Platinum Rule: "Treat others as *they* wish to be treated" (Dolan 2013, 34).

Have you taken a college course to learn about cultural diversity and become more culturally competent? Many colleges offer (and some require) these courses. Take one—it will help prepare you to be an HCO manager.

COMMUNICATION

We now shift to communication, a word for which there are many definitions. The following two definitions have been chosen because together they identify the *process* and expected *outcome* of communication:

1.   Communication is "transmitting a message from a sender to a receiver, through a channel and with the interference of noise" (DeVito 1986, 61).

2.   Communication is "the development of mutual understanding" (Liebler and McConnell 2004, 496).

DeVito's definition identifies elements of the communication process—transmitting, message, sender, receiver, channel, and interference. Liebler and McConnell's definition reflects the desired outcome of communication—achieving mutual understanding. Based on these ideas, this book defines **communication** as transmitting information to someone else to develop shared understanding. Communication involves a sender, message, message transmission, intended receiver(s), and noise that interferes with communication.

Communication is not a management function such as those we studied in prior chapters. Nor is it a way of managing, such as managing in a professional way. Instead, communication is a common activity that just about everyone does throughout the day. It is so common that managers use it continually when they perform their management functions and manage in a professional way.

Communication
Transmitting information to someone else to develop shared understanding.

TYPES OF COMMUNICATION

There are several kinds of communication in HCOs. They vary in how much managers can control them. Some communication is *one-to-one*—a maintenance supervisor talks with a carpenter, for example. Other communication is *one-to-group*—a maintenance supervisor talks with all the maintenance workers on first shift. Some communication is *group-to-group*—the first-shift maintenance workers talk with the second-shift maintenance workers. The more people who are involved, the harder it is for a communicator or manager to control the communication.

Communication is sometimes *intentional* and sometimes *unintentional*. We often communicate intentionally, even thinking ahead about what we intend to say or write. We communicate unintentionally when our actions, behavior, body language, and facial expressions accidentally communicate unconscious feelings and attitudes. **Managers control and shape intentional communication but not unintentional communication.** This concept is important because unintentional communication affects how employees view managers' intentional communication. Managers use formal communication—the official communication of the HCO's organization structure of managers, authority, policies, rules, and documents. HCOs also have informal communication—the unofficial communication among coworkers, peers, friends, carpoolers, relatives, and others outside of the official organization structure. Informal communication might not agree with managers and is usually not controlled by them. This type of communication is more spontaneous and changes more quickly than formal communication does.

Recall from Chapter 4 that the informal organization has its own unofficial communication known as the *grapevine*. Is there a student grapevine at your college or university? Although managers cannot control the grapevine and informal communication in their HCOs, they should not ignore it. By paying attention to it, managers can better understand how employees feel about the HCO, their jobs, a planned change, and many other aspects of the HCO. For example, managers at one medical center regularly checked in with the grapevine to judge how staff felt about going live with a new computer system. Formal messages gave mild support, but informal messages reflected anxiety. So managers gave employees more training and practice in the new system before it went live. An HCO's grapevine is likely to be extensive, but it is not always accurate. It will carry official news, unofficial news, exaggerated news, gossip, inside information, and stories (both fiction and nonfiction). The grapevine used to be mostly oral communication; now organizations have digital grapevines that spread messages much more widely and rapidly.

DIRECTIONS OF COMMUNICATION

Communication flows in all directions in organizations. Vertical communication has always been common because it follows the vertical hierarchy and chain of command. Trends reflect increasing horizontal and diagonal communication. You may want to turn back to Chapter 5 to refresh your memory about different organization structures and see how communications might flow up, down, sideways, or diagonally (Exhibit 15.1).

Managers use **downward communication** with their subordinates to give directions, make assignments, offer feedback, control performance, motivate, and so on. To communicate this way, managers use memos, policy statements, job descriptions, e-mail, formal talks, phone calls, hallway conversations, written instructions, control reports, balanced scorecards, performance appraisals, and many other communication methods.

Downward communication
Communication to someone at a lower level in one's own vertical chain of command or hierarchy.

EXHIBIT 15.1
Directions of Communication in an HCO

Direction	Explanation	Example
Downward	Communication to someone at a lower level in one's own vertical chain of command or hierarchy	A nursing supervisor tells a nurse the work schedule
Upward	Communication to someone at a higher level in one's own vertical chain of command or hierarchy	A housekeeper tells a supervisor about broken equipment
Horizontal	Communication to someone at the same level of an organization and outside of one's own vertical chain of command or hierarchy	The marketing director explains advertising costs to the finance director
Diagonal	Communication to someone at a higher or lower level of an organization and outside of one's own vertical chain of command or hierarchy	A computer repair tech explains a new online security procedure to the warehouse supervisor

Subordinates use **upward communication** with their bosses to provide feedback, describe progress, report problems, give input and advice, and so on. Upward communication methods include written and oral information, e-mail, phone calls, memos, reports, data, and other means.

Employees, including managers, must communicate upward to keep their boss informed. This communication includes informing one's supervisor about bad news, which may be hard to do. Some people use vague words to communicate negative news and only hint at a problem. For example, they may say, "We're a little behind" instead of directly stating that the HCO is two months behind on a six-month project! That form of communication does not help. In the long run, it will harm the HCO and people involved. Managers respect employees for being professional enough to keep their boss informed by honestly reporting news (good and bad).

Employees and managers use **horizontal communication** to communicate with their counterparts at the same level of the HCO. This type of communication is between people who are not in a supervisor–subordinate relationship (recall the discussion of mutual adjustment from Chapters 4 and 5). Also called *lateral* or *sideways* communication, horizontal communication helps coordinate work between departments. It breaks down silos that develop when only vertical communication exists. Horizontal communication is essential for interprofessional patient care, project teams, and other collaboration. Oral and online conversations, memos, texts, e-mail, and phone calls are some ways people communicate horizontally.

Employees and managers also use **diagonal communication**. This type of communication has become more common as organizations have become more organic and adopted a culture of "we are all on the same team." It uses fast, simple methods, such as texts, face-to-face conversations, phone calls, and e-mail rather than prepared reports and memos. Diagonal communication is useful for sharing information, input, and expertise throughout an organization.

Changes in the external environment are leading HCOs to be more open with communication rather than locked into vertical patterns. For example, HCO managers in Bowling Green, Kentucky, may use groups, task forces, and project teams of employees drawn from multiple departments throughout an HCO. These groups and teams can bring together employees who are in diagonal relationships with each other in the organization chart. Open communication is in line with the trend for organizations to be more natural, horizontal, adaptive, and collaborative with information communicated throughout the organization.

Upward communication
Communication to someone at a higher level in one's own vertical chain of command or hierarchy.

Horizontal communication
Communication to someone at the same level of an organization and outside of one's own vertical chain of command or hierarchy.

Diagonal communication
Communication to someone at a higher or lower level of an organization and outside of one's own vertical chain of command or hierarchy.

THE COMMUNICATION PROCESS

The purpose of communication is to create shared understanding. However, sometimes communication creates *mis*understanding. Surely everyone has experienced a

Exhibit 15.2
Communication
Model

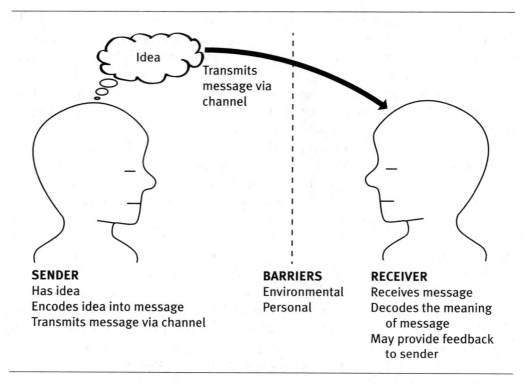

SENDER
Has idea
Encodes idea into message
Transmits message via channel

BARRIERS
Environmental
Personal

RECEIVER
Receives message
Decodes the meaning
of message
May provide feedback
to sender

communication breakdown. Breakdowns result from ineffective communication methods, and they lead to misunderstandings that can spread like bad germs to confuse people, waste valuable resources, and cause harm in HCOs. To be effective in their jobs, managers must understand how communication occurs and how to create effective communication. The communication model in Exhibit 15.2 can help you understand these concepts.

Recall that communication is transmitting information to someone else to develop shared understanding. The model in Exhibit 15.2 shows two people. The person on the left (sender) has an idea and wants the person on the right (receiver) to understand and share that same idea. **Communication must transmit the idea from the sender's mind to the receiver's mind.** Here are the essential elements of communication:

◆ *Idea:* thought, opinion, or feeling in the sender's mind

◆ *Sender:* person who has an idea to communicate with someone else

◆ *Message:* the sender's idea encoded (expressed) in words, icons, symbols, visuals, speech, body language, behaviors, or actions

◆ *Channel:* method/media (e.g., e-mail, phone call, text message, published report, speech) to transmit a message from sender to receiver

◆   *Receiver:* person(s) to whom a message is communicated

◆   *Barriers:* biases, distractions, and other obstacles that impede communication

The following is an example of how the elements of the communication model work together to communicate:

1. Sara Sender has an idea in her mind that she wants to communicate to Rob Receiver so that the same idea is in his mind. Then they will share understanding of Sara's idea.

2. Sara considers how to encode her idea into a message and how to transmit the message using channels. She considers possible barriers (environmental and personal) that could interfere with her encoding and sending the message or interfere with Rob receiving and decoding her message.

3. Sara chooses two channels—e-mail and phone call—to transmit her message to Rob.

4. Sara encodes her idea into words. She again considers possible barriers between herself and Rob when encoding her idea. When using the e-mail channel, she adds a smiley face symbol ☺ to reflect how she feels.

5. Rob receives the messages from Sara via e-mail and a phone call.

6. Rob decodes (interprets) the content and feeling of the messages. He figures out what these messages mean to him.

7. Rob now has an idea in his mind that came from Sara. They have shared understanding.

Suppose Rob wants Sara to know that he received her messages. He also wants to be sure that he accurately understands Sara. To accomplish these tasks, he decides to send feedback. The feedback begins a new communication. Rob now becomes the sender, and Sara becomes the receiver. Rob follows steps 1–7 to send a message to Sara. Sara receives and decodes Rob's feedback message. Sara is happy to know Rob has the same idea in his mind as she has in her mind. She sends Rob a quick e-mail to confirm they both understand her idea the same way!

Communication may happen with—or without—feedback from the receiver to the sender. Notice that in this example, the receiver (Rob) did provide feedback to the sender (Sara) regarding her message to him. In fact, Sara then provided feedback to Rob regarding his message to her. **Feedback from the receiver to the sender helps ensure shared understanding in communication.** It might even help avoid serious mistakes. Imagine a nurse in Grand Rapids, Michigan (during a busy day) listening on the phone (with background noise) to a physician (who is in a hurry) state a medication order that sounds like *4 ml . . .* or maybe it was *40 ml.* The nurse restates the order to give feedback to the physician of how she understands the order. They confirm that they share the same idea: *4 ml.* Yet sometimes receivers do not provide feedback. Do you reply to every text you get? How much feedback is given when an HCO puts a billboard on Interstate 81?

To plan a communication, which does the sender decide first—the encoded message or the channel to send the message? Think about how you have communicated. Often, the channel (e.g., text message, phone call, PowerPoint slide) is decided first, and then the actual message is created and encoded. Alternatively, a manager might encode a message first, such as crafting a message in Microsoft Word and revising it so that it has the right tone and content. Then, the manager decides how to transmit the message—text now for some employees and then the HCO's weekly online newsletter for all employees. The chosen communication channels (methods) affect how senders encode their ideas. The reverse is also true: How a message is encoded affects which channels to use.

Encoding Messages

Messages may be encoded verbally or nonverbally (Exhibit 15.3).

Verbal encoding
Using written or spoken words to represent ideas.

Verbal encoding uses words to encode and represent ideas. A manager encodes her ideas into a message with written or spoken words to represent ideas in her mind. This encoding depends on language and variations based on dialects, slang, acronyms, grammar, and linguistics.

"When I use a word, it means just what I choose it to mean," said Humpty Dumpty. That makes it easy for Mr. Dumpty, but not for people he communicates with. Encoding ideas with words can be tricky because words may mean different things to different people. A mother tells her son to "be home before dark" without realizing he will interpret *dark* differently than she does. Language is often imprecise, and words have multiple meanings. When encoding ideas into a message, managers should think about how the receiver might decode or interpret that message and should strive for shared understanding with clear, direct words and, if necessary, repetition of the idea.

EXHIBIT 15.3
Encoding, Channels, and Barriers in Communication

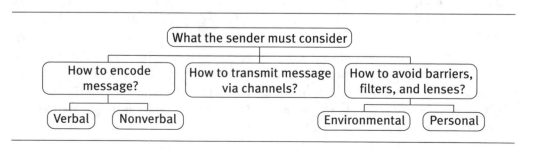

Problems arise in HCOs when a sender encodes a message with healthcare slang (e.g., "She coded so we bagged her") or acronyms (e.g., "MI" for myocardial infarction) that not everyone understands. Slang and acronyms are commonly used in HCOs. Although the receiver (of a message) can look up unknown slang and abbreviations, some receivers will just guess the meaning or skip that part of a message. Oops, we just lost shared understanding!

Nonverbal encoding is done without words. **Nonverbal encoding includes diagrams, charts, icons, pictures, attire, objects, body language, touch, behavior, and actions** (Drafke 2009; Hellriegel and Slocum 2011). Managers sometimes use nonverbal visual materials along with words because words may be imprecise and misinterpreted. Words may be inadequate to encode some ideas, which is reflected in the saying "A picture is worth a thousand words." PowerPoint presentations often combine words with visual symbols to strengthen understanding.

Recall from earlier in this chapter that a professional manager behaves in ways that earn trust, confidence, and respect. Professionalism includes how you present yourself—communicate nonverbal messages about yourself—to others. Have you ever seen someone who looked excited and someone else who looked tired? Nonverbal messages in gestures, facial expressions, handshakes, eye contact, and other **body language** communicate (sometimes unintentionally) feelings and attitudes. When manager Serika smiles, stands up straight, and moves quickly, other employees think she is happy and excited about her work. If she frowns, slouches, and trudges along, her employees think she is unhappy and tired of her work. **Employees observe and follow what managers do, so managers should consider how they present themselves and are perceived by others.** If a nonverbal message (body language) conflicts with words, receivers generally believe the nonverbal message (Drafke 2009).

You get only one chance to make a first impression, and it happens quickly. One communications expert claims that "people decide ten things about you within ten seconds of meeting you" based on your appearance and behavior (Bjorseth 2007, 52). Visit your college career center for advice on making a good first impression. Perhaps staff can videotape you in a pretend meeting and then review the tape to offer feedback. "Ryan, when you met Mrs. Mantoni, you stood up, smiled, and made eye contact. Very good! You looked professional!" Some colleges offer an "Etiquette and Dining 101" course to help students develop self-presentation skills before going to job interviews.

Communication Channels

How do managers transmit messages? They use **channels** of communication. **Channels are the methods and media that carry an encoded message from sender to receiver.** How you encode a message affects how you transmit the message, and vice versa, so think about them together when deciding how to communicate. HCO managers use phone calls, texts,

Nonverbal encoding
Representing ideas without using words, such as by using diagrams, charts, icons, pictures, attire, objects, body language, touch, behavior, and actions.

Body language
Communication by posture, facial expressions, gestures, eyes, and mouth.

Channels
Methods and media that transmit a message from sender to receiver(s).

speeches, websites, teleconferences, posters, tweets, YouTube videos, personal conversations, reports, blogs, intranet newsletters, and other communication channels.

Channels differ in information richness; the richer a channel is, the more quickly it creates understanding in receivers (Ledlow and Stephens 2009). Exhibit 15.4 shows some channels in descending order of information richness. The richer channels (media) enable more rapid feedback, personalization, language variety, and frequent verbal cues (e.g., a louder voice) and nonverbal cues (e.g., a frown) to add information. **Channels that convey both verbal and nonverbal information are richest in information and thus create understanding more quickly and accurately than those that are less information-rich.** However, all channels have pros and cons, which are explained next.

Channels such as speeches, phone calls, face-to-face discussions, video conferences, and a shouted "Yo dude!" all transmit messages of spoken words. These channels convey a speaker's tone of voice, pauses, and pronunciations. As a result, they transmit information about feelings and emotion. These types of channels enable immediate feedback, questions and answers, and clarification, so managers use these channels to direct, instruct, motivate, train, lead, and control (Dunn 2010). However, not all messages delivered through spoken channels are understood. Consider casual, spontaneous conversation. Little time is spent encoding, transmitting, or decoding messages in casual conversation, which reduces understanding between speaker and receiver. Some channels for spoken messages take time to prepare and transmit, such as formal speeches and video conferences, which improves understanding.

Channels such as e-mail, formal reports, texts, memos, and handwritten notes taped to a wall transmit messages of written words. Advantages of such communication include a record of the communication for later use and consistency so that everyone gets the same

Exhibit 15.4
Information Richness of Some Communication Channels (in Descending Order)

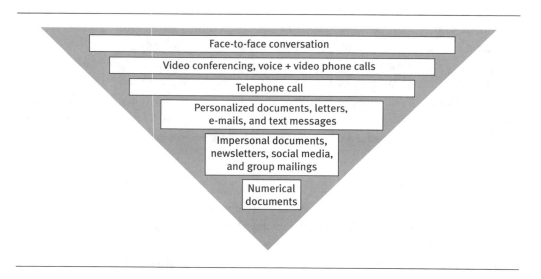

- Face-to-face conversation
- Video conferencing, voice + video phone calls
- Telephone call
- Personalized documents, letters, e-mails, and text messages
- Impersonal documents, newsletters, social media, and group mailings
- Numerical documents

message (Dunn 2010). These channels usually allow more time to carefully encode and decode, which improves shared understanding. Thus, technical information and details that must be exact are conveyed in written documents that have been precisely encoded and then proofread. Channels with written messages usually provide slower feedback than channels with verbal information, although texting and online chat have helped written channels become faster. However, by emphasizing speed and brevity, these digital channels transmit less content. Consequently, receivers may "read between the lines" to add content and thereby decode messages incorrectly.

Written channels are less rich than spoken channels because they do not convey as much emotional information, though senders may use emoticons such as ☺ and ☹ as well as different font effects and styles to convey feelings. When using a smartphone, talking is a richer channel than texting because it better expresses the sender's feelings. Written media are viewed as more formal than oral media, and online writing is less formal than writing on letterhead with proper grammar and spelling. Which channels should a manager use in an HCO? It depends. Like many other aspects of managing, no single approach is always best. Managers must assess the situation and judge which method is best. What would fit with the HCO's culture? Which channel(s) would work best for the people who will receive and have to decode the message? Which channels would avoid a communication breakdown?

Face-to-face conversation is best for personal, sensitive, and complex communication, such as mental health counseling. Pick information-rich channels for spoken words and body language when you want to understand emotions and get the receiver's visual cues for immediate feedback. Simple channels may be used for routine communication, such as reminders to order supplies. Use more information-rich personal channels, such as a face-to-face meeting, when explaining the reason an employee was not promoted. Individual communication is often time-consuming and costly for communicating with groups, so other channels may be preferred, such as digital newsletters, tweets, and speeches. These channels are less information-rich but also require less cost and less time. **Multiple channels of communication can help ensure the correct message gets through, although too much communication can be a problem.** Communication overload causes "selective receiving," in which intended receivers select which messages to receive and which to ignore. Managers can ask stakeholders which channels and media they prefer. Some hospitals ask physicians for their preferred ways to communicate.

Decoding Messages

For correct communication to occur, receivers must receive messages and accurately decode (interpret) those messages. They must play back voicemail, observe nonverbal cues, read texts, and listen to a speech. The receiver has to assign meaning to words. She must interpret facial expressions and gestures. Senders can improve communication by encoding and transmitting messages in ways that make it easy for the receiver to receive and decode the message.

Management and communication require effective listening to receive and decode messages, yet listening often is not done well—perhaps because schools teach writing, reading, and speaking, but they do not teach listening. Here are some useful tips to improve listening skills (Bjorseth 2007):

1. First, pay attention.

2. Listen for content (the meaning of the words) and for feeling (the emotions of the speaker).

3. Avoid the urge to speak; do not interrupt.

4. Be open-minded about the content rather than judging the content as soon as you hear it.

5. Ask questions that show your interest and that encourage the speaker to keep talking.

6. Provide feedback to the speaker.

(→) **TRY IT, APPLY IT**

You can develop listening ability to improve how well you receive and decode spoken messages. Doing so will make you a better manager. Consider the six listening techniques previously mentioned. Which are typical of how you listen? Which are not? Identify the listening techniques you want to improve and then practice them. Make a reminder note for yourself. Ask friends to give you listening feedback. After talking with someone, think about how well you listened, based on these guidelines. With practice, you can make these guidelines part of how you listen.

Barriers, Filters, and Lenses

Barriers can distort, reduce, and even block communications at all stages of encoding, sending, receiving, and decoding. There are two types of barriers—environmental and personal. Environmental barriers arise from the environment(s) in which communication takes place. Because the sender and receiver may be in different environments, both environments should be considered to avoid barriers and communication breakdowns

(Drafke 2009). Personal barriers arise from the people who communicate—the sender and receiver(s). Here too, both must be considered to avoid communication problems.

Have you ever been talking with a friend while walking in a city but suddenly could not hear because of an ambulance siren? Have you ever been unable to read in bad lighting? Have you ever missed a cell phone call because you were in a "dead zone"? These situations involve communication barriers created by the environment in which people try to communicate. HCO managers create and confront communication barriers because of their work environment. Electronic equipment and devices make distracting noises. A manager blocks communication when she works behind a closed door. You cannot avoid all barriers, but you can anticipate and avoid some of them.

People create personal barriers to communication. Personalities, emotions, moods, beliefs, and biases can impede communication. To begin with, personal barriers affect our willingness to even send or receive a message. Then they affect how we talk, write, hear, read, and interpret what others say and write. Emotions such as fear, anger, love, joy, resentment, and relief affect how we send and receive communications. If we distrust a manager, we filter out what he says. Filtering may occur unconsciously and be hard to avoid. Cultural differences, studied earlier in this chapter, lead to different attitudes and styles for speaking, listening, writing, reading, body language, personal space, preferred communication channels, and timeliness of response to a message. Disabilities with vision, hearing, and dexterity also may interfere with communication. Excessive multitasking can create a personal barrier for accurate communication. **Senders and receivers should try to avoid communication barriers to avoid communication breakdowns.**

HERE'S WHAT HAPPENED
Representatives of HCOs, schools, churches, businesses, youth groups, social agencies, and other organizations came together to plan how to reduce tobacco use by adolescents and teenagers in a small metropolitan area. Everyone agreed on the goal and wanted to help. When they met for the first time, personal barriers to communication emerged. People had different communication styles. Some people knew each other well whereas others were strangers. Some people had time for a long meeting with lots of discussion, but others were in a hurry. Some people who were talkative during a private phone call hesitated to speak in a group. Representatives of small HCOs did not feel at ease with the leader of a big HCO. The group leaders had to decrease personal communication barriers to increase communication.

TIPS FOR EFFECTIVE COMMUNICATION
As a manager, you can use the following suggestions to improve your communication at work (Borkowski 2009; Drafke 2009; Dunn 2010; Moussa 2012):

◆ Create an organizational culture that values and rewards good communication.

◆ Be accessible and open to communication; visit employees' work areas and have an open office door.

◆ Learn about differences in communication that come with cultural diversity.

◆ Seek and pay attention to verbal and nonverbal feedback when communicating.

◆ Prepare to communicate by removing distractions, organizing ideas, anticipating barriers, and choosing how to encode and transmit your message so that the receiver will understand.

◆ When communicating with varied stakeholders, customize the communication content and process to fit different stakeholders.

◆ Be careful how you communicate when you feel strong emotions.

◆ Empathize; put yourself in the receiver's situation.

◆ Use multiple channels and repetition when necessary.

◆ Read and listen for meaning and feeling (content and emotion).

◆ Practice and develop communication skills; pay attention to role models; obtain training if necessary.

Finally, to communicate effectively, use good emotional intelligence and cultural competence, which were explained earlier in this chapter.

ONE MORE TIME

Managers at all levels of HCOs should strive for a high degree of professionalism in which their character and conduct live up to ethical and professional standards. Professionalism involves forming effective relationships with other people, being accountable for one's actions and behavior, lifelong learning, and service to the community and profession. It requires managers to be dependable, honest, fair, competent, and respectful. Emotional intelligence and cultural competence are important for professionalism and management. Emotional intelligence is the ability to recognize and understand emotions in oneself and others and use this awareness to manage behavior and relationships. Cultural competence is knowledge, skills, and attitudes to understand and interact well with people who are culturally different from oneself.

Managers at all levels of HCOs communicate to create shared understanding with other people. Communication is used to perform the five basic management functions and ten management roles. Formal communication in an HCO is the official communication of the organization structure (e.g., managers, authority, rules, documents). Informal communication (the grapevine) is outside of the official organization structure. Although managers do not control informal communication, they should pay attention to it. Formal communication in an organization goes in all directions—mostly vertically and horizontally, but also diagonally. Workers develop their own informal communication patterns.

Communication involves an idea, sender, message, channel, receiver, and barriers that interfere with communication. The sender encodes (verbally or nonverbally) an idea into a message and then transmits it through channels (media) to the receiver. The receiver decodes (interprets) the message by reading, listening, and observing. Barriers can distort, reduce, and even block communications at all stages of the process. Environmental barriers arise from the environment in which communication takes place. Personal barriers arise from the people who communicate—the sender and receiver. To avoid communication breakdowns, managers must assess the communication situation and decide how to encode and send the message. The receiver may provide feedback to the sender to ensure effective communication and shared understanding.

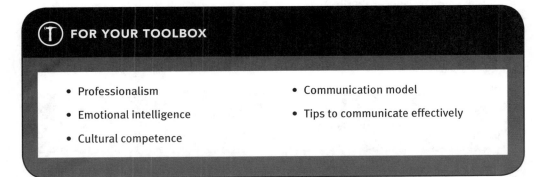

(T) FOR YOUR TOOLBOX

- Professionalism
- Emotional intelligence
- Cultural competence
- Communication model
- Tips to communicate effectively

FOR DISCUSSION

1. In your own words, what is professionalism? Why is it important for HCO managers?

2. In your own words, what is emotional intelligence? Why is it important for HCO managers?

3. In your own words, what is cultural competence? Why is it important for HCO managers?

4. Discuss in detail how communication occurs using the communication model in this chapter.

5. In your experience, which parts of the communication model have caused problems? How could you avoid those problems?

6. Discuss how nonverbal communication is important for managers.

CASE STUDY QUESTIONS

These questions refer to the Integrative Case Studies at the back of this book.

1. Taking Care of Business at Graceland Memorial Hospital case: Based on how professionalism is explained in this chapter, to what extent does Mr. Prestwood demonstrate professionalism? How about Ms. Thompson?

2. I Can't Do It All case: Using what you learned in this chapter, describe the emotional intelligence of people in this case.

3. Disparities in Care at Southern Regional Health System case: Explain how professionalism and cultural competence will be important for Tim Hank as he tries to reduce healthcare disparities.

4. Nowhere Job case: Using the communication model presented in this chapter, describe causes of Ernest's communication problems. Then use the model to suggest improvements.

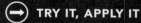 TRY IT, APPLY IT

Think of communication in your classroom. List at least five environmental barriers and five personal barriers that could interfere with communication in the classroom. How can these barriers be avoided?

A MANAGEMENT EXAMPLE: PARTNERS HEALTHCARE

PARTNERS HEALTHCARE: CONNECTING HEART FAILURE PATIENTS TO PROVIDERS THROUGH REMOTE MONITORING

Andrew Broderick

Reprinted with permission from The Commonwealth Fund.
Case Studies in Telehealth Adoption, January 2013.

OVERVIEW

Partners HealthCare (Partners), an integrated health system in Boston, is undergoing a mission-driven, system-level transformation by aligning the organization with external forces shaping the future organization, financing, and delivery of health care. Its strategic initiatives center on making patient care more affordable and accountable through providing integrated, evidence-based, patient-centered care. Partners' strategy implementation group has been looking at performance improvement in a number of priority conditions. These initially included diabetes, acute myocardial infarction, coronary artery bypass graft surgery, stroke, and colorectal cancer, but other conditions will be added to the initial care redesign portfolio over time. Care redesign initiatives are working to move the organization from an episodic and specialty approach to a longitudinal, condition-based, and patient-focused orientation. These include determining how technology can contribute toward improving care quality and cost-effectiveness and identifying strategies for their successful introduction into practice.

A key strategic priority at Partners has been to reduce 30-day readmissions to improve quality of care and patient satisfaction, and to minimize Partners' financial risk for potential reductions in Medicare payments. Initiatives that work toward meeting those goals include: providing patients with critical information at discharge to promote safer transitions, using transitions teams and health coaches, participating in the Center for Medicare and Medicaid Services' care coordination pilot demonstrations, and programs that connect chronic care patients with specialized outpatient care services.[1] Health information technologies, including patient-centered telehealth technologies, serve as a strategic tool across many of these process improvement initiatives. In the future, widespread use of connected health solutions at Partners will be driven by structural changes like new reimbursement models and the introduction of patient-centered medical homes.

Partners' Center for Connected Health (CCH)[2] leads the development of patient-centered telehealth solutions and remote health services for a variety of chronic health conditions, potentially leading to reductions in preventable readmissions. The shared goal of these telehealth solutions is to improve outpatient care management. Partners' experience with the implementation of technology into workflow and care management practices indicates that the technology has a positive impact on patient activation and engagement in self-care and plays a critical role in realizing better clinical outcomes. This evidence is critical in demonstrating to providers that this new program supports behavior changes that lead to improved care and quality outcomes. However, Partners' experience indicates that organizations must be prepared for potential implementation delays imposed by the current fee-for-service environment's adverse impact on staff behavior. To overcome workforce resistance, organizations must demonstrate to clinicians and other staff that new programs will support care and quality outcomes.

BACKGROUND

Boston-based Partners HealthCare is an integrated health system. In addition to the two academic medical centers, Brigham and Women's Hospital and Massachusetts General Hospital, the Partners' system includes community and specialty hospitals, community health centers, a physician network, home health and long-term care services, and other health-related entities. The spectrum of care offered at Partners includes prevention and primary care, hospital and specialty care, rehabilitation, and home care services. As one of the nation's leading medical research organizations and a principal teaching affiliate of Harvard Medical School, the nonprofit organization employs more than 50,000 physicians, nurses, scientists, and caregivers.

Partners' mission includes a commitment to its community and the recognition that increasing value and continuously improving quality are essential to maintaining operational excellence. Partners is also dedicated to enhancing patient care, teaching, and research and to taking a leadership role as an integrated health care system. The organization also prizes technology adoption and innovation to drive improvements in operations, productivity, and patient care. Its success to date in the large-scale adoption of electronic health record (EHR) and computerized physician order entry (CPOE) systems attests to the organizational culture of openness, preparedness, and ability to adapt to change. Such attributes have helped to ensure that the rollout of new technologies is minimally disruptive and seamless to workflow.

Partners has launched efficient care redesign efforts for five conditions—diabetes, acute myocardial infarction, coronary artery bypass graft surgery, stroke, and colorectal cancer—that reflect its shift toward longitudinal, condition-, and patient-focused orientation in care. The care redesign initiative is being led by Partners Community HealthCare (PCH), the management services organization for the Partners' network of physicians and hospitals. PCH encompasses more than 5,500 employed and affiliated physicians and seven acute care hospitals within the system. If opportunities for using technology-enabled strategies to aid in redesigned care have been identified, Partners' Center for Connected Health will lead the design and development of patient-centered telehealth solutions and remote health services. PCH will help introduce them into practice across the Partners' network.

PERFORMANCE IMPROVEMENT INITIATIVES THAT REDUCE PREVENTABLE READMISSIONS

A top strategic priority at Partners is to reduce 30-day readmissions to improve the quality of patient care and patient satisfaction and minimize risk for reductions in Medicare payments. In a survey of Massachusetts hospitals, more than 10 percent of patients were reported to have been readmitted for the same or unrelated complaints within 30 days.[3] Processes that ensure seamless transitions from hospital to other care settings are essential. These include improvements in educating patients and caregivers, reconciling medications carefully before and after discharge, communicating with receiving clinicians, and ensuring prompt outpatient follow-up. Exhibit 1 illustrates 30-day readmission rates for heart failure, acute myocardial infarction, and pneumonia at selected Partners' hospitals.[4] Partners is currently pilot-testing several programs addressing patient safety,[5] experience,[6] and quality,[7] with a goal of reducing 30-day readmission rates for patients at high risk of readmission. These include programs that target critical failures in communication and information exchange during care transitions across settings and caregivers.

THE CENTER FOR CONNECTED HEALTH'S ROLE IN ADVANCING PATIENT-CENTERED TECHNOLOGY

In 1995, Partners established Partners Telemedicine to use consumer-ready technologies to enhance the patient–physician relationship and deliver remote care. This entity later evolved to become the Center for Connected Health. "Connected health" signifies new patient-centered technology strategies and care models that use information and

	Brigham & Women's Hospital	Faulkner Hospital	Mass. General Hospital	Newton-Wellesley Hospital	North Shore Medical Center	U.S. National Rate
Acute myocardial infarction	21.1%	21.1%	22.1%	20.8%	18.6%	19.8%
Heart failure	23.7	27.0	23.7	23.8	22.8	24.8
Pneumonia	20.4	20.0	19.0	17.1	18.6	18.4

Partners HealthCare Data Period: July 1, 2007–June 30, 2010.

Partners HealthCare Source: Hospital Compare.

Reference Point Source: U.S. National Rate for Heart Failure, Acute Myocardial Infarction, and Pneumonia for Medicare Patients.

communications technology—cell phones, computers, networked devices, and simple remote monitoring tools—to support the health care needs of patients in community-based settings without disrupting their day-to-day lives. CCH solutions help providers and patients manage chronic conditions, maintain health and wellness, and improve adherence, engagement, and clinical outcomes. To date, CCH has generated more than 100 scholarly publications and helped more than 30,000 patients. In 2011, CCH collected its one millionth vital life sign from program participants.[8]

CCH's programs use a combination of remote monitoring, social media, and data management applications to enhance patient adherence and engagement to realize improvements in care quality and cost outcomes. The center also supports mobile health initiatives, including a prenatal care text-messaging program for expectant mothers, and wellness programs, such as Step It Up and Virtual Coach, that emphasize activity and exercise among elementary school children and overweight people, respectively. The center offers video-based, real-time consultations and an online second-opinion service, Partners Online Specialty Consultations. CCH recently spun off a health service company, Healthrageous, to provide self-management tools that offer personalized support and motivation in health and lifestyle management.

CCH focuses on applying technologies to conditions that have standard clinical measures of success or offer a clear business case in terms of the potential cost savings or return on investment. For example, the Medicare payment reductions associated with 30-day readmissions provides the heart failure program with a clear business case in terms of the negative financial implications from poor care outcomes. For management of diabetes, HbA1c is a well-accepted clinical marker used to measure success. One program that has been successfully piloted and implemented at scale across Partners is the Connected

Cardiac Care Program (CCCP). It provides home telemonitoring and patient education over a four-month period to enable patients to collect frequent readings and become more engaged in their care.

Exhibit 2 outlines two connected models of care that are currently being deployed at Partners to address congestive heart failure, as well as diabetes and hypertension.

EXHIBIT 2.
Connected Health Models of Care at Partners

The Diabetes Connect and Blood Pressure Connect programs offer patients and their care providers a way to track their blood sugar or blood pressure readings and to collaborate on establishing a shared care plan between office visits. These programs differ from the Connected Cardiac Care Program (CCCP), which uses a centralized telemonitoring model. Diabetes Connect and Blood Pressure Connect operate on a distributed model where each practice comes up with its own structure and protocols for managing patients. Nurses, certified diabetes educators, pharmacists, or primary care physicians can monitor patients' data. The driver to adopt is greater provider efficiency and quality outcomes, and less focus on cost savings. The programs help manage patients by providing structured data frequently and engaging patients actively in their care management. Both programs are available at several primary care practices affiliated with Massachusetts General and Brigham and Women's Hospitals, and through the Partners Community HealthCare network of physicians and hospitals.

Connected Health Program	Summary Description
Connected Cardiac Care Program	A centralized telemonitoring and self-management and preventive care program for heart failure patients that combines telemonitoring capabilities with nurse intervention and care coordination, coaching, and education. The daily transmission of weight, heart rate, pulse, and blood pressure data by patients enables providers to more effectively assess patient status and provide "just-in-time" care and patient education. The program has led to an approximate 50 percent reduction in heart failure–related hospital readmissions for participants.
Diabetes Connect Blood Pressure Connect	Provide practices with tools for the self-management and monitoring of patients with diabetes and hypertension. A recent clinical study with 75 enrolled patients found that participants in Diabetes Connect achieved an average drop in HbA1c of 1.5 percent, while 22.3 percent of participants enrolled in Blood Pressure Connect achieved a 10mmHg or greater drop in systolic blood pressure, compared with 16.7 percent among nonparticipants.

SOURCE: Center for Connected Health.

CARE OUTCOMES

Remote monitoring improves the health of ambulatory patients who have been recently hospitalized for heart failure and leads to reductions in hospital readmissions. A 2006 pilot study of CCCP with 150 heart failure patients, with an average age of 70, who had been admitted to Massachusetts General Hospital and received six months of follow-up care did not reach statistical significance. However, the results indicated a positive trend in reducing readmissions (Exhibit 3). Sixty-eight patients received usual care for heart failure; the remaining 82 patients were offered remote monitoring. Forty-two patients accepted and 40 declined to participate. The remote monitoring group had a lower rate of all-cause readmissions compared with usual-care patients and nonparticipants. Patients in the remote monitoring group also had fewer heart failure–related readmissions. However, all-cause emergency room (ER) visits were higher among the remote-monitoring group than for usual care and nonparticipating patients. This higher frequency of reporting to the ER may be a result of closer monitoring.

EXHIBIT 3.
Remote Monitoring CCCP Pilot Results at Six-Month Follow-Up

	Control (n=68) Mean rate (± standard deviation)	Intervention (n=42) Mean rate (± standard deviation)	Nonparticipant (n=40) Mean rate (± standard deviation)	P-value
Hospital readmissions				
• All-cause	0.73 (±1.51)	0.64 (±0.87)	0.75 (±1.05)	.75
• Heart failure–related	0.38 (±1.06)	0.19 (±0.45)	0.42 (±0.93)	.56
Emergency room visits				
• All-cause	0.57 (±1.43)	0.83 (±1.08)	0.65 (±1.0)	.10
• Heart failure–related	0.25 (±1.02)	0.26 (±0.49)	0.35 (±0.80)	.31
Length of stay				
• All-cause	10.64 (±9.7)	9.16 (±9.00)	13.2 (±13.4)	.85
• Heart failure–related	8.52 (±8.3)	10.57 (±12.5)	10.78 (±9.1)	.78

SOURCE: A. Kulshreshtha, J. C. Kvedar, A. Goyal et al., "Use of Remote Monitoring to Improve Outcomes in Patients with Heart Failure: A Pilot Trial," *International Journal of Telemedicine and Applications*, published online May 19, 2010.

PROCESS EFFICIENCIES

Initial studies of CCCP that involved patients receiving skilled nursing care from a home care provider found that introducing telemonitoring not only affected care outcomes but also indicated a trend toward a decreasing need for nurse visits. The studies did not have a large enough sample to definitively demonstrate cost savings, nor did they indicate that telemonitoring would replace home visits. However, telemonitoring was seen as providing a critical adjunct to patient care and workload efficiency for nurses. The impact was significant enough to support adoption of telemonitoring as part of the care plan for heart failure patients. This led Partners in 2007 to fund the program's expansion systemwide for all heart failure patients that met the inclusion criteria. To date, more than 1,200 patients have been enrolled. Exhibit 4 shows that the proportion of enrollees in CCCP with one or more heart failure hospitalizations in the year following disenrollment was 13.3 percent compared with 39.8 percent one year prior to enrollment.

USER SATISFACTION

Eleven research studies were conducted at Partners-affiliated hospitals to measure patient perceptions of connected health technologies; namely, if patients feel empowered to better

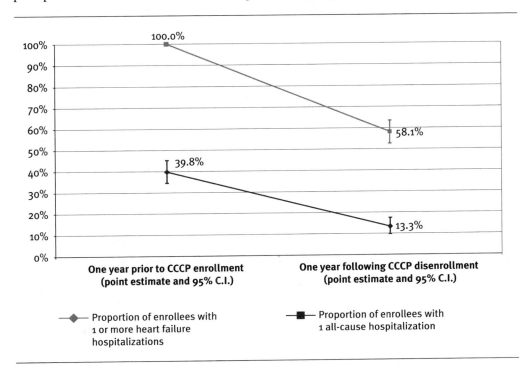

EXHIBIT 4.

Proportion of Connected Cardiac Care Program Enrollees with One or More Hospitalizations

Data include 332 CCCP enrollments among 301 unique patients discharged from the CCCP program prior to July 1, 2009. Results are similar within more recent cohorts of enrollees discharged from the program prior to October 1, 2009, and prior to January 1, 2010.

manage their care, if they have increased satisfaction with care, and if their overall health is improved.[9] Patients in CCCP reported the program increased their confidence and improved their understanding of heart failure and helped them avoid hospitalizations (Exhibit 5). Of the 20 participants in the pilot's remote monitoring group who returned the satisfaction survey, high levels of program satisfaction were recorded (93%). All patients reported that the equipment was easy to use, resulted in greater confidence to self-manage, and helped them stay out of the hospital. In general, once patients are enrolled in the program, less than 10 percent opt out of the program. Those that do drop out usually do so because of personal factors, such as preferences, and not as a result of problems with the technology. Diabetic patients report that blood sugar monitoring was most valuable when they were newly diagnosed or trying to regain control of their diabetes. Electronic communication between providers and patients outside of scheduled office visits was perceived as important in improving diabetes management.

THE CONNECTED CARDIAC CARE PROGRAM

CCCP is developing new ways to help patients at risk for hospitalization to manage their heart disease, by integrating technology into remote patient care and supporting self-monitoring. Contract changes to the Medicare payment structure for the home care industry—in which Medicare provided a prospective payment rate for up to 60 days of service—presented an impetus to create CCCP. Partners HealthCare at Home (PCAH),

EXHIBIT 5.
Results of Connected Cardiac Care Program Patient Satisfaction Survey

- 98% of patients reported learning more information about heart failure because of being enrolled in the CCCP

- 85% reported they felt in control of their health because of the program

- 85% reported they were able to gain control over their heart failure while in the program

- 82% reported they were able to stay out of the hospital because of the program

- 82% reported they were able to avoid the emergency room because of the program

- 77% reported they will continue to check their weight daily

- 64% reported they are confident that they can independently manage their heart failure

- 77% reported they would like their treatment providers to offer this program to other heart failure patients

NOTE: A subset of CCCP participants returned the satisfaction survey (n=93).
SOURCE: Center for Connected Health.

one of the region's largest home care providers, partnered with the Center for Connected Health to develop CCCP, and provides all of the telemonitoring nurses and clinical support for the program. PCAH, which is recognized as a top-performing agency by the Centers for Medicare and Medicaid Services, offers medical, therapeutic, and supportive home-based services for patients who are recovering from a hospitalization, managing chronic illness, or those who need assistance to remain in their own homes.

CCCP's core components are care coordination, education, and development of self-management skills through telemonitoring. Patients use equipment—a home monitoring device with peripherals to collect weight, blood pressure, and heart rate measurements, and a touch-screen computer to answer questions about symptoms—on a daily basis for four months. Telemonitoring nurses monitor these vitals, respond to out-of-parameter alerts, and guide patients through structured biweekly heart failure education (Exhibit 6). This concentrated effort is effective in meeting the primary goal of reducing hospital readmissions.

PCAH was initially interested in using telehealth under the new Medicare reimbursement model to leverage staff across more patients. Heart failure was targeted as a priority condition because of the high costs involved in caring for heart failure patients and the potential savings from preventing unnecessary admissions to hospitals. The support of Partners' senior leadership was critical to the program's expansion. In particular, the leadership's interest in connected health solutions as a way to augment care delivery systemwide and its commitment of funds to support the development of the program have been critical to scaling CCCP across Partners' network.

CCCP allows patients to monitor their physiological health on a daily basis and provides a virtual link to their health care team from their home. Daily monitoring, "just-in-time" teaching—based on the immediacy of interventions in response to monitored patient data—and weekly structured education sessions help patients become aware of their daily behaviors. This impact leads to changes in behavior and the development of new self-management skills. The CCCP team provides the technology, support, and training. It also installs equipment in patients' homes and shows them how to use it. PCAH and other clinical partners provide the expertise for successfully designing and implementing the technology for use in care practices.

There is no cost to patients to enroll or for use of the equipment. The program is open to all patients with a Partners' affiliated primary care physician or cardiologist. Patients are referred by hospital case managers, nurse practitioners, primary care physicians, cardiologists, and other clinicians. Since the inception of CCCP in 2006, the program has included eligible patients from across the Partners HealthCare system on an opt-out basis.

Evaluations of CCCP have been limited to before and after evaluations rather than randomized controlled trials. Such assessments have shown a positive, sizable effect in reducing readmissions, which increased the comfort level among Partners senior leadership with the intervention. There has also been ongoing iterative research using small groups

EXHIBIT 6.

Key Features of the
Connected Cardiac
Care Program

√ Four-month home telemonitoring of congestive heart failure patients by a telemonitoring nurse

√ Intervention by telemonitoring nurse based on physician orders

√ Interactive patient education and lifestyle management

√ Reports posted in electronic health record with email alerts to physicians and nurse practitioners

√ No cost to the patient

√ Open to patients with a Partners' affiliated primary care physician or cardiologist

Who is eligible?	Who is *not* eligible?
• Patients age 18 and older with a diagnosis of heart failure	• Patients currently receiving skilled home care services***
• Patients considered to be at high risk for hospitalization	• Patients with end-stage renal disease on dialysis
• Patients who have a Partners' affiliated primary care physician or cardiologist	• Patients with organ transplant • Patients in hospice
• Patients covered by Medicare, Medicaid, or certain patients in the safety net*	• Patients with an active cancer diagnosis • Patients who reside in nursing homes
• Patients able to speak and read English**	• Patients who do not have a stable environment to conduct the monitoring
• Patients mentally competent and willing**	• Patients with any physical disability that precludes use of telemonitoring equipment
• Patients with a traditional phone line	

* Limited funding available for some patients with commercial insurance.

** Or those with a primary caregiver willing to assume responsibility for telemonitoring.

*** Exception: Partners' Health at Home skilled Medicaid and commercial patients.

SOURCE: Partners HealthCare System, Connected Cardiac Care Program, http://www.connected-health.org/media/224132/cccp summary 6 2 11.doc.

of people to assess the intervention and identify the need for modifications. CCH has also been working with PCH to test effective adoption and the role of financial incentive mechanisms to facilitate spread. CCH's in-house analysis estimates that the program has generated total cost savings of more than $10 million since 2006 for the more than 1,200 enrolled patients (Exhibit 7).

Exhibit 7.
Reducing Hospital
Readmissions with
the Connected
Cardiac Care
Program

Program outcomes

√ 51% reduction in heart failure hospital readmissions*

√ 44% reduction in non–heart failure hospital readmissions*

√ Improved patient understanding of heart failure and self-management skills

√ High levels of clinician and patient acceptance and satisfaction

Savings**

A case study prepared by the Center for Connected Health outlines the following cost savings:

Cost of CCCP:	$1,500 per patient
Total savings from reduction in hospitalizations:	$9,655 per patient
Total net savings:	$8,155 per patient
Total savings:	$10,316,075 for 1,265 monitored patients since 2006

* N=332 patients

** This program targeted reductions in unplanned heart failure and non–heart failure related admissions. The savings realized factor involves the cost of running the program, including marketing, referral management, telemonitoring nurse support, and technology.

SOURCE: Center for Connected Health.

LESSONS LEARNED IN TAKING CCCP FROM PILOT TO SCALE

Partners' experience with connected health technologies and with successfully implementing telehealth-enabled programs across the provider network highlights the significant potential value of transforming care delivery, improving care outcomes, and lowering costs. Social processes are as important in ensuring program success as are the technical factors. Key social factors include leadership support and the championing of technology, the integration of patient data into the workflow to enable providers to more effectively assess patient status and provide just-in-time care and education, and using personal health data to help educate and motivate patients to make necessary lifestyle changes. Even though it has not always been met with immediate success, the organization has persevered to introduce telehealth-enabled care management solutions, to generate evidence of impact, and to use that evidence to advocate for broader deployment across the provider network. This experience imparts important lessons for the successful planning, implementation and deployment of telehealth-enabled care management programs at scale and for identifying future opportunities for continued program advances in patient care management.

PATIENT ACTIVATION AND ENGAGEMENT ARE CRITICAL TO PROGRAM SUCCESS

With the decision by PCAH to use telehealth to leverage staff across more patients in response to Medicare reimbursement changes, CCH became a strategic partner to PCAH. CCH and PCAH collaborated in the design of the technology-enabled clinical program, the selection of the technology, and the staffing of the operational model. Both parties market and perform outreach of CCCP to patient referral sources. There was a low level of adoption in the initial phase of the program. Nurses at first saw CCCP as driving a wedge between them and their patients. They resisted the introduction of the program and the replacement of the more traditional high-touch approach to care. An important factor in overcoming that initial pushback from staff—and an important lesson for the adoption of patient-centered technology in general—is the positive impact the technology has once it's placed in patients' hands. With CCCP, patients felt more connected and nurses learned to develop relationships with patients accordingly with the help of technology. Another important insight in terms of adoption is that patients need to be aware that the provider is engaged in order for them to regularly use the technology as a self-management tool.

AUTOMATIC ENROLLMENT OF PATIENTS IMPROVES CLINICIAN INVOLVEMENT AND SATISFACTION

As the program was extended beyond home care throughout the Partners system, pushback came from other sources, primarily primary care physicians and cardiologists, such that physician referrals and enrollment into the program were challenged. The program struggled initially but the key watershed point came with the decision to change patient enrollment to an opt-out process. Once a patient is identified for enrollment in CCCP, clinicians are responsible for notifying CCCP that they do not want the patient in the program. As a result, enrollment has increased, readmission rates have declined, and satisfaction levels among doctors have increased as benefits in patient care became evident. The refusal rate to participate among doctors went from 10 percent to less than 1 percent.

DATA CAN MOTIVATE AND EMPOWER CLINICIANS AND PATIENTS

Outcomes in controlled trials, as well as in before-and-after studies, have consistently demonstrated an approximate 50 percent drop in cardiac-related readmissions for patients enrolled in CCCP. One drive of that outcome is patients learning self-management skills and receiving constant feedback about how lifestyle factors affect health outcomes. Another is just-in-time care, whereby remote monitoring and intervention by nurses sends a strong message to patients that they are accountable. CCH's commitment to research allows the organization access to the data and studies to counter resistance and arguments from clinicians about the impact on quality and patient experience. CCH is also able to prepare the business case and concomitant cost-savings argument. But the traditional business case approach cannot convey the full impact that other factors, such as patient experience and staff satisfaction, have on improved health outcomes and higher quality of care.

New Technology-Enabled Solutions Do Not Fit Old Policy Frameworks

CCH faces challenges in optimizing the impact of connected health programs on care outcomes. The current fee-for-service environment can present a mental barrier for clinicians, and pilots involving financial incentives that reward provider engagement have not led to significant behavior change. Many doctors view the move toward a patient-centered medical home as requiring more staff, such as nurses and pharmacists, rather than an opportunity for leveraging technology in support of fewer staff. While the widespread use of connected health solutions will require structural changes in the form of reimbursement and new care models like the patient-centered medical home, a significant amount of work remains to be done in promoting the use of technology to leverage existing staff across more patients.

Implications For U.S. Health Care Organizations

Being in an integrated delivery network that owns a home care service business has allowed Partners to be ahead on the adoption curve with telehealth relative to other health systems. Organizations—particularly ones lower on the adoption curve—that are considering technology-enabled solutions will need to address the following issues: establishing acceptance that the technology can clinically make a difference, identifying the method by which the organization will implement and integrate the technology, determining whether a one-size-fits-all approach will be feasible across the network or system, and evaluating whether the prevailing financial system can support an economical approach to scaling.

From an organizational readiness perspective, it is critical to recognize the role of champions who understand workflow and also to understand the requirements for successfully integrating solutions into practice. To gain buy-in from staff, it is important to put the data in the hands of motivated individuals, like clinicians who want to help their patients. It is also important to aggregate external data, integrate it with clinical health information systems, and communicate it to patients and providers alike. Data cannot be maintained in separate data silos and must be placed in the EHR to be meaningful and useful in clinical decision support. Patients need access to the patient portal, with the ability to retrieve clinical information and perform administrative functions. CCH has invested significant resources in developing a platform to support the integration and management of data, which will also serve as a platform for the development and implementation of other applications.

However, recognizing that not all systems are equal in the U.S. health care delivery system, CCH's experience also points to common pitfalls to avoid rather than just best practices to adopt. A common mistake is attempting to shoehorn a connected health program into the traditional care model. Technologies such as telemonitoring can be disruptive to workflow and represent a change in the way care is delivered. Organizations often tend to view connected health solutions as simply requiring a technical interface to existing programs rather than a redesign of the care delivery model. Partners' experience indicates that connected health requires a different mind-set to program design and execution. Otherwise, there is a low likelihood that it will change practice and lead to desired outcomes. Looking forward, Partners is developing a predictive algorithm as a screening strategy of a hospitalized patient's risk for readmission. This will help contribute toward a more aggressive segmentation of the population and tiering of the program to meet the needs of more acute patients on discharge and to manage them so they can exit the program.

Dedicating staff members to the implementation and oversight of the program is more critical than the technology itself in understanding why programs sometimes fail. But often, many technology-enabled solutions in health care fail to recognize the need for solutions that are social in nature rather than solely technological. In the current fee-for-service environment, organizations have to also be prepared for the delays that payment system can impose on staff behavior. Organizations must show clinicians that connected health programs will support care and quality outcomes, while planning workflow changes very carefully and taking the time and making the effort to work methodically and systematically through issues that may arise. Finally, it takes time to integrate technology into health delivery and to allow staff to adapt to the new work model. As a result, structure, coordination, planning, and setting goals, as well as expectations, for the program are critical preparatory steps for success.

NOTES

1. Partners HealthCare System, Quality, Safety and Efficiency, http://qualityandsafety.partners.org/.

2. Partners HealthCare System, Center for Connected Health–Changing Healthcare Delivery, http://www.connected-health.org/.

3. Partners HealthCare System, Annual Report 2010, http://www.partners.org/Assets/Documents/AboutUs/PartnersHealthCare_2010AnnualReport.pdf.

4. Partners HealthCare System, Efficiency: 30-Day Readmission Rate to Discharging Hospital for AMI/HF/PNE, http://qualityandsafety.partners.org/measures/readmissionv2.aspx?id=93.

5. Partners HealthCare System, Report Card: Patient Safety Measures, http://qualityandsafety.partners.org/measures/overview.aspx?id=2.

6. Partners HealthCare System, Report Card: Patient Experience, http://qualityandsafety.partners.org/measures/overview.aspx?id=17.

7. Partners HealthCare System, Report Card: Quality Measures for Clinical Conditions, http://qualityandsafety.partners.org/measures/highquality.aspx?id=3.

8. "Center for Connected Health Reaches Milestone of One Million Vital Signs Collected from Patients via Remote Monitoring," Partners HealthCare press release, Oct. 20, 2011, http://www.connected-health.org/media-center/press-releases/center-for-connected-health-reaches-milestone-of-one-million-vital-signs-collected-from-patients-via-remote-monitoring.aspx.

9. "Center for Connected Health Presents Growing Evidence of the Benefits of Technology to Improve Patient Satisfaction and Empowerment," Partners HealthCare press release, April 8, 2008, http://www.connected-health.org/media-center/press-releases/center-for-connected-health-presents-growing-evidence-of-the-benefits-of-technology-to-improve-patient-satisfaction-and-empowerment.aspx.

INTEGRATIVE CASE STUDIES

These case studies enable you to apply and integrate what is learned throughout the book. At the end of each chapter are questions for some of these cases. Several chapters are required to fully resolve the problems in each case, so each case has questions from several chapters. By answering questions from several chapters for a single case, you will develop your ability to use and combine management tools and methods from throughout the book. You may also make up more questions to strengthen your ability to apply management theories, methods, principles, models, and tools to real-world healthcare organizations and situations.

Three cases—"Decisions, Decisions," "'I Can't Do It All!'," and "Taking Care of Business at Graceland Memorial Hospital"—are reprinted, with permission, from *Managing Health Services: Cases in Organization Design and Decision Making* by Deborah E. Bender with Julie Curkendall and Heather Manning (Health Administration Press 2000). Three cases—"Nowhere Job," "Ergonomics in Practice," and "Disparities in Care at Southern Regional Health System"—are reprinted, with permission, from *Health Services Management: Cases, Readings, and Commentary* by Ann Scheck McAlearney and Anthony R. Kovner (Health Administration Press 2013).

CASE: DECISIONS, DECISIONS

BACKGROUND AND CASE OVERVIEW

University Memorial Hospitals (UMH) is located in a small, Midwestern college town, which is home to a large state university and teaching hospital. UMH is a 571-bed, state-owned, teaching medical center that employs over 4,000 people. As the primary public hospital in its state, UMH provides tertiary care and specialty services to patients from numerous urban and rural communities. The mission of UMH is to provide high-quality patient care, to educate healthcare professionals, to advance health research, and to provide community service. The Planning department's multiple responsibilities include strategic planning, facility planning, and program development.

ORGANIZATIONAL PROBLEM

"Where am I supposed to leave my kids while I'm helping Dr. Smith with patients?" Mary Rogers, a recently hired nursing assistant, asked Tom Martin, manager of the Planning department at UMH. "Here in University Town," she continued, "the daycare facilities are too expensive and inconvenient. Sometimes I have to take time off from work to care for my children. Can't you in Planning do something to remedy that?"

About a year ago, an employee mentioned the idea of a daycare center for hospital employees. Since then, Mr. Martin had been approached repeatedly by aggravated employees, such as Mrs. Rogers, who were dissatisfied with the inadequate supply and high cost of daycare facilities in University Town. As the number of families with two fully employed parents increased, UMH employees faced greater difficulty in finding suitable care for their children during work hours. Mr. Martin realized that UMH must respond to the changing environment and act as a leader in meeting the needs of its employees. UMH, however, needed to consider a variety of issues before committing to the massive project of building a daycare center.

The CEO of UMH assigned Mr. Martin and Planning the task of determining the advantages and disadvantages of creating a daycare center. Given the large number of UMH employees, the daycare center would have to be able to accommodate a large number of children. If the project seemed feasible, Mr. Martin would also be responsible for developing an acceptable business plan to be presented to UMH's board of directors. He contemplated various ways of approaching this project and decided to create a subcommittee to discuss the pertinent issues and formulate a report for the board. Both UMH and University employees would be invited to participate on the subcommittee to account for the various employee perspectives.

Mr. Martin and his subcommittee considered the possibility of a joint venture between the hospital and the University to build a daycare center in a mutually convenient location. If this option were pursued, UMH and the University would need to collaborate and discuss numerous issues including who would manage the facility, where it would be located, how many slots would be allocated to University versus UMH employees, and what criteria would be used to grant participation to employees.

Mr. Martin wanted to make the best proposal possible for the board, and he was not sure whether he should even recommend building the center. He wondered if UMH overlooked any options that could more effectively meet the daycare needs of employees. He knew the organization needed to respond to the changing environment. In recent months, UMH had consistently experienced increased absenteeism and decreased employee morale. Mr. Martin wondered if the appropriate action was to build a daycare center or if a different approach held the solution.

CASE: DISPARITIES IN CARE AT SOUTHERN REGIONAL HEALTH SYSTEM

Tim Hank leaned back in his chair and closed his eyes. While he had been afraid the reports might have bad news, he now had to figure out what to do with this new information. Flipping through the first binder on his desk, reporting results of the recent Robert Wood Johnson Foundation–sponsored assessment of the cardiovascular care provided by his organization, he was increasingly concerned. Southern Regional Health System was based in Jackson, Mississippi, an area known for a highly diverse population and high poverty rates. Black and Hispanic residents in the area were about three times more likely to live in poverty than were whites. Unemployment was also a big problem that affected whites and nonwhites differently—in the Jackson area, black residents were two and a half times more likely to be unemployed and Hispanics over twice as likely to be unemployed as white residents. Beyond poverty and employment differences, though, was the issue of different care given to different patients. This issue of disparities in care was receiving increasing national attention, but Hank had thought the care they provided at Southern Regional was "color blind." Given the health system's mission of providing "excellent quality of care for all," he assumed that the care was equitably delivered across patients and patient populations.

Apparently, this was not the case. This first report showed that there were indeed disparities in the care provided by Southern Regional. Data on heart care had been collected by race and ethnicity for the past year, and these baseline data showed differences. For instance, using the four core measures for heart failure that the Centers for Medicare & Medicaid Services currently collects and reports, only 41 percent of patients were receiving all recommended heart failure care, and the numbers were worse based on race and ethnicity. The analysis showed that while 68 percent of whites received all recommended care, the comparable number among nonwhites was 27 percent. For one measure—the percentage of heart failure patients receiving discharge instructions—only 65 percent of Hispanic patients received the information, compared to 85 percent of non-Hispanic patients. Also troubling Hank was the fact that none of these measures was close to 100 percent—this certainly wasn't the type of care he'd want offered to his own family. Yet he truly didn't understand how his hospital could be providing such disparate care.

The second binder on his desk offered little information to ease his concern. This report, the "Assessment of Organizational Readiness to Change" for Southern Regional Health System, showed that few individuals in his hospital were aware of the nationwide problem of disparities in care, and even fewer were aware that such an issue might be problematic within their own hospital. Now he had the data for Southern Regional that showed significant gaps in care provided to African American and Hispanic patients relative to white patients, but the accompanying readiness-to-change evaluation showed a strong tendency among hospital employees and physicians to resist any proposed changes and instead "go with the flow." Hank knew that his ability to bring the issue of disparate care to the forefront of hospital concerns and successfully make strides to reduce these disparities would be a legacy he would love to leave. Yet he didn't know how he could possibly begin to address this issue at Southern Regional Health System.

CASE: ERGONOMICS IN PRACTICE

Riverlea Rehabilitation Hospital's administrators had recently begun to notice high levels of absenteeism, workers' compensation claims, and time off from work associated with back and other injuries suffered by their workers. Staff were prone to injuries when patients lost their balance while being moved—especially when staff were required to use their own bodies to prevent patient falls. Patients, in turn, could be injured when staff were unable to secure the patients due to the overwhelming physical load or because of preexisting injuries or deficits in staff members' physical strength. Tim Montana, the administrative director, had heard that the new system of patient lifting devices planned for installation at Riverlea Hospital could effectively reduce both the number of workers' injuries and associated workers' compensation claims and absenteeism rates, but the new system was expensive. Montana believed the lift system's cost would be worth the benefits, but he wanted to make sure.

The new lift system had been designed so that patients could be placed in a harness and moved from a bed to a chair, the bathroom, or anywhere else in the room. It was meant to be used consistently, and consistent use was apparently associated with reduced risk of injury to both staff and patients.

To prove that the new lift system helped address the problems associated with the musculoskeletal injuries reported by Riverlea nursing staff, Montana enlisted a team of researchers from the local school of public health. Montana wanted to be able to provide quantifiable evidence that the new system had made a positive impact at Riverlea.

During Montana's meeting with the research team, Dr. Jason Terry, the lead environmental health services researcher, explained that the best approach to evaluating the impact of the lift system would be to undertake a longitudinal study of the health of Riverlea personnel. As Terry explained, the research team could first collect baseline information using existing injury data, then supplement these data by collecting new information about work practices, shifts, and musculoskeletal symptoms among the target workers. After installation of the new lift system hospital wide, the researchers could collect follow-up data to assess the system's efficacy.

Montana convinced the rest of Riverlea's administrative team that a research study was justified, and approved the budget request to support the investigation. Baseline data were collected before the lift system was installed, and plans for the follow-up assessment were made. However, Montana observed the implementation and initial use of the lift system at Riverlea and was concerned about the process. He and his team had seen evidence that many staff members were using the devices incorrectly, were using them intermittently, or were not using them at all. Well aware that improper use of the system would bias any research data collection process, Montana decided to ask the engineering department to check whether the lift system was operating as planned. After a week of study, the engineering personnel reported to Montana that the lifts themselves were functioning properly, so that was not the problem.

Montana next asked individual staff members for their opinions about the lift system. After only a handful of conversations, Montana realized that there were plenty of opinions about the lift system, and most of these were negative. Staff appeared unconvinced about the value of the lift system, and instead were delighted to tell Montana stories about how they had managed to "work around" the system to lift their patients in the "usual way." Montana still believed that the lift system could have a positive impact at Riverlea, but he knew that current use patterns were inconsistent and inappropriate. He knew he had to do something to intervene, but he didn't know where to start.

CASE: "I CAN'T DO IT ALL!"

BACKGROUND AND CASE OVERVIEW

Based in Walnut Creek, California, Healthdyne is a health maintenance organization (HMO) that provides healthcare to the northern California Bay Area. It serves approximately 1.2 million enrollees composed mainly of upper-class, white-collar professionals. Healthdyne occupies a relatively small corner of the market, but is quickly gaining prominence in the area and has developed a solid financial footing with bright prospects. It is located in a growing community, with a 15 to 20 percent annual growth rate projected for the next five years.

For the past 20 years, Healthdyne's former president, Amanda Huggins, has successfully carried out the organizational mission—to provide more affordable and better quality healthcare for its members by setting the statewide standard for excellence and responsiveness. As one of the key players in the organization since its inception, Ms. Huggins is a recognized expert in the managed care industry. Corporate legend has it that her motto was "It doesn't happen without my signature!" Upon Ms. Huggins's retirement, Arnold Brice was recruited to take her place.

ORGANIZATIONAL PROBLEM

When Mr. Brice, who is the former CEO of Atlantic Healthcare, was brought in as president, he inherited an executive staff composed of the vice presidents of the marketing, finance, and professional services departments as well as a medical director, all of whom were capable of fulfilling their managerial responsibilities. However, within a few weeks of joining Healthdyne, Mr. Brice perceived a serious flaw with his staff—none of the vice presidents would make a decision, not even on routine matters such as personnel questions, choice of marketing media, or changing suppliers. The vice presidents frequently presented him with issues in their areas of responsibility and requested that he make the decision. This troubled Mr. Brice. Before long, the situation seriously impeded his efforts to engage in strategic planning for the HMO.

At a regular staff meeting, when every member of his staff had an issue that required his attention, Mr. Brice finally blew up. The catalyst to this incident was this question from the Finance vice president: "What font do you want this in?"

Waving his arms in exasperation, Mr. Brice shouted, which is very uncharacteristic of him, "I cannot do it all! You are going to have to make these decisions yourselves."

The meeting broke up with the staff looking very puzzled and Mr. Brice realizing that he had to make serious changes.

CASE: NOWHERE JOB

Jack Ernest works for a young and growing healthcare company. The company has successfully developed a market niche by contracting with colleges and universities to manage and operate their campus health centers. Ernest has been hired to develop the operational structure for a new product that will link students' managed care health insurance coverage to services provided by their campus health centers. This new product will result in cost savings as well as improved service delivery. It is a new concept in the industry and while Ernest does not have significant healthcare experience, he does have a great deal of energy and enthusiasm, and he is expected to learn on the job.

Ernest has not been given a formal job description. He was originally given a list of performance objectives verbally, but these objectives have been subsequently changed without his input, and there have been no new objectives put in place. Ernest's work environment is unusual in that he mostly works out of a home office, with occasional trips to the corporate office 70 miles away. Ernest reports directly to the corporate medical director of the company, but this director is located in Miami, 1,200 miles away. Communication with his boss occurs almost exclusively by e-mail, telephone, or fax.

Ernest has made progress toward achieving organizational objectives, but he is now facing obstacles that are largely caused by his isolation from others in the company. He is not informed when changes are made to project objectives, nor are the underlying reasons for these changes ever explained to him. Ernest finds that his isolation limits his ability to grow professionally, and he has trouble contributing to the work of the company because he is unable to describe his company's needs accurately to outside vendors without being properly informed himself.

Ernest has asked to have a formal job description and stated performance objectives based on the format suggested by a human resources consultant hired by the company, but he has received no response. Meanwhile, Ernest has been asked to complete the contracts he has negotiated with several outside vendors, and he is told he now reports to an outside consultant who has been hired to help coordinate technical operations, including information systems. This outside consultant tells Ernest not to proceed with these contracts the very day after the CEO tells him to complete them.

Ernest attempts to contribute to the sales and marketing efforts of his company by proposing that the company sponsor an institute at a prestigious university, and he wants to contribute his time and energy to make this project a success. He is told it is a good idea, but the vice president of sales and marketing does not keep his commitment to respond to Ernest's proposal. Ernest sends reminders and continues to develop the idea with the university. He is trying to expand his job responsibilities to include business development, but he knows he needs the support of others in his organization to make a meaningful contribution.

CASE: TAKING CARE OF BUSINESS AT GRACELAND MEMORIAL HOSPITAL

BACKGROUND AND CASE OVERVIEW

Graceland Memorial Hospital is a not-for-profit, community hospital located in a medium-sized urban area in the Midwest. The only other hospital that serves this community is a large, tertiary care teaching hospital affiliated with a major university medical center.

When Jack Prestwood, vice president of Human Resources at Graceland, read the current Occupational Safety and Health Administration (OSHA) regulations, he knew that he needed to comply with them. Under the newly formed OSHA regulations, Graceland is required to enforce the correct usage of respiratory masks and conduct respiratory fit-testing to prevent the transmission of communicable diseases. In the past, Graceland employees who had frequent contact with patients who suffered from airborne communicable diseases were not fitted for a correctly sized respiratory mask. Therefore, to prevent large OSHA fines for noncompliance with the new regulations, Graceland's administration concluded that it must update its own regulations.

ORGANIZATIONAL PROBLEM

Mr. Prestwood called Janet Bowers, director of Employee Health, into his office one morning to ask, "Janet, are you familiar with the new OSHA regulations for respiratory mask fit-testing?"

"I certainly am, Jack," replied Ms. Bowers. "After reading about the OSHA update in Employee Health Weekly, I called our two health equipment supply companies yesterday afternoon to get an idea of the costs involved with mask fit-testing. I knew that I would need the information sooner or later since the hospital will obviously have to comply with the new regulations."

"Sounds great, Janet. What did you find out?" asked Mr. Prestwood.

"It seems that both companies will give us a discount for a large order of the masks. They will also provide training to Employee Health and Infection Control staffs for proper use of the new masks," Ms. Bowers continued.

"It looks like you've done your homework, Janet. Let's schedule a meeting with the Infection Control staff about this," Mr. Prestwood suggested.

Mr. Prestwood arranged the meeting the next day with Ms. Bowers and Erika Thompson, the director of Infection Control, to discuss the updated OSHA regulations and the proposed compliance change. To Mr. Prestwood and Ms. Bowers' surprise, Ms. Thompson objected to implementing the change.

"Why should we have to undergo such a major policy change since the other hospitals in the area are not making any changes in their infection control policies?" Ms. Thompson complained. "That's only going to require more work for my staff and for me.

I really don't think that the change is worth the cost of its implementation. I recommend that we keep things as they are. The current policies have worked just fine for the past couple of years. If other hospitals begin to make the change, then maybe we could decide to update our policies."

After the meeting with Ms. Thompson, Mr. Prestwood was very frustrated. As a vice president, he had a legal and moral obligation to implement changes for compliance. Although few hospitals had begun to implement the new safety measures within their Infection Control departments, he was concerned about the potential risk of following in their footsteps. Graceland had always been known as a leader, but now he was thinking of dragging behind with the pack. But there could be fines to pay; after all, the new guidelines were the law, and if there was an accident, the consequences could be worse! He did not understand why Ms. Thompson's response to the situation was different from others in the past.

To find a solution to the dispute, Mr. Prestwood arranged another meeting with Ms. Bowers and Ms. Thompson, but this time he also invited Margaret Ridell, vice president of Medical Staff Affairs, and two doctors on the medical staff. All, except for Ms. Thompson, agreed with Mr. Prestwood's recommendation. Ms. Thompson, who represented the aggregate view of Infection Control, still would not voice her support for the policy change. After two hours of intense discussion, no clear resolution had been reached. Mr. Prestwood decided that he would have to look at other avenues by which to get the new fit-testing requirement in place.

REAL-WORLD APPLIED INTEGRATIVE PROJECTS

Healthcare organizations (HCOs) have to implement big projects and accomplish important goals. For example, many of them must become more eco-friendly, reduce costs, increase productivity, enhance customer satisfaction, raise employee satisfaction, prevent medical errors, merge with another HCO, create a satellite facility, or improve population health.

There are plenty of ways to become more eco-friendly, such as reducing energy use, recycling waste, and carpooling to work. But how do managers get their HCOs to save energy, recycle, and carpool? Costs can be reduced in many ways, such as by doing procedures right the first time and by not wasting supplies. But how do managers make their organizations and employees do it right the first time and not waste supplies? Customer satisfaction may be enhanced by more compassionate employees and reduced wait times. How do managers make employees more compassionate? We can think of good ideas to help an HCO be eco-friendly, reduce costs, enhance customer satisfaction, and so on. But how can managers bring those good ideas to life and make them happen in their HCOs with their employees?

Managers cannot just wave a magic wand and expect employees to do these things. Instead, managers must apply management theories, principles, models, techniques, and tools from this book. For example, managers could use principles from Chapters 2 and 4 to assign responsibility to specific jobs for reducing energy. Managers could use Chapter 3 to revise the organization's mission to emphasize that the HCO will be green and eco-friendly. To help an HCO become eco-friendly, a student might say, "Let's have a green team." OK, next, let's use Chapter 6 to form an *effective* green team. And let's use motivation theories and methods from Chapter 10 to influence workers so they actually do carpool and reduce energy usage. Chapter 14 has useful methods for managing change so that an HCO can become more green and eco-friendly. Students can be challenged to identify, apply, and integrate many management theories, principles, models, techniques, and tools from this book to help an HCO achieve a major goal and implement a major project.

Listed below are ten real-world projects that many HCOs are involved in. Later, when students become managers, they probably will be involved in many of these projects.

1. Manage an HCO to become a more green and eco-friendly HCO

2. Manage an HCO to become a more culturally competent HCO

3. Manage an HCO to increase productivity

4. Manage an HCO to enhance customer satisfaction

5. Manage an HCO to improve employee satisfaction

6. Manage an HCO to prevent medical errors

7. Manage an HCO to merge with another HCO

8. Manage an HCO to create and open a satellite facility

9. Manage an HCO to improve population health

10. Manage an HCO to reduce costs

The instructor may vary assignments using some of these suggestions:

◆ Students work alone or in groups.

◆ Students are required to use at least 10 different chapters or 20 different management tools.

◆ Students work on a project week-by-week, chapter-by-chapter during classes as a learning activity, or students work on a project as a semester-long integrative cumulative assignment due late in the semester.

◆ Students make presentations in class or prepare written reports.

◆ Students explain how to implement these projects for various types of HCOs, such as a medical group practice, nursing home, health insurance company, hospital, medical supply company, outpatient diagnostic test center, or primary care clinic.

USEFUL WEBSITES FOR HEALTHCARE MANAGEMENT

Agency for Healthcare Research and Quality	www.ahrq.gov
American College of Health Care Administrators	www.achca.org
American College of Healthcare Executives	www.ache.org
American College of Physician Executives	www.acpe.org
American Health Information Management Association	www.ahima.org
American Hospital Association	www.aha.org
American Medical Association	www.ama-assn.org
American Nurses Association	www.nursingworld.org
American Organization of Nurse Executives	www.aone.org
American Public Health Association	http://apha.org

American Society for Healthcare Human Resources Administration	www.ashhra.org
Association for Benchmarking Health Care	www.abhc.org
Association of American Medical Colleges	www.aamc.org
Association of University Programs in Health Administration	www.aupha.org
Baldrige Performance Excellence Program	www.nist.gov/baldrige/
Center for Healthcare Governance	www.americangovernance.com
Centers for Disease Control and Prevention	www.cdc.gov/datastatistics/
Centers for Medicare & Medicaid Services	www.cms.gov
The Commonwealth Fund	www.commonwealthfund.org
Community Connections	www.ahacommunityconnections.org
Consumer Assessment of Healthcare Providers and Systems	www.cahps.ahrq.gov
Disparities Solutions Center	www2.massgeneral.org/disparitiessolutions/
Healthcare Financial Management Association	www.hfma.org
Healthcare Leadership Alliance	www.healthcareleadershipalliance.org
Healthy People 2020	www.healthypeople.gov/2020/
Institute for Diversity in Health Management	www.diversityconnection.org
Institute for Healthcare Improvement	www.ihi.org
Institute for Patient- and Family-Centered Care	www.ipfcc.org
Institute of Medicine	www.iom.edu

The Joint Commission	www.jointcommission.org
Kaiser Family Foundation	www.kff.org
Leadership Health Care	www.healthcarecouncil.com/leadership_health_care.aspx
Lean Hospitals	www.leanhospitals.org
The Leapfrog Group	www.leapfroggroup.org
Medical Group Management Association	www.mgma.org
Medicare Hospital Compare	www.medicare.gov/hospitalcompare/
National Association for Healthcare Quality	www.nahq.org/membership/ leadership/devmodel.html
National Business Coalition on Health	www.nbch.org
National Center for Healthcare Leadership	www.nchl.org
National Committee for Quality Assurance	www.ncqa.org
National Database of Nursing Quality Indicators	www.nursingquality.org
National Patient Safety Foundation	www.npsf.org
National Quality Forum	www.qualityforum.org
Planetree	www.planetree.org
Project Management Institute	www.pmi.org
The Schwartz Center for Compassionate Healthcare	www.theschwartzcenter.org

YOUR MANAGEMENT TOOLBOX

These management tools, methods, theories, models, and concepts will be especially useful to you in your healthcare management career. The chapter from which the tool is drawn is indicated in parentheses.

Adams's equity theory (10)

Administrative theory (2)

Alderfer's ERG theory (10)

Approaches to creating and maintaining ethics (11)

Bar graph (bar chart) (12)

Behavior theory (9)

Benchmarks (12)

Bureaucratic theory (2)

Business plan (3)

Cause-and-effect (fishbone) diagram (12)

Code of ethics (11)

Collaborative leadership (9)

Communication model (15)

Complex adaptive systems theory (2)

Conflict resolution styles and guidelines for choosing a style (13)

Contingency theory (2)

Continuum of care (1)

Control chart (12)

Coordination mechanisms (4)

Cultural competence (15)

Differences between managers and physicians (9)

Divisional form (5)

Emotional intelligence (15)

Environment divided into ten sectors (1)

Evidence-based decision making (13)

Five approaches for who makes a decision (13)

Flowchart (12)

Force field model with determinants of health (1)

Functional form (5)

GLOSSARY

Administrative theory: An integrated set of ideas to organize work, positions, departments, supervisor–subordinate relationships, hierarchy, and span of control to design an organization.

Appraising performance: Evaluating the job performance of workers and discussing those evaluations with the workers.

Authority: Power formally given to a job position to make decisions, take actions, and direct and expect obedience from subordinates.

Autonomy: An ethical principle that includes individual privacy, freedom of choice, and self-control.

Balanced scorecards: Reports with performance measures for finances, customer service, internal business processes, and growth/learning; other kinds of measures may be used.

Behavior theory: Leadership theory that considers what a leader actually does and how a leader behaves.

Benchmark: The best level of performance for a group.

Beneficence: An ethical principle that includes doing good, not doing harm, and promoting the welfare of others.

Body language: Communication by posture, facial expressions, gestures, eyes, and mouth.

Bounded rationality: Limits to human rational decision making.

Cause-and-effect (fishbone) diagram: A tool that visually identifies which factors might affect performance.

Centralization: How high or low in an organization the authority exists to make a decision.

Channels: Methods and media that transmit a message from sender to receiver(s).

Collaborative leadership: Leadership used to form alliances, partnerships, and other forms of interorganizational relationships.

Committee: A formal group that is established with an official mandate, is linked to the organizational hierarchy, and is accountable for its mandate.

Communication: Transmitting information to someone else to develop shared understanding.

Compensating staff: Determining and giving wages, salaries, incentives, and benefits to workers.

Compensation: Wages, salaries, incentives, and benefits for employees.

Complex adaptive system: A system with so many unpredictable changing parts and interactions that it cannot be fully understood and is thus more like a biological organism (natural system) than a machine (mechanical system).

Conflict of interest: A situation in which a person's self-interest interferes with that person's trusted obligation to another person, organization, profession, or purpose.

Content theories: Motivation theories that focus on human needs and unmet needs that all people have.

Contingency theory: Theory that there is no single best way to organize; the best way depends on factors that differ from one situation to another.

Contingent: Dependent on something.

Continuum of care: The full range of healthcare, beginning with prenatal care and continuing to end-of-life care.

Control: To monitor performance and take corrective action if performance does not meet expected standards.

Controlling: Monitoring performance and adjusting if necessary so that goals and objectives are achieved.

Coordination: How different work units (e.g., departments) are connected to work together toward a common purpose.

Cultural competence: The knowledge, skills, and attitudes needed to understand and interact well with people who are culturally different from oneself.

Culture: The values, norms, guiding beliefs, and understandings shared by members of an organization and taught to new members as the correct way to think, feel, and behave.

Decision making: Choosing from among alternatives to determine and implement a course of action.

Delegate authority: Share authority from one position to a lower-level position.

Departmentalization: Organization of jobs into departments, bureaus, divisions, sections, offices, and other formal work groups.

Designing jobs and work: Determining work tasks to be done by a job, along with working conditions, rules, schedules, supervision, and qualifications.

Diagonal communication: Communication to someone at a higher or lower level of an organization and outside of one's own vertical chain of command or hierarchy.

Differentiation: Differences among departments in how the departments are set up and how their workers think and feel.

Directing: Assigning work to workers and motivating them to do the work.

Disparities: Differences in health problems, health status, and use of health services among people who differ in ethnicity, gender, and other characteristics.

Division of work: How work is separated into smaller, more specialized activities.

Divisional form: Organizes departments and positions to focus on particular groups of customers or services.

Downward communication: Communication to someone at a lower level in one's own vertical chain of command or hierarchy.

Emotional intelligence: Ability to recognize and understand emotions in yourself and others, and then use this awareness to manage your behavior and relationships.

Environment: The world in which one exists and that exists beyond oneself. Environment can include people, organizations, laws, societies, natural events, external forces, and many other elements outside of oneself.

Ethical dilemma: A situation in which any decision or course of action will have an undesirable ethical outcome.

Ethics: Values and moral principles about what is right and wrong.

Evidence-based decision making: Making decisions based on systematically finding, evaluating, and applying the best relevant evidence to a clearly defined problem.

External equity: Fairness compared to other jobs outside the organization.

External recruitment: Seeking job applicants from outside the organization.

Flowchart: A tool that identifies and shows in sequence the flow of steps required to complete a process; also called a process map.

Formal organization: The official organization as approved by managers and stated in written documents.

Functional form: Organizes departments and positions according to the functions workers perform and the abilities they use.

Gantt chart: Graphic arrangement of tasks (needed to complete a project) in sequence with start and end dates for each task.

Garbage can decision making: Seemingly random organizational decision making resulting from evolving streams of problems, solutions, participants, and decision-making opportunities.

Goal: An important, specific, intended target or desired outcome that can be measured to determine how well it was achieved.

Group: Social interaction between two or more people in a stable arrangement who have common goals or interests and who perceive themselves as a group.

Groupthink: Group members quickly, politely, and superficially reach agreement without considering diverse ideas; usually done to maintain group harmony.

Health: A state of complete physical, mental, and social well-being; not merely the absence of disease or infirmity.

Healthcare: Services that promote health, prevent health problems, diagnose and treat health problems to cure them, and improve quality of life.

Heredity: Genes, traits, and characteristics inherited from parents.

Hiring staff: Recruiting and selecting workers for jobs, which may include reassigning existing workers by promotion or transfer.

Horizontal communication: Communication to someone at the same level of an organization and outside of one's own vertical chain of command or hierarchy.

Human relations: A type of management based on psychology and sociology that considers employees' feelings and behaviors, especially in groups.

Implement: Make happen, carry out, perform, put into effect.

Incremental change: Small, minor evolutionary change.

Inertia: An object at rest tends to stay at rest and an object in motion tends to continue its motion; this principle applies to work in organizations.

Informal organization: Workers' own unwritten rules, procedures, expectations, agreements, and communication networks (e.g., the grapevine).

Integrator: A person who works full-time coordinating the work of several departments toward a common purpose.

Internal equity: Fairness compared to other jobs inside the organization.

Internal recruitment: Seeking job applicants from inside the organization.

Intuition: Knowing or deciding based on experience, hunches, or unconscious processes rather than on rational thinking and reasons.

Job: A group of activities and duties that entail natural units of work that are similar and related; may be performed by more than one person.

Job description (also position description): States the job title and work to be done; usually includes the authority, reporting relationships, and minimum qualifications to perform the job; may include the equipment and materials used, working conditions, work schedule, mental and physical demands, interactions with others, and salary range.

Justice: An ethical principle that includes fairness and equality.

Knowledge management: A system for finding, organizing, and making available an organization's knowledge, including its experience, understanding, expertise, methods, judgment, lessons learned, and know-how.

Labor union: An outside organization that represents specific groups of employees and negotiates on their behalf with managers for workers' schedules, work conditions, compensation, and terms of employment.

Leadership: A process through which an individual attempts to intentionally influence people to accomplish a goal.

Lean production: Design of work processes to reduce waste, increase efficiency and speed, and thereby produce more value for customers.

Liaison: A job that includes responsibility to coordinate one department with another department.

Lifestyles: Patterns of attitudes and behaviors that make up one's way of living.

Line of authority: The vertical chain of command, authority, and formal communication up and down an organization.

Line work: Work that contributes directly to achieving an organization's purpose and main goals.

Management: The process of getting things done through and with people.

Managerial ethics: Ethics that guide right and wrong in the practice of management.

Matrix form: Combines the functional and divisional organization forms to obtain advantages of both forms.

Mechanistic: Emphasizing specialized, rigidly defined tasks; strict hierarchy, control, rules, and authority; and vertical communication and interaction.

Medical care: Diagnosis and treatment in the care of patients, sometimes limited to care by physicians and sometimes more broadly including care by nurses, therapists, and others who care for patients.

Medical ethics: Ethics that guide right and wrong in the practice of medicine.

Mission: The purpose of an organization; why the organization exists.

Modular form: Outsources much work to other organizations and connects them with contracts and electronic information systems.

Moral distress: A situation in which an organization's constraints prevent a person from doing what she thinks is ethically right.

Motivation: Desire and willingness of a person to expend effort to reach a particular goal or outcome.

Mutual adjustment: Workers who do not have a supervisor–subordinate relationship exchange information and alter their work if needed to fit with each other.

Nonprogrammed decisions: Decisions that are new, unusual, hard to define, and hard to diagnose; they present fuzzy alternatives with uncertain cause and effect.

Nonverbal encoding: Representing ideas without using words, such as by using diagrams, charts, icons, pictures, attire, objects, body language, touch, behavior, and actions.

Norms: Behaviors and attitudes expected of people in a group, organization, or society.

Onboarding: The process of helping new hires adjust to social and performance aspects of their new jobs quickly and smoothly.

Opportunities: Favorable events, elements, and situations in the environment that an organization could exploit for its strategic gain.

Organic: Emphasizing shared common tasks; teamwork; loose hierarchy, control, rules, and authority; and horizontal communication and interaction.

Organization chart: Visual portrayal of vertical hierarchy, departments, span of control, reporting relationships, and flow of authority.

Organization structure: The reporting relationships, vertical hierarchy, spans of control, groupings of jobs into departments and an entire organization, and systems for coordination and communication.

Organizations: Social entities that are goal directed, designed as deliberately structured and coordinated activity systems, and linked to the external environment.

Organizing: Arranging work into jobs, teams, departments, and other work units; arranging supervisor–subordinate relationships; assigning responsibility, authority, and other resources.

Outcome measures: Measures of results and effects.

Parallel form: Starts with a functional structure to produce the routine work and then adds a parallel structure to organize for multidepartmental approaches to solving complex problems.

Plan-Do-Check-Act (PDCA) cycle: A control model in which managers plan goals, do things to implement plans, check implementation, and act to improve implementation to achieve goals.

Planning: Deciding what to do and how to do it.

Planning for staff: Forecasting the organization's future staffing requirements and deciding how to ensure the needed workers are available.

Point-factor method: Assigns points to a job based on how that job rates on a common set of factors used to rate all jobs; points are used to determine pay for a job.

Politics: The use of power to influence decisions.

Population health: Measuring a community's health outcomes and the factors that cause them, and then using those measures to coordinate the community's people and organizations to improve health.

Position: Consists of duties and responsibilities that are performed by only one person.

Power: The ability to influence others to bring about desired outcomes.

Procedural justice: A process to resolve ethical conflicts based on fair procedures that consider competing values of all affected groups.

Process measures: Measures of the work that is done, how it is done, and the activities performed.

Process theories: Motivation theories that focus on the context in which work is done and how people think and feel about work.

Professional bureaucracy: Organization, coordination, and authority are based on highly specialized education, training, and expertise, with less reliance on authority from a job position.

Professional ethics: Ethics that guide right and wrong for a profession, such as the nursing profession.

Professionalism: The ability to align personal and organizational conduct with ethical and professional standards.

Programmed decisions: Decisions that are well defined, routine, recurring, easily diagnosed, and easily solved with standard rules, formulas, and procedures.

Project management: The application of knowledge, skills, tools, and techniques to project activities to meet project requirements.

Protecting staff: Ensuring that workers have proper work conditions and that their opinions are considered by managers.

Radical change: Large, major revolutionary change.

Reengineering: Redesigning and improving work processes that involve multiple departments that must work together to accomplish a result.

Refreeze: Lock in change and make it the new correct way of doing things.

Satisfice: To decide on a satisfactory alternative that will suffice, although it might not be the best.

Scientific management: A type of management that uses standardization, specialization, and scientific experiments to design jobs for greater efficiency and production.

Servant leadership: Leadership that emphasizes that a leader should serve the followers by listening, mentoring, teaching, and helping.

Six Sigma: Performance improvement that aims to reduce variation and defects in work processes.

Skill theory: Leadership theory that considers the skills and abilities of leaders.

Social responsibility: Ethics that guide right and wrong for the good of society.

Span of control: How many subordinate workers a manager is directly responsible for; how many workers report directly to that manager. (Sometimes called *span of supervision*.)

Specialization: The width of the range of tasks and work done by an employee or department.

Staff work: Work that uses specialized skills, abilities, and expertise to support line workers and thereby indirectly contribute to the organization's purpose.

Staffing: Obtaining and retaining people to fill jobs and do work.

Stakeholders: People and organizations that have a stake (interest) in what an HCO does and that could affect the HCO.

Strategic planning: Deciding how the organization wants to position itself in its future environment and relative to competitors, and then deciding how to achieve that position.

Strategic thinking: The mental process of analyzing and synthesizing information to create a strategy to achieve a goal.

Strategy: A pattern of ideas used to attain and sustain competitive advantage over rivals.

Strengths: An organization's abilities, assets, and competencies that create strategic advantages.

Structure measures: Measures of resources, staff, equipment, competencies, inputs, facilities, and characteristics of the organization; how the organization is set up.

Subculture: Culture of a distinct part of an organization (e.g., a department or team) that exists within the organization's culture.

Supervision: Workers have a supervisor–subordinate relationship in the chain of command, and they inform each other.

SWOTs: Strengths, weaknesses, opportunities, and threats.

System: A set of interrelated parts that function as a whole to achieve a common purpose.

Team: A group with specific complementary abilities, strong commitment to common goals, and shared accountability for goal achievement.

Theory X: Leader assumes people dislike work, are lazy and stupid, are motivated by rewards from others, lack self-discipline, want security, and do not want responsibility.

Theory Y: Leader assumes people like meaningful work, are creative and capable, are motivated by rewards from within oneself, have self-control, can direct themselves, and want responsibility.

Theory Z: Leader emphasizes concern for workers, develops long-term cooperative relationships, gradually provides growth opportunities for workers, and promotes individual and collective responsibility.

Threats: Unfavorable events, elements, and situations in the environment that could harm an organization.

Training and developing staff: Enabling employees to acquire new knowledge, skills, attitudes, and behaviors for current and future jobs.

Trait theory: Leadership theory that considers the traits and characteristics of leaders.

Transactional leadership: Leadership based on transactions in which workers perform tasks to achieve goals and then the leader gives workers pay and other rewards.

Transformational leadership: Leadership based on inspiration, the greater good for everyone, people's need for fulfillment, innovation, and revitalizing the organization with change.

Unfreeze: Create dissatisfaction with the current situation and motivate people to change.

Unity of command: Arrangement in which a worker takes commands from and is responsible to only one boss.

Upward communication: Communication to someone at a higher level in one's own vertical chain of command or hierarchy.

Values: Deeply held fundamental beliefs and ideals.

Verbal encoding: Using written or spoken words to represent ideas.

Vision: What the organization wants to be in the long-term future.

Weaknesses: An organization's flaws, shortcomings, and liabilities that create strategic disadvantages.

REFERENCES

Abrahamson, E. 2000. "Change Without Pain." *Harvard Business Review* 78 (4): 75–79.

Adams, J. S. 1963. "Toward an Understanding of Inequity." *Journal of Abnormal and Social Psychology* 67: 422–36.

Alderfer, C. 1972. *Existence, Relatedness, and Growth*. New York: Free Press.

Alterman, E. 2001. *It Ain' t No Sin to Be Glad You' re Alive: The Promise of Bruce Springsteen*. Boston: Back Bay.

American College of Healthcare Executives (ACHE). 2014. "Career Resource Center." Accessed May 26. www.ache.org/carsvcs/ycareer.cfm.

———. 2013. *ACHE Healthcare Executive Competencies Assessment Tool 2014*. Accessed September 8, 2014. www.ache.org/pdf/nonsecure/careers/competencies_booklet.pdf.

———. 2011. *Code of Ethics*. Amended November 14. www.ache.org/abt_ache/code.cfm.

Baird, C. H., and G. Parasnis. 2011. "From Social Media to Social Customer Relationship Management." *Strategy & Leadership* 39 (5): 30–37.

Baldwin, G. 2011. "Social Media: Friend or Foe?" *Health Data Management* 19 (9): 24–31.

Banner Health. 2009. "Banner Health Cultivates Nurses to Lead the Way in Innovative Care." *American Nurse Today* 4 (4): 11.

Barnard, C. 1938. *The Functions of the Executive.* Cambridge, MA: Harvard University Press.

Barton, P. L. 2010. *Understanding the US Health Services System*, fourth edition. Chicago: Health Administration Press.

Bauer, T. N. 2010. "Onboarding New Employees: Maximizing Success." Society for Human Resource Management Foundation. Published May 27. www.shrm.org/about/foundation/products/Documents/Onboarding%20EPG-%20FINAL.pdf.

Benne, K., and P. Sheats. 1948. "Functional Roles of Group Members." *Journal of Social Issues* 4 (2): 41–49.

Benson, K., and C. Hummer. 2014. "Creating a Culture of Professionalism." In *New Leadership for Today's Health Care Professionals: Concepts and Cases,* edited by L. G. Rubino, S. J. Esparza, and Y. S. Reid Chassiakos, 77–88. Burlington, MA: Jones & Bartlett Learning.

Bertalanffy, L. von. 1968. *General System Theory: Foundations, Development, Applications.* New York: George Braziller.

Bewley, L. W. 2008. "Power and Politics." In *Health Organizations: Theory, Behavior, and Development,* edited by J. A. Johnson, 137–48. Sudbury, MA: Jones & Bartlett.

Birk, S. 2014. "Creating a Culture of 'We': Investing in Physician Leaders." *Healthcare Executive* 29 (1): 10–18.

———. 2013. "The Future of Physician Leadership." *Healthcare Executive* 28 (1): 8–16.

———. 2010. "The New Quality-Cost Imperative: Systemwide Improvements Can Yield Financial Gains." *Healthcare Executive* 25 (2): 14–24.

————. 2009. "Creating a Culture of Safety." *Healthcare Executive* 24 (2): 14–22.

Biro, M. M. 2013. "7 Hottest Trends in HR Technology." *Forbes*. Published October 6. www.forbes.com/sites/meghanbiro/2013/10/06/7-hottest-trends-in-hr-technology/.

Bjorseth, L. 2007. "Ten Principles of Communication." *Healthcare Executive* 22 (5): 52–55.

Blake, R. R., and J. S. Mouton. 1964. *The Managerial Grid: The Key to Leadership Excellence*. Houston: Gulf Publishing.

Blum, H. L. 1983. *Planning for Health*. New York: Human Sciences Press.

Bodinson, G. W. 2005. "Change Healthcare Organizations from Good to Great." *Quality Progress* 38 (11): 22–29.

Borkowski, N. 2011. *Organizational Behavior in Health Care,* second edition. Sudbury, MA: Jones & Bartlett.

————. 2009. *Organizational Behavior, Theory, and Design in Health Care*. Sudbury, MA: Jones & Bartlett.

Borkowski, N., and B. P. Deppman. 2014. "Collaborative Leadership." In *New Leadership for Today's Health Care Professionals: Concepts and Cases,* edited by L. G. Rubino, S. J. Esparza, and Y. S. Reid Chassiakos, 193–203. Burlington, MA: Jones & Bartlett Learning.

Bplans. 2014. "Home Health Care Services Business Plan." Accessed July 17. www.bplans.com/home_health_care_services_business_plan.

Briner, R. B., D. Denyer, and D. M. Rousseau. 2009. "Evidence-Based Management: Concept Cleanup Time?" *Academy of Management Perspectives* 23 (November): 19–32.

Broscio, M. A. 2013. "Behavioral Interviewing: 'Back to the Future.'" *Healthcare Executive* 28 (4): 56–57.

Brown, M. P., and R. L. Fink. 2012. "Human Resource Outsourcing in Health Care: Strategic, Cost, and Technical Considerations." *Southern Business Review* 37 (1): 51–60.

Buell, J. M. 2014. "Essential Strategies for Hospital-Physician Relations." *Healthcare Executive* 29 (1): 20–31.

Bureau of Labor Statistics, US Department of Labor. 2014. "Medical and Health Services Managers." *Occupational Outlook Handbook, 2014–15 Edition*. Published January 8. www.bls.gov/ooh/management/medical-and-health-services-managers.htm.

Burns, J. 1978. *Leadership*. New York: Harper & Row.

Burns, T., and G. M. Stalker. 1961. *The Management of Innovation*. London: Tavistock.

Calayag, J. 2014. "Physician Engagement." *Healthcare Executive* 29 (2): 28–36.

Cardinal Health. 2014. "Vendor-Managed Inventory." Accessed September 8. www.cardinal.com/us/en/Hospitals/MaterialsAndPurchasing/Vendor-managedInventory.

Carroll, L. 1946. *Alice's Adventures in Wonderland*, special edition. New York: Random House.

Charns, M. P., and G. Young. 2012. "Organization Design and Coordination." In *Shortell & Kaluzny's Health Care Management: Organization Design and Behavior,* sixth edition, edited by L. R. Burns, E. H. Bradley, and B. J. Weiner, 64–90. Clifton Park, NY: Delmar Cengage Learning.

Connelly, M. D., and M. J. O'Brien. 2007. "Reorganize for Effective Communication." *Healthcare Executive* 22 (2): 54–59.

Connolly, C. 2009. "For This Health System, Less Is More." *Washington Post*, March 31.

Cooper, A. 2013. "Using Social Networks to Help Patients Self-Care." *Nursing Times* 109 (10): 22–24.

Costa, J. 2009. "Team Building and Development." In *Health Organizations*, edited by J. Johnson, 311–30. Sudbury, MA: Jones & Bartlett.

Daft, R. L. 2013. *Organization Theory & Design,* eleventh edition. Mason, OH: South-Western Cengage.

———. 2010. *Organization Theory and Design,* tenth edition. Cincinnati, OH: South-Western Cengage.

Darling, H. 2014. "Large Employers' Responses to Healthcare Reform: Trends and Outlook." In *Futurescan 2014: Healthcare Trends and Implications 2014–2019*, edited by D. Seymour, 41–46. Chicago: Society for Healthcare Strategy & Market Development and Health Administration Press.

Deckard, G. J. 2011a. "Contemporary Leadership Theories." In *Organizational Behavior in Health Care,* edited by N. Borkowski, 209–30. Sudbury, MA: Jones & Bartlett.

———. 2011b. "Contingency Theories of Leadership." In *Organizational Behavior in Health Care,* edited by N. Borkowski, 191–208. Sudbury, MA: Jones & Bartlett.

DeVito, J. A. 1986. *The Communication Handbook: A Dictionary.* New York: Harper & Row.

DeVore, S. D., and K. Figlioli. 2010. "Lessons Premier Hospitals Learned About Implementing Electronic Health Records." *Health Affairs* 29 (4): 664–67.

Diez Roux, A. V. 2012. "Conceptual Approaches to the Study of Health Disparities." *Annual Review of Public Health* 33: 41–58.

DiMaggio, P. J., and W. W. Powell. 1983. "The Iron Cage Revisited: Institutional Isomorphism and Collective Rationality in Organizational Fields." *American Sociological Review* 48 (2): 147–60.

Dolan, T. C. 2013. "Aspirations of a Servant Leader." *Healthcare Executive* 28 (6): 30–38.

Donabedian, A. 1966. "Evaluating the Quality of Medical Care." *Milbank Memorial Fund Quarterly* 44 (2): 166–206.

Drafke, M. W. 2009. *The Human Side of Organizations*, tenth edition. Upper Saddle River, NJ: Pearson Education.

Dreachslin, J. L., and D. Kiddy. 2006. "From Conflict to Consensus." *Healthcare Executive* 21 (6): 9–14.

Drucker, P. F. 1967. *The Effective Executive.* New York: Harper & Row.

Dunn, R. 2010. *Dunn and Haimann's Healthcare Management*, ninth edition. Chicago: Health Administration Press.

Dye, C. F. 2010. *Leadership in Healthcare,* second edition. Chicago: Health Administration Press.

Dye, C. F., and A. N. Garman. 2015. *Exceptional Leadership: 16 Critical Competencies for Healthcare Executives*, second edition. Chicago: Health Administration Press.

Elkins, E., J. Melton, and M. Hall. 2014. "Transformational Leadership." In *New Leadership for Today's Health Care Professionals: Concepts and Cases,* edited by L. G. Rubino, S. J. Esparza, and Y. S. Reid Chassiakos, 209–21. Burlington, MA: Jones & Bartlett Learning.

Esparza, S., and L. Rubino. 2014. "A Call for New Leadership in Health Care." In *New Leadership for Today's Health Care Professionals: Concepts and Cases,* edited by L. G. Rubino, S. J. Esparza, and Y. S. Reid Chassiakos, 1–19. Burlington, MA: Jones & Bartlett Learning.

Evans, R. M. 2009. "Culture Values and Ethics." In *Health Organizations: Theory, Behavior, and Development*, edited by J. A. Johnson. Sudbury, MA: Jones & Bartlett.

Fallon, L. F., and C. R. McConnell. 2014. *Human Resource Management in Health Care: Principles and Practices,* second edition. Burlington, MA: Jones & Bartlett.

Fayol, H. 1916. *General and Industrial Management.* London: Pittman.

Flood, A. B., J. S. Zinn, and W. R. Scott. 2006. "Organizational Performance: Managing for Efficiency and Effectiveness." In *Health Care Management: Organization Design and Behavior*, fifth edition, edited by S. M. Shortell and A. D. Kaluzny, 415–54. Clifton Park, NY: Thomson Delmar Learning.

Fos, P. J., and D. J. Fine. 2005. *Managerial Epidemiology for Healthcare Organizations*, second edition. San Francisco: Jossey-Bass.

Fottler, M. D. 2008a. "Job Analysis and Job Design." In *Human Resources in Healthcare*, third edition, edited by B. J. Fried and M. D. Fottler, 163–95. Chicago: Health Administration Press.

———. 2008b. "Strategic Human Resources Management." In *Human Resources in Healthcare*, third edition, edited by B. J. Fried and M. D. Fottler, 1–26. Chicago: Health Administration Press.

Fottler, M. D., S. J. O'Connor, M. J. Gilmartin, and T. A. D'Aunno. 2006. "Motivating People." In *Health Care Management: Organization Design and Behavior*, fifth edition, edited by S. M. Shortell and A. D. Kaluzny. Clifton Park, NY: Thomson Delmar Learning.

French, J., and B. Raven. 1959. "The Bases of Social Power." In *Studies in Social Power*, edited by D. Cartwright, 150–67. Ann Arbor, MI: University of Michigan Press.

French, W. L. 2007. *Human Resources Management*, sixth edition. Boston: Houghton Mifflin Company.

Freshman, B., and L. Rubino. 2002. "Emotional Intelligence: A Core Competency for Healthcare Administrators." *The Healthcare Manager* 20 (4): 1–9.

Fried, B. J. 2008. "Performance Management." In *Human Resources in Healthcare*, third edition, edited by B. J. Fried and M. D. Fottler, 257–80. Chicago: Health Administration Press.

Fried, B. J., and M. Gates. 2008. "Recruitment, Selection, and Retention." In *Human Resources in Healthcare*, third edition, edited by B. J. Fried and M. D. Fottler, 197–235. Chicago: Health Administration Press.

Fried, B. J., T. G. Rundall, and S. Topping. 2000. "Groups and Teams in Health Services Organizations." In *Health Care Management: Organization Design and Behavior*, fourth edition, edited by S. M. Shortell and A. D. Kaluzny, 154–90. Clifton Park, NY: Thomson Delmar Learning.

Fried, B. J., S. Topping, and A. C. Edmondson. 2012. "Teams and Team Effectiveness in Health Services Organizations." In *Shortell & Kaluzny's Health Care Management Organization Design and Behavior,* sixth edition, edited by L. R. Burns, E. H. Bradley, and B. J. Weiner, 121–62. Clifton Park, NY: Delmar Cengage Learning.

Friedman, L. H., and A. R. Kovner. 2013. *101 Careers in Healthcare Management*. New York: Springer.

Gantt, H. 1919. *Organizing for Work*. New York: Harcourt, Brace and Howe.

Gertner, E. J., J. N. Sabino, E. Mahady, L. M. Deitrick, J. R. Patton, M. K. Grim, J. F. Geiger, and D. Salas-Lopez. 2010. "Developing a Culturally Competent Health Network: A Planning Framework and Guide." *Journal of Healthcare Management* 55 (3): 190–204.

Gilbert, J. 2013. "What Drives an Ethical Culture?" *Healthcare Executive* 28 (5): 48–49.

Gilbreth, F. B., and L. Gilbreth. 1917. *Applied Motion Study*. New York: Sturgis & Walton Company.

Gill, S. 1987. "Can Doctors and Administrators Work Together?" *Physician Executive* 13 (5): 11–16.

Glandon, G. 2014. "Assuring the Health of the Nation." Association of University Programs in Health Administration. Posted January 13. http://network.aupha.org/network/blogsmain/blogviewer/?BlogKey=e2ba0914-e7ba-464d-979e-3e28ff126849.

Gleick, J. 1998. *Chaos: Making a New Science*. New York: Penguin.

Goleman, D. 1998. *Working with Emotional Intelligence*. New York: Random House.

Green, A. 2013. "What Does It Mean to Be Professional at Work?" *U.S. News and World Report.* Published July 22. http://money.usnews.com/money/blogs/outside-voices-careers/2013/07/22/what-does-it-mean-to-be-professional-at-work.

Gulick, L., and L. Urwick. 1937. *Papers on the Science of Administration.* New York: Institute of Public Administration, Columbia University.

Haeberle, K., J. Herzberg, and T. Hobbs. 2009. "Leading the Multigenerational Workforce." *Healthcare Executive* 24 (5): 62–67.

Hammer, M. 1996. *Beyond Reengineering: How the Process-Centered Organization is Changing Our Work and Our Lives.* New York: HarperCollins.

Hamric, A. B., E. G. Epstein, and K. R. White. 2014. "Moral Distress and the Healthcare Organization." In *Managerial Ethics in Healthcare: A New Perspective,* edited by G. L. Filerman, A. E. Mills, and P. M. Schyve, 137–58. Chicago: Health Administration Press.

Haraden, C., and A. Frankel. 2004. "Shuttling Toward a Safety Culture: Healthcare Can Learn from Probe Panel's Findings on the Columbia Disaster." *Modern Healthcare* 34 (1): 21.

Harris, M. S. 2013. "Efficacy of Utilizing a Novel Education-Entertainment Strategy to Increase Health Information Seeking Behaviors Among African-American Patients and the Feasibility of Its Incorporation into Healthcare Settings." *Journal of Community Medicine & Health Education* 3 (3): 210.

Haynes, V. D. 2008. "What Nurses Want." *Washington Post*, September 13, D01.

Healthcare Financial Management Association (HFMA). 2009. "Engaging Physicians for Supply Chain Savings." *HFM* 63 (5): 1–8.

Hellriegel, D., and J. W. Slocum. 2011. *Organizational Behavior,* thirteenth edition. Mason, OH: South-Western Cengage Learning.

Herzberg, F. 1966. *Work and the Nature of Man.* New York: World Publishing Company.

Hoff, T., and K. W. Rockmann. 2012. "Power, Politics, and Conflict Management." In *Shortell & Kaluzny's Health Care Management Organization Design and Behavior,* sixth edition, edited by L. R. Burns, E. H. Bradley, and B. J. Weiner, 188–220. Clifton Park, NY: Delmar Cengage Learning.

Holland, J. H. 1992. *Adaptation in Natural and Artificial Systems.* Cambridge, MA: MIT Press.

Honaman, J. C. 2013. "The Jobs of Tomorrow." *Healthcare Executive* 28 (3): 76–78.

Hostetter, M. 2008. "Case Study: Implementing Developmental Screening at Oxford Pediatrics." *Quality Matters.* Published September 15. www.commonwealthfund.org/ Content/Innovations/Case-Studies/2008/Sep/Case-Study--Implementing-Developmental-Screening-at-Oxford-Pediatrics.aspx.

Institute for Healthcare Improvement (IHI). 2014. "IHI Triple Aim Initiative." Accessed May 27. www.ihi.org/offerings/Initiatives/TripleAim/Pages/default.aspx.

Institute of Medicine (IOM). 2001. *Crossing the Quality Chasm: A New Health System for the 21st Century.* Washington, DC: National Academies Press.

Ivanitskaya, L. V., S. Glazer, and D. A. Erofeev. 2009. "Group Dynamics." In *Health Organizations: Theory, Behavior, and Development*, edited by J. A. Johnson, 109–36. Sudbury, MA: Jones & Bartlett.

Jacob, S. 2013. "Baylor, Scott & White First Tackled Cultural Fit in Merger Due Diligence." *Dallas/Fort Worth Healthcare Daily.* Published October 30. http://healthcare.dmagazine. com/2013/10/30/baylor-scott-white-first-tackled-cultural-fit-in-merger-due-diligence.

Jorna, H, and S. A. Martin Jr. 2014. "Coordinating Care to Provide Effective Population Health Management." In *Futurescan 2014: Healthcare Trends and Implications 2014–2019*, edited by D. Seymour, 5–10. Chicago: Society for Healthcare Strategy & Market Development and Health Administration Press.

Kaiser Family Foundation. 2013. "Focus on Health Reform: Summary of the Affordable Care Act." Modified April 23. http://kaiserfamilyfoundation.files.wordpress. com/2011/04/8061-021.pdf.

Kaplan, R. S., and D. P. Norton. 1996. "Linking the Balanced Scorecard to Strategy." *California Management Review* 39 (1): 53–79.

Kash, B. A., A. Spaulding, C. E. Johnson, and L. Gamm. 2014. "Success Factors for Strategic Change Initiatives: A Qualitative Study of Healthcare Administrators' Perspectives." *Journal of Healthcare Management* 59 (1): 65–81.

Katz, D., and R. Kahn. 1966. *The Social Psychology of Organizations*. New York: John Wiley & Sons, Inc.

Katz, R. L. 1974. "Skills of an Effective Administrator." *Harvard Business Review* 52 (5): 90–102.

———. 1955. "Skills of an Effective Administrator." *Harvard Business Review* 33 (1): 33–42.

Kellermann, A. L., and S. S. Jones. 2013. "What It Will Take to Achieve the As-Yet-Unfulfilled Promises of Health Information Technology." *Health Affairs* 32 (1): 63–68.

Khan, A. 2011. "Managing Virtual Teams in Healthcare Systems." *Middle East Health*. Uploaded November 15. www.middleeasthealthmag.com/nov2011/feature7.htm.

Kindig, D. A. 2014. "What Is Population Health?" *Improving Population Health*. Accessed May 27. www.improvingpopulationhealth.org/blog/what-is-population-health.html.

Kivland, C. 2014. "Your Future Gets Brighter with Emotional Intelligence." *Healthcare Executive* 29 (1): 72–75.

Kotter, J. P. 1996. *Leading Change*. Cambridge, MA: Harvard Business School Press.

Kovner, A. R., D. J. Fine, and R. D'Aquila. 2009. *Evidence-Based Management in Healthcare*. Chicago: Health Administration Press.

Kraft, D. 2013. "Where Technology Can Take Healthcare." *Forbes*. Published February 5. www.forbes.com/sites/matthewherper/2013/02/05/forbes-health-summit-how-technology-will-change-health-care.

Lawrence, P. R., and J. W. Lorsch. 1969. *Organization and Environment*. Homewood, IL: Richard D. Irwin.

Leatt, P., J. R. Kimberly, and R. Baker. 2006. "Organization Design." In *Health Care Management: Organization Design and Behavior*, fifth edition, edited by S. M. Shortell and A. D. Kaluzny. Clifton Park, NY: Thomson Delmar Learning.

Ledlow, G. R. 2009. "Conflict and Interpersonal Relationships." In *Health Organizations: Theory, Behavior, and Development*, edited by J. A. Johnson, 149–65. Sudbury, MA: Jones & Bartlett.

Ledlow, G. R., and M. N. Coppola. 2009. "Leadership Theory and Influence." In *Health Organizations: Theory, Behavior, and Development*, edited by J. A. Johnson, 167–92. Sudbury, MA: Jones & Bartlett.

Ledlow, G. R., and J. Stephens. 2009. "Decision Making and Communication." In *Health Organizations: Theory, Behavior, and Development*, edited by J. A. Johnson, 213–32. Sudbury, MA: Jones & Bartlett.

Lewin, K. 1951. *Field Theory in Social Science*. New York: Harper & Row.

Liebler, J. G., and C. R. McConnell. 2004. *Management Principles for Health Professionals*, fourth edition. Sudbury, MA: Jones & Bartlett.

Likert, R. 1961. *New Patterns of Management*. New York: McGraw-Hill.

Locke, E. A. 1968. "Effects of Knowledge of Results, Feedback in Relation to Standards, and Goals on Reaction-Time Performance." *American Journal of Applied Psychology* 81: 566–74.

Longenecker, C. O., and P. D. Longenecker. 2014. "Why Hospital Improvement Efforts Fail: A View from the Front Line." *Journal of Healthcare Management* 59 (2): 146–57.

Longest, B. B., and G. J. Young. 2006. "Coordination and Communication." In *Health Care Management: Organization Design and Behavior*, fifth edition, edited by S. M. Shortell and A. D. Kaluzny. Clifton Park, NY: Thomson Delmar Learning.

Luke, R. D., S. L. Walston, and P. M. Plummer. 2003. *Healthcare Strategy: In Pursuit of Competitive Advantage.* Chicago: Health Administration Press.

Malvey, D., M. Fottler, and J. Sumner. 2013. "The Fear Factor in Healthcare: Employee Information Sharing." *Journal of Healthcare Management* 58 (3): 225–37.

Maslow, A. H. 1954. *Motivation and Personality.* New York: Harper & Row.

May, E. L. 2014. "The Power of Analytics." *Healthcare Executive* 29 (2): 18–26.

———. 2013. "Managing Your Career in Transformative Times." *Healthcare Executive* 28 (6): 10–18.

Mayo, E. 1945. *The Social Problems of an Industrial Civilization.* Boston: Graduate School of Business Administration, Harvard University.

McCarthy, D., and A. Cohen. 2013. *The Colorado Beacon Consortium: Strengthening the Capacity for Health Care Delivery Transformation in Rural Communities.* The Commonwealth Fund. Published April. www.commonwealthfund.org/~/media/files/publications/case-study/2013/apr/1686_mccarthy_colorado_beacon_consortium_case_study.pdf.

McClelland, D. C. 1985. *Human Motivation.* Glenwood, IL: Scott-Foresman.

McDaniel, R. R., and M. E. Jordan. 2009. "Complexity and Post-Modern Theory." In *Health Organizations: Theory, Behavior, and Development*, edited by J. A. Johnson, 63–86. Sudbury, MA: Jones & Bartlett.

McGregor, D. M. 1960. *The Human Side of Enterprise.* New York: McGraw-Hill.

McIlwain, T. F., and M. Ugwueke. 2014. "Strategic Thinking Leaders." In *New Leadership for Today's Health Care Professionals: Concepts and Cases*, edited by L. G. Rubino, S. J. Esparza, and Y. S. Reid Chassiakos, 113–36. Burlington, MA: Jones & Bartlett Learning.

McKinney, M. 2011. "About That Quality Chasm: 10 Years After IOM Report, Authors See Progress, But . . ." *Modern Healthcare* 41 (8): 38–39.

McSweeney-Feld, M. H., and N. Rubin. 2014. "Human Resource Considerations at the Top." In *New Leadership for Today's Health Care Professionals: Concepts and Cases,* edited by L. G. Rubino, S. J. Esparza, and Y. S. Reid Chassiakos, 95–109. Burlington, MA: Jones & Bartlett Learning.

Meyer, J. W., and B. Rowan. 1977. "Institutionalized Organizations: Formal Structure as Myth and Ceremony." *American Journal of Sociology* 83 (2): 340–63.

Miller, A. R., and C. Tucker. 2013. "Active Social Media Management: The Case of Health Care." *Information Systems Research* 24 (1): 52–70.

Mills, A. E. 2014. "Ethics and the Healthcare Organization." In *Managerial Ethics in Healthcare: A New Perspective,* edited by G. L. Filerman, A. E. Mills, and P. M. Schyve, 19–50. Chicago: Health Administration Press.

Mintzberg, H. 1990. "The Manager's Job: Folklore and Fact." *Harvard Business Review* 68 (2): 163–76.

———. 1983a. *Power In and Around Organizations.* Englewood Cliffs, NJ: Prentice-Hall.

———. 1983b. *Structure in Fives: Designing Effective Organizations.* Englewood Cliffs, NJ: Prentice-Hall.

Molinari, C., and L. Shanderson. 2014. "The Culturally Competent Leader." In *New Leadership for Today's Health Care Professionals: Concepts and Cases,* edited by L. G. Rubino, S. J. Esparza, and Y. S. Reid Chassiakos, 57–72. Burlington, MA: Jones & Bartlett Learning.

Moorhead, S., M. Johnson, M. Maas, and E. Swanson (eds.). 2013. *Nursing Outcomes Classification (NOC): Measurement of Health Outcomes,* fifth edition. St. Louis, MO: Elsevier Mosby.

Moussa, M. 2012. "Communication." In *Shortell & Kaluzny's Health Care Management Organization Design and Behavior,* sixth edition, edited by L. R. Burns, E. H. Bradley, and B. J. Weiner, 163–87. Clifton Park, NY: Delmar Cengage Learning.

Myers, S. A., and C. M. Anderson. 2008. *The Fundamentals of Small Group Communication.* Thousand Oaks, CA: Sage Publications.

Nelson, W. A. 2005. "An Organizational Ethics Decision-Making Process." *Healthcare Executive* 20 (4): 8–14.

Nelson, W. A., and T. Lahey. 2013. "The Ethics of Mandatory Flu Shots." *Healthcare Executive* 28 (6): 42–46.

Nembhard, I. M., J. A. Alexander, T. J. Hoff, and R. Ramanujam. 2009. "Why Does the Quality of Health Care Continue to Lag? Insights from Management Research." *Academy of Management Perspectives* 23 (1): 24–42.

Nester, B. A. 2014. "Physician–Hospital Alignment: An Essential Ingredient in Value Production." In *Futurescan 2014: Healthcare Trends and Implications 2014–2019*, edited by D. Seymour, 17–22. Chicago: Society for Healthcare Strategy & Market Development and Health Administration Press.

Neuman, W. 2007. "Safety Violations Cited for Deaths in Subway Work." *New York Times,* August 2.

Neumeister, L. 2010. "Novartis Hit with $250M Gender Bias Damages." *MSNBC.com.* Updated May 19. www.msnbc.msn.com/id/37233213/ns/business-us_business.

Noe, R., J. Hollenbeck, B. Gerhart, and P. Wright. 2015. *Human Resource Management: Gaining a Competitive Advantage,* ninth edition. Chicago: McGraw-Hill Higher Education.

Olden, P. C. 2012. "Managing Mechanistic and Organic Structure in Health Care Organizations." *Health Care Manager* 31 (4): 357–64.

Olden, P. C., and M. L. Diana. 2009. "Classical Theories of Organization." In *Health Organizations: Theory, Behavior, and Development*, edited by J. A. Johnson, 29–46. Sudbury, MA: Jones & Bartlett.

Olden, P. C., and J. Haynos. 2013. "How to Create a Health Care Organization That Can Succeed in an Unpredictable Future." *Health Care Manager* 32 (2): 193–200.

Olden, P. C., and K. Hoffman. 2011. "Hospitals' Health Promotion Services in Their Communities: Findings from a Literature Review." *Health Care Management Review* 36 (2): 104–13.

Olden, P. C., and W. C. McCaughrin. 2007. "Designing Healthcare Organizations to Reduce Medical Errors and Enhance Patient Safety." *Hospital Topics* 85 (4): 4–9.

Ouchi, W. 1981. *Theory Z.* Reading, MA: Addison-Wesley.

Parrington, M. 2014. "Healthcare Reform and Incorporating Mission, Values, and Culture in Provider Affiliations." In *Futurescan 2014: Healthcare Trends and Implications 2014–2019*, edited by D. Seymour, 23–26. Chicago: Society for Healthcare Strategy & Market Development and Health Administration Press.

Peters, T., and R. Waterman. 1982. *In Search of Excellence.* New York: Harper & Row.

Pointer, D. D. 2006. "Leadership: A Framework for Thinking and Acting." In *Health Care Management: Organization Design and Behavior*, fifth edition, edited by S. M. Shortell and A. D. Kaluzny. Clifton Park, NY: Thomson Delmar Learning.

Polzer, J. T., M. A. Neale, and J. L. Illes. 2006. "Conflict Management and Negotiation." In *Health Care Management: Organization Design and Behavior*, fifth edition, edited by S. M. Shortell and A. D. Kaluzny, 148–70. Clifton Park, NY: Thomson Delmar Learning.

Porter, M. E. 1985. *Competitive Advantage: Creating and Sustaining Superior Performance.* New York: Free Press.

Project Management Institute (PMI). 2013. *A Guide to the Project Management Body of Knowledge (PMBOK Guide)*, fifth edition. Newtown Square, PA: Project Management Institute.

Reinertsen, J. 2014. "Leadership for Quality." In *The Healthcare Quality Book*, third edition, edited by M. S. Joshi, E. R. Ransom, D. B. Nash, and S. B. Ransom. Chicago: Health Administration Press.

Ricker, J. 2012. "Patient-Centered Care: What It Means and How to Get There." *Health Affairs Blog*. Published January 24. http://healthaffairs.org/blog/2012/01/24/patient-centered-care-what-it-means-and-how-to-get-there.

Roberts, S. J., and T. Roach. 2009. "Social Networking Web Sites and Human Resource Personnel: Suggestions for Job Searches." *Business Communication Quarterly* 72 (1): 110–14.

Roethlisberger, F. G., and W. J. Dickson. 1939. *Management and the Worker.* Cambridge, MA: Harvard University Press.

Rorty, M. V. 2014. "Introduction to Ethics." In *Managerial Ethics in Healthcare: A New Perspective,* edited by G. L. Filerman, A. E. Mills, and P. M. Schyve, 1–18. Chicago: Health Administration Press.

Rosenau, P. V., and R. Roemer. 2008. "Ethical Issues in Public Health and Health Services." In *Introduction to Health Services*, seventh edition, by S. J. Williams and P. R. Torrens, 321–44. Clifton Park, NY: Thomson Delmar Learning.

Schoen, C., S. Guterman, M. A. Zezza, and M. K. Abrams. 2013. "Confronting Costs: Stabilizing U.S. Health Spending While Moving Toward a High Performance Health Care System." Commonwealth Fund Commission on a High Performance Health System. Published January 10. www.commonwealthfund.org/Publications/Fund-Reports/2013/Jan/Confronting-Costs.aspx.

Schwalbe, K., and D. Furlong. 2013. *Healthcare Project Management*. Minneapolis, MN: Schwalbe Publishing.

Scott, G. 2009. "Teamwork." *Healthcare Executive* 24 (2): 46–47.

Shier, G., M. Ginsburg, J. Howell, P. Volland, and R. Golden. 2013. "Strong Social Support Services, Such as Transportation and Help for Caregivers, Can Lead to Lower Health Care Use and Costs." *Health Affairs* 32 (3): 544–51.

Silversin, J., and M. J. Kornacki. 2000. *Leading Physicians Through Change: How to Achieve and Sustain Results*. Tampa, FL: American College of Physician Executives.

Simon, H. 1957. *Models of Man.* New York: John Wiley & Sons.

Skinner, B. F. 1969. *Contingencies of Reinforcement: A Theoretical Analysis.* New York: Appleton-Century-Crofts.

Slee, D. A., V. N. Slee, and H. J. Schmidt. 2008. *Slee's Health Care Terms*, fifth edition. Sudbury, MA: Jones & Bartlett.

Slovensky, R., and W. H. Ross. 2012. "Should Human Resource Managers Use Social Media to Screen Job Applicants? Managerial and Legal Issues in the U.S.A." *Info* 14 (1): 55–69.

Smith, H. L., B. J. Fried, D. Van Amerongen, and J. D. Laughlin. 2008. "Compensation Practices, Planning, and Challenges." In *Human Resources in Healthcare,* third edition, edited by B. J. Fried and M. D. Fottler, 281–318. Chicago: Health Administration Press.

Spath, P. L. 2013. *Introduction to Healthcare Quality Management*, second edition. Chicago: Health Administration Press.

Stempniak, M. 2012. "AHA Nova Awards." American Hospital Association. Accessed September 8, 2014. www.aha.org/content/12/2012novaawards.pdf.

Stoto, M. A. 2013. "Community Health Needs Assessments—An Opportunity to Bring Public Health and the Healthcare Delivery System Together to Improve Population Health." *Improving Population Health*. Published April 16. www.improvingpopulationhealth.org/blog/2013/04/index.html.

Swayne, L. E., W. J. Duncan, and P. M. Ginter. 2009. *Strategic Management of Health Care Organizations,* sixth edition. San Francisco: Jossey-Bass.

Tallia, A. F., K. C. Stange, R. R. McDaniel, V. A. Aita, W. L. Miller, and B. F. Crabtree. 2003. "Understanding Organizational Designs of Primary Care Practices." *Journal of Healthcare Management* 48 (1): 45–59.

Taylor, F. W. 1911. *The Principles of Scientific Management.* New York: Harper & Brothers.

———. 1903. *Shop Management.* New York: Harper & Row.

Thomas, K. W., and R. H. Kilman. 1974. *Thomas-Kilman Conflict-Mode Instrument.* Tuxedo, NY: Xicom, Inc.

Tuckman, B. W. 1965. "Developmental Sequence in Small Groups." *Psychological Bulletin* 63 (6): 384–99.

Tuckman, B. W., and M. A. C. Jensen. 1977. "Stages of Small Group Development Revisited." *Group and Organizational Studies* 2: 419–27.

Tyson, B. J. 2014. "The Quest for Affordability in Healthcare." In *Futurescan 2014: Healthcare Trends and Implications 2014–2019*, edited by D. Seymour, 27–31. Chicago: Society for Healthcare Strategy & Market Development and Health Administration Press.

US Census Bureau. 2012. "U.S. Census Bureau Projections Show a Slower Growing, Older, More Diverse Nation a Half Century from Now." Published December 12. www.census.gov/newsroom/releases/archives/population/cb12-243.html.

US Small Business Administration. 2014. "Create Your Business Plan." Accessed June 3. www.sba.gov/category/navigation-structure/starting-managing-business/starting-business/writing-business-plan.

Vroom, V. H. 1964. *Work and Motivation.* New York: John Wiley and Sons.

Waldrop, M. M. 1992. *Complexity: The Emerging Science at the Edge of Order and Chaos.* London: Viking.

Warren, K. 2014. "Quality Improvement: The Foundation, Processes, Tools, and Knowledge Transfer Techniques." In *The Healthcare Quality Book*, third edition, edited by M. S. Joshi, E. R. Ransom, D. B. Nash, and S. B. Ransom, 83–107. Chicago: Health Administration Press.

Weber, M. 1947. *The Theory of Social and Economic Organization.* Translated by A. M. Henderson and T. Parsons; edited by T. Parsons. New York: Oxford University Press.

———. 1946. *From Max Weber: Essays in Sociology.* Translated and edited by H. Gerth and C. W. Mills. New York: Oxford University Press.

Weiner, B. J., H. Amick, and S. D. Lee. 2008. "Review: Conceptualization and Measurement of Organizational Readiness for Change." *Medical Care Research and Review* 65 (4): 379–436.

Weiner, B. J., and C. D. Helfrich. 2012. "Complexity, Learning, and Innovation." In *Shortell & Kaluzny's Health Care Management Organization Design and Behavior*, sixth edition, edited by L. R. Burns, E. H. Bradley, and B. J. Weiner, 221–48. Clifton Park, NY: Delmar Cengage Learning.

Weiner, B. J., C. D. Helfrich, and S. R. Hernandez. 2006. "Organizational Learning, Innovation, and Change." In *Health Care Management: Organization Design and Behavior*, fifth edition, edited by S. M. Shortell and A. D. Kaluzny. Clifton Park, NY: Thomson Delmar Learning.

Welch, S. 2010. "Understand Physician Culture to Facilitate Change." *Healthcare Executive* 25 (3): 92–95.

Wetlaufer, S. 2001. "The Business Case Against Revolution." *Harvard Business Review* 79 (2): 112–21.

White, E. 2005. "Learning to Be the Boss." *Wall Street Journal*, November 21, B1.

White, K. R., and J. R. Griffith. 2010. *The Well-Managed Healthcare Organization,* seventh edition. Chicago: Health Administration Press.

Winterhouse Institute. 2010. "Mayo Clinic: Design Thinking in Health Care." Yale School of Management: Design and Social Enterprise Case Series. Published November 23. http://nexus.som.yale.edu/design-mayo.

Woodward, J. 1965. *Industrial Organization: Theory and Practice.* London: Oxford University Press.

———. 1958. *Management and Technology.* London: H. M. Stationery Office.

World Health Organization (WHO). 1946. *Preamble to the Constitution of the World Health Organization as adopted by the International Health Conference, New York, 19–22 June, 1946; signed on 22 July 1946 by the Representatives of 61 States (Official Records of the*

World Health Organization, No. 2, P. 100) and entered into force on 7 April 1948. Geneva, Switzerland: WHO.

Zazzali, J. L., J. A. Alexander, S. M. Shortell, and L. R. Burns. 2007. "Organizational Culture and Physician Satisfaction with Dimensions of Group Practice." *Health Services Research* 42 (3, Part I): 1150–76.

Zuckerman, A. M. 2005. *Healthcare Strategic Planning,* second edition. Chicago: Health Administration Press.

ABOUT THE CHAPTER OPENER QUOTES

Chapter 1: From Grazier, K. 2003. "Interview with Philip A. Newbold." *Journal of Healthcare Management* 48 (1): 2–5.

Chapter 2: From CC-M Productions. 2010. *Cultural Transformation Discussion Guide Volume 24: A New Way of Thinking.* Washington, DC: CC-M Productions, Inc, page 11. Accessed May 1. http://forecast.umkc.edu/ftppub/ba541/DEMINGLIBRARY/DLVol24-25.PDF.

Chapter 5: Louis Sullivan's quote comes from his article "The Tall Office Building Artistically Considered" in *Lippincott's Magazine,* March 1896. His expression was originally stated as "form ever follows function" and was later shortened.

Chapter 7: This common business slogan also appears on page 63 of Peter Drucker's book *Managing in a Time of Great Change* (2009, Harvard Business School Press).

Chapter 9: The quote is the title of a paper presented by Dr. Steven Ronik (CEO, Henderson Mental Health Center, Fort Lauderdale, Florida) at a Bruce Springsteen Symposium presented by the Pennsylvania State University and held at Monmouth University, New Jersey, September 9–11, 2005.

Chapter 11: From Peters, T., and R. Waterman. 1982. *In Search of Excellence.* New York: Harper & Row, 291.

Chapter 14: This quote comes from an 1867 speech Disraeli gave in Edinburgh. The full quote is "Change is inevitable. In a progressive country change is constant."

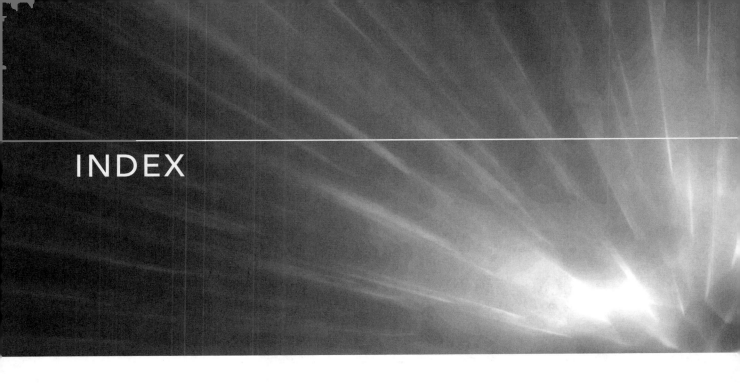

INDEX

Note: Italicized page locators refer to exhibits.

cians, organizational decisions, and, 249; physicians *vs.*, *176,* 176–77, 178; political tactics used by, 196; protecting staff and role of, 156; recruitment of employees and, 133; reinforcement theory used by, 194, 195; salaries for, 155; specialized areas for, *14;* staffing and responsibilities of, 124; tasks organized into jobs and positions by, 62–63; three-step control method for, 230–32, 235–38, 240; work organization in healthcare organizations and, 60–61
Mandate: for group, 105
Mandela, Nelson, 165
Market analysis: in business plan, 51
Marketing: groups and teams within, 105
Marketing and sales details: in business plan, 51
Market sector: external environment and, 9
Maslow, Abraham: hierarchy of needs theory of, 182, *183,* 183–85, *184,* 200
Massachusetts General Hospital, 314; Connected Health models of care available at, *313;* within Partners HealthCare system, 310; 30-day readmission rates for AMI, heart failure, and pneumonia at, *312*
Mathematical formulas, 253
Matrix form of organization structure, 80, 84–86, 98; advantages and disadvantages of, 86; definition of, 84; organization chart for, *85;* variations in, 85–86
Mayo, Elton: human relations and, 23–24
Mayo Clinic: project management and, 47
McClelland, David: learned needs theory of, 182, 185–86, 200
McConnell, C. R.: communication defined by, 294, 295
Measuring performance, 232, 235–36; digital "big data" tools used in, 236; quantitative measures, 232, *232, 233;* scoreboards and dashboards used in, 235–36
Mechanical systems, 58
Mechanistic approach: in management theory, 30
Mechanistic organizations, 80, 273; definition of, 69
Mechanistic structure: change impeded by, 273; environment and, *70;* stable environment and, *70,* 76
Media: as stakeholders, 41, *41*
Mediators: conflict resolution and, 264
Medical care: definition of, 4; hospital board of directors and delegation of, 95; standardized, 68
Medical errors: organizational culture and, 208

Medical ethics, 223; definition of, 213; in healthcare organizations, *213*
Medical expertise: physician's power and influence based on, 75, 96
Medical faculty, 95
Medical Group Management Association, 8; ethical guidance provided through, 216; website for, 82, 341
Medical group practices: organizational culture in, 210; services provided by, 7
Medical hierarchy: surgeons in, 75
Medical–management committees, 96
Medical practices: management support for groups and teamwork in, 102
Medical records: data for graphics and, 235
Medical services: disparities linked to, 5; in force field model of health, *3,* 4, 5, 16
Medical specialties: groups and teams within, 105
Medical staff: hierarchy of, in hospitals, 96; physicians and, in healthcare organizations, 94–97, 99; structure of, in hospitals, 95
Medical supply firms, 8
Medicare: contract changes to payment structure for home care industry and, 316; hospital patient satisfaction linked to reimbursement from, 131, 135, 145, 310, 311; new reimbursement model for leveraging staff across more patients, 317, 320; payment reductions associated with 30-day readmissions, 312
Medicare Hospital Compare: website for, 341
Medicine: blending of management and, 75; blurred boundary between administration and, 96; division of work in, 21
Meetings: effective, managers' guidelines for, 119–20
Membership in groups, 105, 106–8, 120
Memorial Healthcare System (Broward County, Florida): data analytics used in, 236
Mental demands: job descriptions and, 131
Mental health, 3
Mental health clinics: management support for groups and teamwork in, 102
Mentoring, 147; effective groups and teams and, 118; onboarding and, 158
Mentors: leadership styles and, 171
Mergers, 93, 174, 205; change and, 269; organizational culture and, 210; procedural justice and, 223
Merit increases, 152
Merit pay systems, 129
Message(s): in communication, 295; in communication model, 298, *298,* 299, 307; decoding, 303–4, 307; encoding, 300–3, 307